Gisela Dallenbach-Hellweg

Magnus von Knebel Doeberitz

Marcus J. Trunk

Color Atlas of Histopathology of the Cervix Uteri

Gisela Dallenbach-Hellweg
Magnus von Knebel Doeberitz
Marcus J. Trunk

Color Atlas of Histopathology of the Cervix Uteri

Second Edition

With 239 Figures and 4 Tables

Springer

Professor Dr. med.
Gisela Dallenbach-Hellweg
Private address:
Ludolf-Krehl-Strasse 57
D-69120 Heidelbeg
Tel. +49 -6221-471461

Dr. med. Marcus J. Trunk
Head of Pathology
MTM Laboratories AG
Im Neuenheimer Feld 583
D-69120 Heidelberg
Email: trunk@mtm-laboratories.com

Professor Dr. med.
Magnus von Knebel Doeberitz
Institute of Molecular Pathology
University of Heidelberg
Im Neuenheimer Feld 220
D-69120 Heidelberg
Email: knebel@med.uni-heidelberg.de &
mvkd@aol.com

Library of Congress Control Number: 2005926890

ISBN 978-3-540-25188-0 Springer Berlin Heidelberg New York
1st Edition ISBN 978-3-540-52295-9 Springer Berlin Heidelberg New York

Springer is a part of Springer Science+Business Media
springeronline.com

Editor: Gabriele Schröder, Heidelberg, Germany
Desk Editor: Ellen Blasig, Heidelberg, Germany
Production: ProEdit GmbH, 69126 Heidelberg, Germany
Cover: Frido Steinen-Broo, EStudio Calamar, Spain
Typesetting: K. Detzner, 67346 Speyer, Germany

Printed on acid-free paper 24/3151 ML 5 4 3 2 1 0

Preface to the Second Edition

The new edition of this atlas integrates all significant advances made in the past 15 years in molecular pathology, tumor virology, and genetics of cervical cancer. It emphasizes the importance of these advances in facilitating its pathological diagnosis and in optimizing clinical management and prognosis. A new chapter on immunohistochemistry has been added, which includes refined detection methods, e.g., the overexpression of $p16^{INK4a}$ as a molecular marker in the early differential diagnosis of premalignant lesions. The section on etiology and pathogenesis in human papillomavirus-induced neoplasia has been incorporated to represent new insights into the sequences of cellular and nuclear deregulation at the molecular level. All chapters have been revised to include the newest advances and relevant experiences in how to interpret and manage cervical disease; they are supported by the addition of 35 new microphotographic illustrations. The tumor nomenclature is adapted to the latest edition of the WHO classification; the morphology code of the international classification of diseases for oncology (ICD-O) has been added. We have also updated the list of references by adding recent relevant publications.

Again, the staff of Springer-Verlag deserve our thanks for their patience and skill in preparing the manuscript and in reproducing the microphotographs.

Heidelberg, February 2005

Gisela Dallenbach-Hellweg,
Magnus von Knebel Doeberitz,
and Marcus J. Trunk

Preface to the First Edition

During the past decade our understanding of the histopathology of the cervix uteri has changed greatly. Because of the lifestyles of the modern permissive society, cervical viral infections have become epidemic, resulting in inflammatory and precancerous lesions that were uncommon but now are seen mainly in the younger age groups with increasing frequency. Then too, progress in molecular biology and immunohistochemistry has enabled us to distinguish subtypes of papilloma viruses, to proceed in understanding their action within the genome, and to trace the infected metaplastic and neoplastic-transformed cells to their histogenetic origins. The resultant refined classification of cervical neoplasias has helped to predict clinical outcome and to choose type of therapy.

This atlas is intended for all pathologists, to aid them in their routine diagnostic work. We hope it explains just how comprehensive, important and complex the histopathology of the cervix uteri has become during the last few years. It covers all pertinent differential diagnostic aspects and describes in detail how to reach the correct diagnosis. The atlas is also meant for the clinician, to guide him in his often difficult decision of how to provide optimal care for the frequently young patient, who desires children but is at risk for cancer. In particular, the atlas is designed to foster an improved dialogue between the pathologist and the clinician.

The microphotographs were selected from our daily diagnostic material, since they show best the technical variations confronting the clinical pathologist in his daily routine, where effects of specimen transport, differences in tissue fixation, and variations in embedding and staining often compound his diagnostic problems. The various shades of haematoxylin-eosin stains shown by our photographs reflect the differences we have experienced with our material as it comes in daily or is received as referral cases from clinics and institutes. We have not attempted to eliminate the deficiencies of these specimens, since the pathologist using this atlas is entitled to find realistic photographs rather than idealistic ones. We want him to recognize a lesion irrespective of the quality of fixation or intensity of staining.

We express our gratitude to Prof. Dr. Frederick D. Dallenbach for the subtle English translation. We also extend our thanks to the staff of Springer-Verlag for their patience, generosity, and skill in preparing the manuscript and in reproducing our microphotographs.

We find ourselves in an exciting period of molecular biology, during which rapid developments in diagnostic techniques and concepts are clarifying relationships between molecular changes and the pathogenesis of cervical cancer. As is to be expected, some of our statements will be short-lived, forced aside as new facts and information emerge to replace them. In contrast, other statements we have made may grow in importance.

May both the controversial issues and those being accepted with ever-increasing favour contribute to make this atlas a source of stimulus to encourage lively discussions and rewarding ideas.

Mannheim and Copenhagen, July 1990

Gisela Dallenbach-Hellweg
and Hemming Poulsen

Contents

Premalignant Lesions . . . 82

Malignant Tumors . . . 117

Erratum

Figure 197 (page 150) is incorrect. The correct figure is given here.

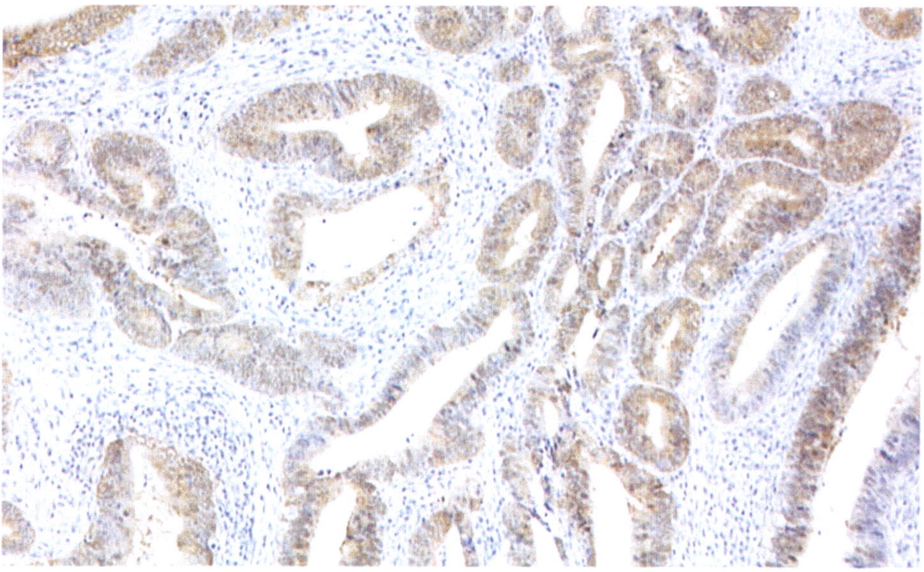

Fig 197. Adenocarcinoma of endocervix, endometrioid type. Diffuse and continuous positive staining reaction for $p16^{INK4a}$ in tumor cells. $p16^{INK4a}$ immunostain

Screening for Cervical Cancer Precursors to Prevent Invasive Disease

In many developed countries a decline in the incidence and mortality of cervical cancer has been observed in the past 30 years. The description of a cytological technique of cervical cancer detection by Papanicolaou in 1941 has given rise to the most successful early detection scheme worldwide. Population-based screening programs or opportunistic screening systems have been implemented in many affluent countries for decades. Due to lack of resources and infrastructure, however, these programs have not been implemented easily in other, less developed parts of the world. The problems encountered in screening for cervical cancer precursors with the aim to prevent invasive carcinoma depend on many different social and political issues, such as lack of patient knowledge, unwillingness of patients to participate in a screening program, or program quality. These issues should be addressed accordingly.

In early cancer detection, different cytological classification schemes, and depending on these, different disease management systems, are used. These different ways of diagnosing and treating diseases are not to be considered as "wrong" or "false," they depend on country-specific conditions. The value of a classification and management system of a disease should be measured on a list of things: if it is meeting the (rightful) expectancies of the patients and their physicians, if it is scientifically correct, and if it can be practiced in line with the medico-legal and medico-economical environment.

In the USA the cytological classification most commonly used is the Bethesda system (Solomon and Nayar 2004), originally developed in and for the USA. Many European countries use different classifications, based on the original Papanicolaou system, of which the Munich nomenclature is the most widely accepted. According to the cytological classifications, the therapeutic consequences vary: for instance, in the USA, cervical intraepithelial neoplasia (CIN 2 and CIN 3 (HSIL) lesions) are removed by surgery, whereas in Europe, especially in Germany and the Netherlands, only CIN 3 lesions are seen as the direct precursor of invasive disease and therefore surgically removed.

New screening and diagnostic techniques that will lead to changes in already existing programs should be implemented only if the existing problems have been addressed and if the new techniques are evaluated with state-of-the-art methods.

Methods of Obtaining and Preparing Cervical Tissue for Histological Examination

Diagnostic or Therapeutic Procedures

Histological examination of the uterine cervix is required for diagnosing a lesion that is suspicious on gross, colposcopic, or cytological examination. In such instances, the extent of the biopsy may depend on the individual situation, but sufficient tissue should always be removed to provide the pathologist with optimal material for examination and for consideration and evaluation of the diagnostic possibilities. Pathologists should never hesitate to ask for more tissue if they believe this will help in reaching a definitive diagnosis.

Depending on the prevailing guidelines and recommendations, there are several options for diagnostic and/or therapeutic procedures that will result in tissue specimens for histological diagnosis. Each method has its own indications and its advantages and disadvantages, which require careful consideration before the application of a method.

In general, there are questions about the interpretability of the specimen and the rate of missing a lesion if the specimen is indeed interpretable. Important for the application of excisional methods is the predictive value of histologically clear margins for the recurrence of disease and the general interpretability of the resection margins, especially if there is a thermal effect on the tissue.

In follow-up for positive cytology results, diagnostic biopsies are considered in most disease management guidelines.

Colposcopically Directed (Punch) Biopsy

This is a purely diagnostic procedure, whose value is strongly dependent on the quality of the colposcopy procedure. To rate a colposcopy as satisfactory, the transformation zone should be completely visible. If a suspicious lesion can be seen on the ectocervix without extension into the endocervix, a (punch) biopsy can be performed and should be taken at the maximum of the lesion, but will be of limited predictive value if the lesion extends to the tissue border. On the other hand, a small biopsy will suffice for preoperative histological verification of a grossly visible invasive neoplasm.

Cold Knife Conization

If the cytology report is positive, but no lesion is visible on gross or colposcopic examination, a cervical conization will be necessary in order to survey the entire squamocolumnar junction. A conization must also be performed if a previous punch biopsy of a grossly suspicious lesion showed that the noninvasive precancerous epithelium had not been completely excised. A biopsy of malignant tumors can never give information about the depth of invasion. If the clinical signs fail to reveal how deeply a tumor has invaded, e.g., a crater is seen, a conization must always be performed. This is the only method on which to base the decision of whether further treatment should consist of simple surgical procedures (enlarged cone or simple hysterectomy) or involve more extensive methods (radical surgery or irradiation). A conization should always contain the entire squamocolumnar junction. Depending upon the age of the patient (Hamperl and Kaufmann 1959), that junction may be localized on the ectocervix, as during the reproductive age, requiring a flat conus, or be up in the endocervical canal, as in old age, requiring an elongated conus (see Fig. 1). Since, however, neoplastic transformation of the endocervical reserve cells may extend into or even start in the endocervical canal, a large and elongated conus is often advisable in young patients, too. The cone should be marked so that the pathologist understands how it was located anatomically; the same marking procedure should be used in all cases. For example, a suture mark at "12 o'clock" will help the pathologist orient the specimen and pinpoint the site of a lesion on either the anterior or posterior lip, or both. Especially when a precancerous lesion

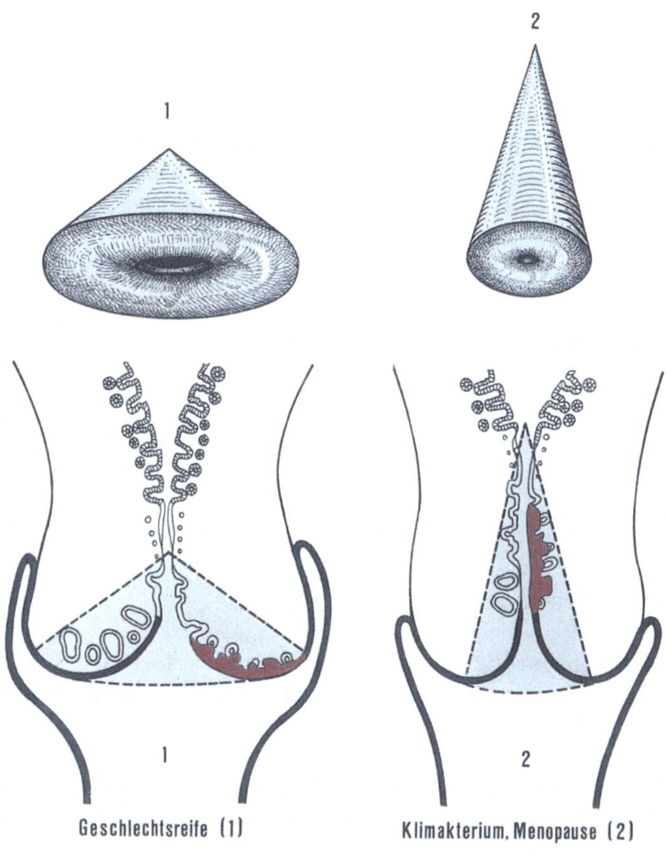

Fig. 1. Location of the squamocolumnar junction indicating zone of possible neoplastic transformation and shape of the conus usually recommended in reproductive age (*1*, for exception see text above) and in old age (*2*) (from Dallenbach-Hellweg 1985)

reaches the excisional margins of the cone, correct localization of the lesion will help the gynecologist in his follow-up treatment of the patient. The lateral margins of a cone may contain cervical glands that project deep into the tissue, possibly with precancerous lesions. Therefore, these parts of the tissue must also be carefully examined. To avoid the possibility of leaving the bottoms of glands behind, many surgeons prefer excising a more cylindrically shaped piece of cervical tissue.

In most instances, precancerous lesions are totally excised by conization and no further operation will be necessary. Accordingly, diagnostic conization serves also as a therapeutic measure. Occasionally cervical conization may be required as a means of treatment, e.g., in patients with resistant vaginal discharge. Here, careful histological examination of the squamocolumnar junction is advisable to ensure that possible precancerous changes are not overlooked.

Loop Electrosurgical Excision Procedure

The term loop electrosurgical excision procedure (LEEP; also known as LLETZ – large loop excision of the transformation zone) indicates use of a wire loop and electric current to remove part of the cervix with the entire transformation zone. For that the entire transformation zone must be visible through the colposcope and the identified lesion must not have extended into the endocervical canal.

It has been shown that LEEP results in the removal of less healthy tissue than does the cold knife conization while providing an equivalent cure rate. This argues for the use of LEEP as opposed to cold knife conization in patients who desire future child bearing (Girardi et al. 1997; Fanning and Padratzik 2002). The disadvantage, however, is the failure to evaluate the coagulated tissue borders: if the neoplastic epithelium reaches the coagulation zone, its complete removal cannot be guaranteed.

A cold knife conization is clearly indicated when:

- The lesion extends into the endocervix
- A previous biopsy indicated a microinvasive carcinoma
- An adenocarcinoma in situ (ACIS) has been suspected in cytology
- A discrepancy exists between cytology, colposcopy and histology of a previous punch biopsy.

Endocervical Curettage

This is also a purely diagnostic procedure, which can be performed if there is an indication for endocervical disease. Endocervical curettage can be performed as part of fractionated abrasio in the search for endometrial disease, whereby the gynecologist performs and collects the cervical scraping before carrying out the endometrial curettage. If malignant transformations are found, the pathologist should attempt from examination of the separately embedded curettings to determine whether the tumor arises only in the cervix, only in the endometrial cavity, or in both.

Simple Hysterectomy

A simple hysterectomy is indicated if the conservative treatment has failed and there is extensive involvement of cervix and vagina. It may also serve as a definitive management of microinvasive carcinoma stage IA2 or of ACIS.

More invasive procedures (radical surgery) may be appropriate but depend on clinical staging and/or type and origin of the tumor in question.

The value of a colposcopically directed biopsy prior to excisional treatment has been debated. The reproducibility and the accuracy of the histological result of this method have been questioned, also the cost-effectiveness and the amount of time between initial positive result and treatment. It has been shown that there is a correlation between the biopsy result and the subsequent histology result, but there is an inherent inaccuracy between the two diagnostic modalities (Barker et al. 2002). Furthermore the correlation between the initial cytology result and the histology result by LEEP can be higher than the correlation between cytology and colposcopically directed biopsy (Berdichevsky et al. 2004). Therefore it is understandable that a "see and treat" protocol with LEEP being performed at the time of colposcopy has been advocated for high-grade lesions detected by cytology (Ferenczy and Wright 1993; Fung et al. 1997). But overtreatment for less severe lesions should be avoided (Dodson and Sharp 1999).

Preparation of the Cervical Specimen

The method used to study a specimen from the uterus depends on the preceding clinical and/or histological diagnoses. If the cervix is not clinically and morphologically suspicious, a tissue section from each lip, including the squamocolumnar junction, will suffice. If a suspicious lesion is found preoperatively, both lips should be sectioned and embedded completely, like a cone specimen. If an invasive carcinoma has been diagnosed preoperatively in a cone specimen, the extent of invasion must be determined histologically, requiring the study of all margins of the conization site, of both parametrial tissues and all lymph nodes surgically excised.

For fixation, a 4% neutral solution of formaldehyde is commonly used and is ideal for most diagnostic procedures. After fixation, a cervical biopsy must be carefully oriented so that it can be properly embedded, and biopsies as well as curettings should be completely embedded. Microtome sections are taken from various levels. Precise orientation of a cervical specimen is essential for evaluating the entire squamocolumnar junction, where most precancerous and carcinomatous lesions originate. For this orientation different techniques have been described (Fig. 2); each has its advantages and disadvantages. We recommend in cone specimens either the circular or the parallel sectioning (Dallenbach-Hellweg 1985). When the anterior lip has been clearly marked, all paraffin blocks made from the cone should be numbered such that a lesion subsequently discovered on microscopic examination can be localized precisely in the cone.

Routine staining of all specimens should include hematoxylin-eosin and a connective tissue stain, for instance, van Gieson's. An additional PAS or alcian blue reaction

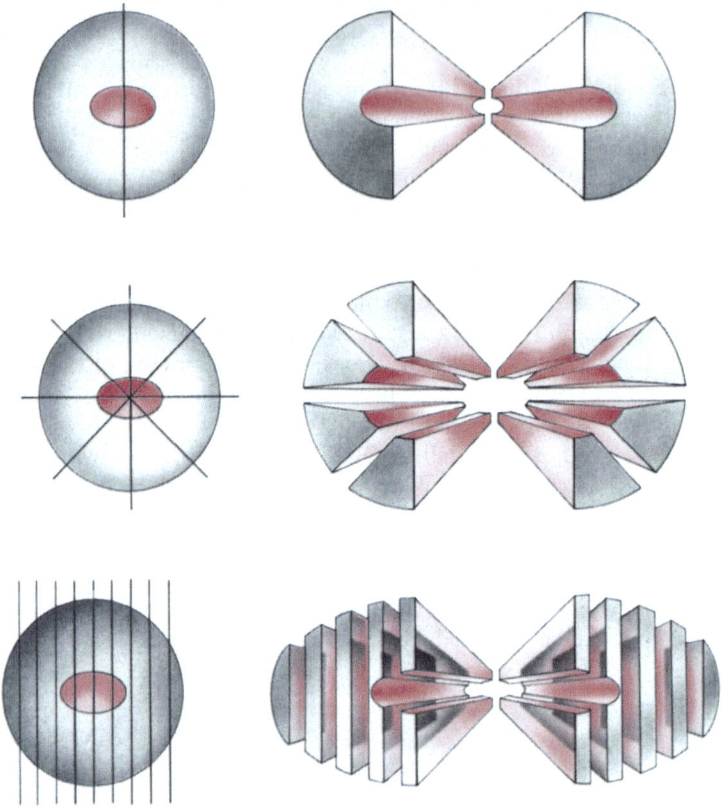

Fig. 2. Various techniques of sectioning a conus for orientation (from Dallenbach-Hellweg 1985)

may be helpful in detecting glycogen or mucopolysaccharides in squamous or glandular epithelial cells to judge the degree of cellular maturation. A reticulum impregnation can be useful in detecting interruptions of the basement membrane in early stromal invasion, or in distinguishing carcinomas from lymphomas.

Immunohistochemistry and In Situ Hybridization

Expression of specific proteins can be monitored in tissue sections using monoclonal antibodies directed against these proteins, whereas the presence or absence of specific nucleic acids (either RNA or DNA) can be monitored by in situ hybridization (ISH) techniques. The latter are also valuable tools to identify either gross chromosomal alterations or the presence or absence of specific microbes like bacteria or viruses.

Immunohistochemistry

There are different techniques for performing immunohistochemistry but all are based on the same principle. An antibody, either monoclonal or polyclonal, directed against the antigen under study, is applied to an appropriately processed tissue section, and labeled, so that its binding site can be detected.

In the simplest method a label is directly bound to this (primary) antibody. If a chromogenic labeling is preferred, an enzyme (either peroxidase or alkaline phosphatase) is employed with a chromogenic substrate. The enzyme acts on the substrate to convert it into an insoluble pigment that precipitates at the site of the bound antibody, revealing where it is located in the cell or tissue. Fluorescent labels bound to the antibody require fluorescent microscopy with ultraviolet illumination and selected filters in order to be visualized.

With an appropriate counterstaining of the tissue section, the labeled antigen can be discretely localized.

To make the method more versatile and sensitive, different techniques have been employed. In routine use the primary antibody is not labeled directly, but indirectly by using a labeled secondary antibody directed against the constant part (Fc portion) of the primary antibody. In more sensitive methods, tertiary complexes involving more labeling molecules are used, e.g., through a biotin-avidin-mediated link a tertiary complex carrying the chromogen may be formed to label the antigen. In newly developed techniques the reagent contains the secondary antibody directed against the primary antibody with several molecules of the enzyme linked by a polymer "backbone." That enhances the labeling and shortens the staining procedure because the secondary antibody step is omitted.

A chromogenic immunohistochemical labeling is stable and can be readily evaluated under routine light microscopy; no special equipment is needed. Specialized equipment is necessary for the evaluation of immunofluorescent stains, and the staining results are not permanent. This method, although precise and sensitive, is therefore impractical for routine studies of cervical pathology.

Caution must be employed for detecting antigens in sections of formalin-fixed and paraffin-embedded tissues. The epitope of the antigen must be unmasked in most instances, because formalin fixation causes proteins to cross-link, preventing antibodies reacting with the epitope of the antigen.

For further technical details, refer to handbooks on microscopic methods in molecular biology. For various groundbreaking reports on immunohistochemical methods with polyclonal and monoclonal antibodies, refer to the historical literature (Moll et al. 1982, 1983; Czernobilsky et al. 1984; Makin et al. 1984; Tsutsumi et al. 1984; Levy et al. 1988).

Reasons for Use

The reasons for using immunohistochemistry in routine practice are manifold. The immunohistochemistry method helps to determine the histogenesis of a given tumor. In most instances that determination depends on the differentiation-related expression of proteins and their location in cell or tissue. The slide-based immunohistochemistry methods are especially suitable for this.

The most important application lies in the differential diagnosis of tumors that may be problematic: for example, how to differentiate CIN from reactive or atrophic epithelia, ACIS from mimics, and endocervical neoplasms from those originating in the upper genital tract. Several lines of evidence also suggest that the use of specific antibodies may improve the reproducibility of the histopathological diagnosis and therefore may play an important role in future quality control measurements.

Cervical Tumor Cell Differentiation

Distinction of Squamous, Glandular and Neuroendocrine Lesions

The distinction of squamous, glandular and neuroendocrine carcinomas of the cervix is clinically significant for at least two reasons. First, a poorly differentiated carcinoma of glandular origin, even with early invasion, is likely to have a worse prognosis than a similar squamous tumor (Benda 1996). Second, neuroendocrine carcinomas are inherently more aggressive than their squamous counterparts and are managed with different protocols (Ambros et al. 1991).

Although all types of cervical epithelial lesions stain positively with pan-cytokeratin antibodies, their reaction to specific types of cytokeratins differs substantially. This is dependent on the cells of origin and modulated during differentiation to the mature type of epithelium or de-differentiation to carcinoma, respectively.

The basal layer of the ectocervix expresses cytokeratins characteristic for simple (glandular) epithelial cells, yet is covered by squamous epithelium with high molecular cytokeratins. Basal cells express CK 18 and 19, the suprabasal cells express CK 4, 5, 10 and 13 in varying degrees. The cytokeratin expression follows thereby a complex pattern correlating to the maturation of the epithelium (or differentiation of the individual cells; Franke et al. 1986).

The bipotential reserve cells of the endocervix contain cytokeratins characteristic for epithelial cells both with squamous and glandular differentiation and are covered by a simple, glandular epithelium. The reserve cells stain positively for CK 17, whereas the (differentiated) columnar cells do not (Martens et al. 2004). Both cell types stain positively for CK 8. Squamous carcinomas of the cervix express mostly CK 13, often combined with CK 8 and 18, and glandular carcinomas of the cervix are more likely to express CK 8 and 18 (Smedts et al. 1992).

p63, a homolog of the tumor suppressor gene p53, is expressed consistently in the nuclei of the basal cell layer of the ectocervical epithelium. p63 is also expressed in endocervical reserve cells, both in normal endocervix and in reserve cell hyperplasia (Quade et al 2001; Martens et al. 2004). On the other hand, it is not expressed in mature epithelium, be it of squamous or glandular origin. p63 is a powerful marker for proliferating cells on their way to squamous differentiation and, when diffusely expressed, excludes a glandular or neuroendocrine differentiation (Wang et al. 2001).

Carcinoembryonic antigen (CEA) is a glycoprotein of heterogeneous composition normally detected in the glycocalix of fetal epithelial cells, particularly those of mucin-secreting glandular nature. It is detectable only in small amounts in the cytoplasm of normal adult cells and benign tumors, but is present in large amount in carcinomas of reserve cell origin, and in mucinous adenocarcinomas. The expression of CEA in reserve cell-derived lesions, either squamous or glandular, indicates malignant transformation, in contrast to benign reserve cell hyperplasia, which is CEA-negative (Tendler et al. 2000).

Expression of chromogranin A, synaptophysin, and various other proteins involved in the formation of neurosecretory granules or CD 56, a neural cell adhesion molecule, can be used as markers of neuroendocrine differentiation, as in neuroendocrine carcinomas of other organs.

The cellular origin of other types of cervical lesions such as melanomas, lymphomas, and mesenchymal tumors can be assessed by using the immunochemical markers established for these tumors in other organ localizations.

CIN versus Reactive/Atrophic Epithelia

Management of preinvasive cervical disease is predicated on confirming a squamous intraepithelial lesion (CIN) by histologic examination and treating those lesions that are classified as high grade (CIN 2 and CIN 3). However, disturbances in maturation and inflammatory-related atypia may mimic CIN, and some CIN lesions may be less conspicuous or difficult to confirm histologically.

$p16^{INK4a}$, a cell cycle control protein, has been shown to be a sensitive and specific marker for CIN, particularly in lesions associated with high-risk human papillomaviruses (HR-HPV) (Sano et al. 1998).

For the evaluation of $p16^{INK4a}$ it is important to observe the distribution of positively stained cells throughout the lesion. Two staining patterns can be distinguished: the "diffuse" and the "focal" expression pattern. A continuous positive staining of cells in the basal and parabasal epithelial layers with variable positive staining in the more superficial layers can be seen in the "diffuse" pattern. The "focal" pattern comprises a staining of isolated cells or small cell groups in more superficial layers, but predominantly not in the basal and parabasal cell layers.

The latter staining pattern can be interpreted as the physiological expression in cells with differentiation irregularities, such as squamous metaplasia and atrophy. Both cytoplasmic and nuclear expression of $p16^{INK4a}$ should be regarded as positive staining (Sano et al. 1998; Klaes et al. 2001; Klaes et al. 2002).

A high expression of the proliferation marker MIB-1 in upper epithelial layers is strongly associated with neoplasia. But MIB-1-positive cell nuclei are occasionally also present in upper epithelial layers of severe reactive and inflammatory change (al-Saleh et al. 1995; Bulten et al. 1996; Kruse et al. 2001; Pirog et al. 2002).

The expression of CEA in reserve cell-derived CIN indicates malignant transformation, in contrast to reserve cell hyperplasia, which is CEA-negative (Tendler et al. 2000).

Adenocarcinoma In Situ versus Mimics

Distinguishing ACIS of the cervix from tubal metaplasia, endometriosis and microglandular hyperplasia may be difficult, but is important because ACIS confers a significant risk of endocervical adenocarcinoma.

A panel of antibodies, comprising $p16^{INK4a}$, CEA, MIB-1, and bcl2 can be a useful adjunct to regular histological stains (see Table 1).

$p16^{INK4a}$ is diffusely positive in ACIS, exhibits focal positivity or is negative in tubal metaplasia, and in endometriosis there may be sometimes widespread, but noncontinuous, scattered positivity. Microglandular hyperplasia is negative for $p16^{INK4a}$ (Cameron et al. 2002; Negri et al. 2003; Ishikawa et al. 2003; Murphy et al. 2004).

ACIS is positive for CEA, in contrast to CEA-negative microglandular hyperplasia, tubal metaplasia or endometriosis (Cina et al. 1997).

ACIS generally shows a high proliferation index with MIB-1. Tubal metaplasia, microglandular hyperplasia, and endometriosis are characterized by a low proliferation index, although some cases of endometriosis may show a moderate proliferative activity (McCluggage et al. 1995; Cina et al. 1997; Cameron et al. 2002).

In ACIS bcl2 is negative or, at most, focally positive. Also, microglandular hyperplasia is negative. In contrast, tubal metaplasia and endometriosis are diffusely positive with bcl2 (McCluggage et al. 1997).

It should be stressed, however, that careful morphological examination should remain the mainstay of diagnosis.

Table 1. Immunohistochemistry of ACIS and mimics

	ACIS	Microglandular hyperplasia	Tubal metaplasia	Endometriosis
$p16^{INK4a}$	++	–	(+)	(+)
CEA	++	–	–	–
MIB-1	++	(+)	(+)	(+)
bcl2	– / (+)	–	++	++

Endocervical Lesions versus Upper Genital Tract Lesions

Determining the site of origin (endometrial versus cervical) of fragments of adenocarcinoma in a curettage or biopsy specimen has important clinical ramifications with regard to treatment options. This includes the primary treatment modality (surgery versus radiation) and type of surgery performed (simple versus radical hysterectomy).

Most primary endocervical adenocarcinomas show a strong, diffuse positivity of 100% of the cells for $p16^{INK4a}$. In endometrial adenocarcinomas, positivity is generally focal and commonly involves less than 50% of the cells. However, occasional endometrial adenocarcinomas of the mucinous type exhibit 100% positivity for $p16^{INK4a}$. Diffuse strong positivity with $p16^{INK4a}$ suggests an endocervical rather than an endometrial origin of an adenocarcinoma (McCluggage and Jenkins 2003; Ansari-Lari et al. 2004). This correlates well with the HR-HPV-related etiology of the endocervical adenocarcinomas.

Vimentin is positive in a characteristic lateral border pattern in the majority of endometrial adenocarcinomas. In contrast, the majority of endocervical adenocarcinomas are negative for this marker (Castrillon et al. 2002; McCluggage et al. 2002; Alkushi et al. 2003).

Estrogen receptor is also expressed in the majority of endometrial adenocarcinomas, whereas endocervical adenocarcinomas are usually negative for this marker (McCluggage et al. 2002; Alkushi et al. 2003).

CEA staining is usually diffusely positive in adenocarcinomas of endocervical origin. It shows weakly focal positivity or is negative in endometrial adenocarcinomas (Castrillon et al. 2002; McCluggage et al. 2002).

In Situ Hybridization

Instead of identifying proteinaceous antigens as in immunohistochemistry, the purpose of ISH is to identify nucleic acids. For that, nucleic acid probes are used instead of antibodies. The microscopic techniques for visualizing and localizing positive labeling results are similar to those for immunohistochemistry.

To detect DNA, nucleic acid probes (for routine use: DNA probes) are allowed to bind to the DNA sequence in question. The probe is linked to digoxigenin, which can be detected by an anti-digoxigenin antibody bound to an enzyme (e.g., alkaline phosphatase). That enzyme converts a chromogenic substrate to insoluble pigment, which precipitates at the bound DNA probe, indicating its presence and its location in the DNA sequence. Similarly fluorescence-based detection methods are also available.

Formerly, the ISH method was widely used to detect microbial DNA, e.g., the viral DNA of HPV (Nagai et al. 1987). Because more sensitive methods have been developed, ISH for microbial DNA detection is no longer used routinely, although it supplies molecular information of didactic value.

In research studies, ISH may be used to locate specific regions in human chromosomes, e.g., in fluorescence in situ hybridization (FISH) or chromogenic ISH. Also there are ISH-based methods for the detection of integration of viral DNA into the chromosomal DNA (Hopman et al. 2004); however, their diagnostic value has to be regarded with great care and these methods are prone to many technical artifacts. FISH methods have also been used extensively to monitor chromosomal alterations in cervical cancer and its precursor lesions. Imbalances of some chromosomal regions were reported to correlate with progression of preneoplasia to invasive cancers. These data, however, still await confirmation in larger clinical trials (Heselmeyer et al. 1996; Heselmeyer et al. 1997).

For further technical details, please refer to handbooks on microscopic methods in molecular biology.

Normal Histology, Regeneration, and Repair

Normal Ectocervix (Figs. 3–9)

A normal ectocervix is covered by a nonkeratinizing stratified squamous epithelium. Its height is influenced by endogenous hormone production and varies accordingly with age and hormonal stimulation.

During reproductive age (Fig. 3) the epithelium is high and well differentiated. It consists of a basal cell layer with elongated nuclei perpendicular to the basal membrane, of one or several layers of small parabasal cells, of a broad intermediate cell zone with abundant cytoplasmic glycogen, and of a covering layer of narrow, superficial cells.

In childhood and in the postmenopausal period (Fig. 4), because hormonal stimulation is lacking, the squamous epithelium is low. Here it consists only of a few layers of small, poorly differentiated epithelial cells. The sparse cytoplasm is devoid of glycogen; stratification may be barely visible or even absent.

Regardless of their differentiation, all cell layers stain positively for broad-spectrum cytokeratins and, except for the basal cells, for cytokeratins 4 and 13 in appropriate im-

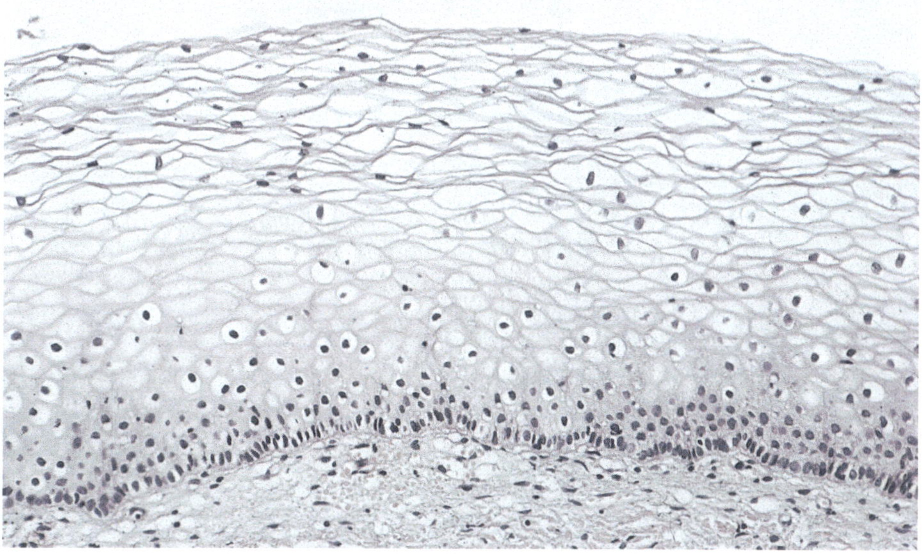

Fig. 3. Normal ectocervix during reproductive age. H&E

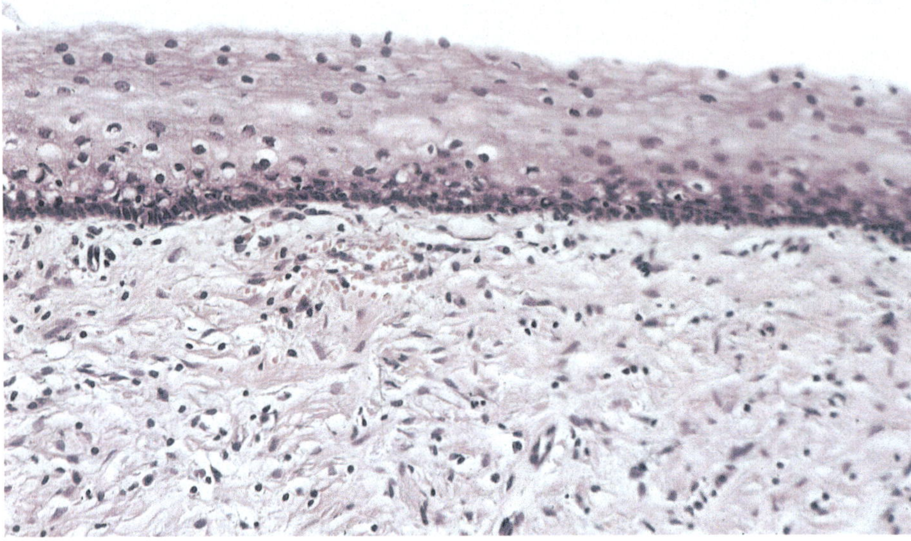

Fig. 4. Normal ectocervix in old age. H&E

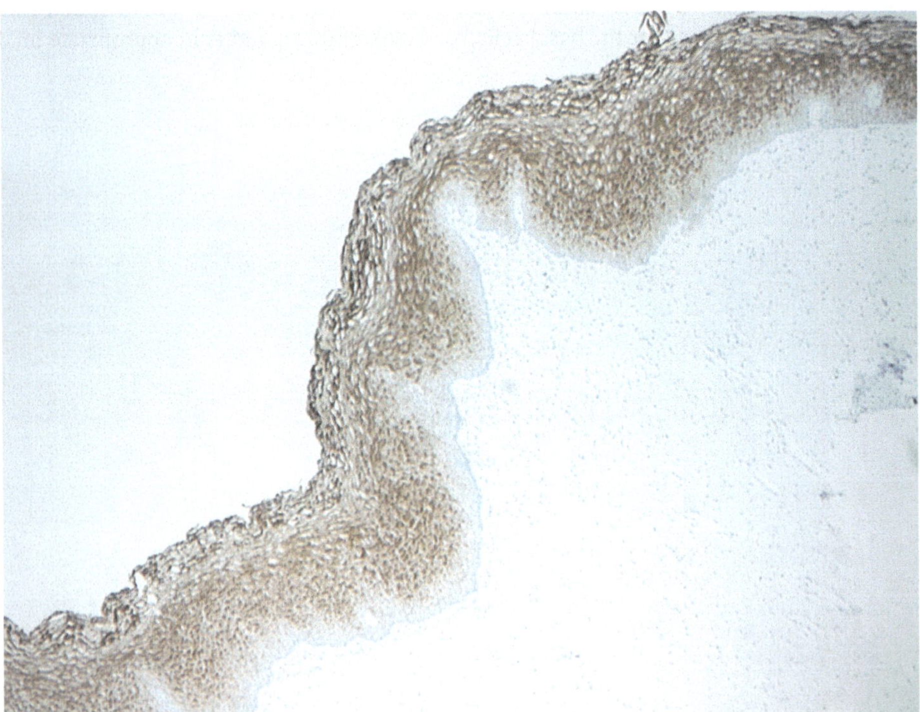

Fig. 5. Normal ectocervix. Immunohistochemical reaction with cytokeratin 13. The basal cell layer shows a negative reaction for CK 13

munohistochemical studies (Fig. 5). Cytokeratin 4 and 13 are normal constituents of epithelial cells in squamous differentiation.

Furthermore, the cell membranes, but not the basal membrane, stain positively with antibodies against E-cadherin (Fig. 6a) and desmoplakin (Fig. 6b). In contrast, the basal cells express cytokeratins of the simple (glandular) epithelial type: 8, 18, and 19 (Fig. 7; Franke et al. 1986).

This variation in the expression of cytokeratins by the basal cells may explain their potential for glandular differentiation and for functioning as the germinal layer of the squamous epithelium (Fig. 9). It may also explain their potential to elongate and ramify as protrusions downwards into the underlying fibrous stroma (Fig. 8).

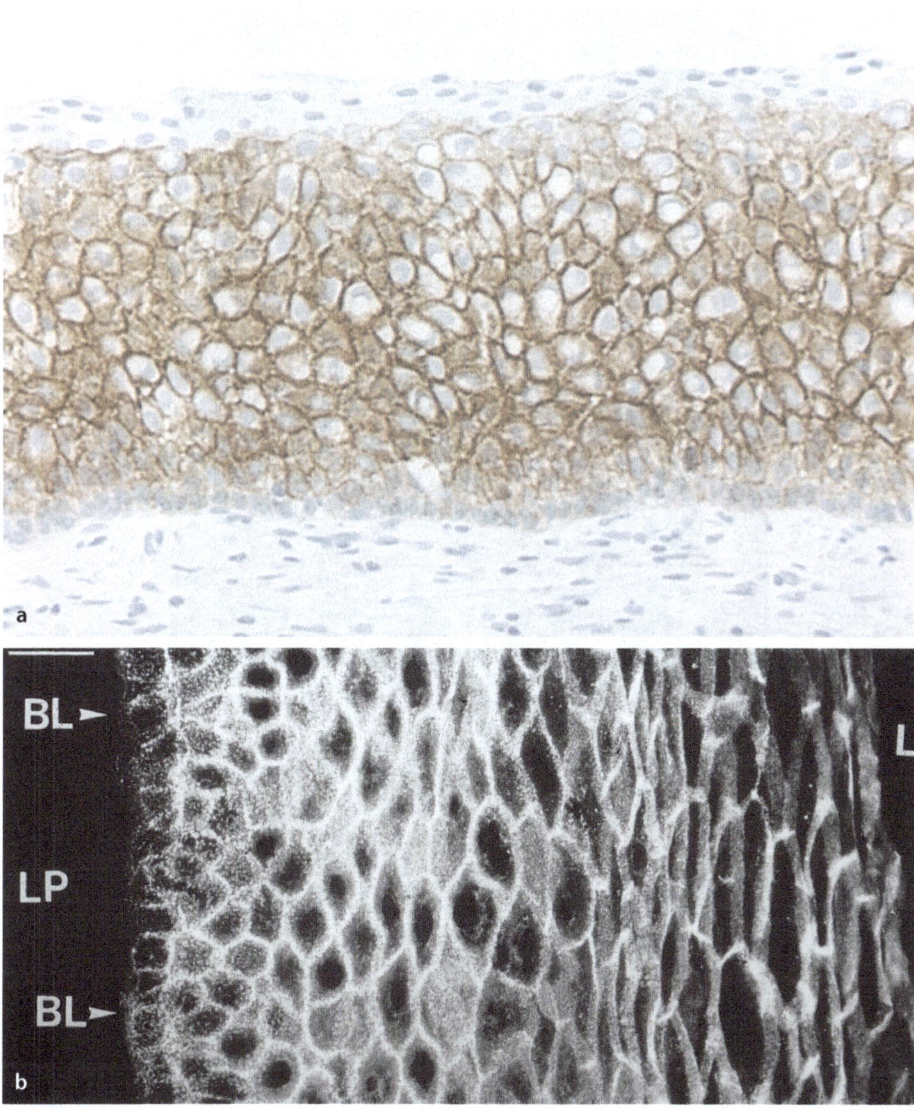

Fig. 6. Normal ectocervix. **a** Immunohistochemical reaction with antibody against E-cadherin. **b** Immunohistochemical reaction with antibody against desmoplakin (from Franke et al. 1986)

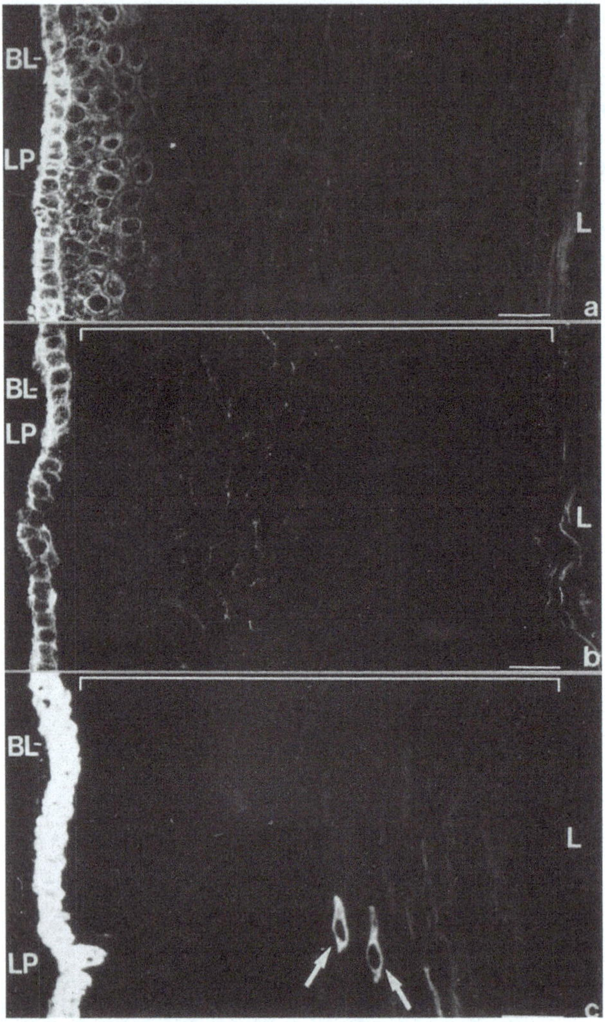

Fig. 7a–c. Normal ectocervix. Immunohistochemical reaction with cytokeratin PKK 1 (**a**), 18 (**b**), and 19 (**c**). *BL* basal lamina, *LP* lamina propria, *L* lumen (from Franke et al. 1986)

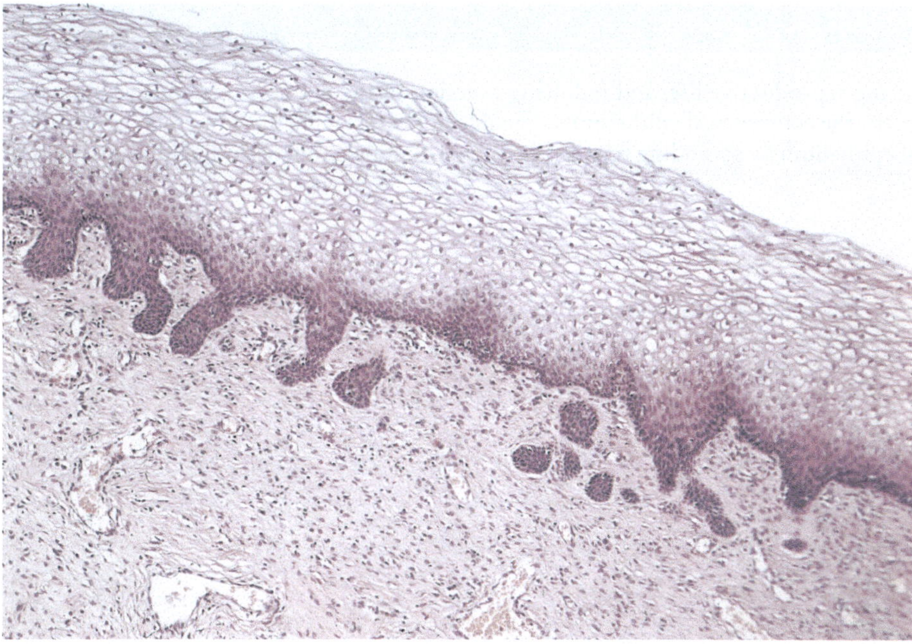

Fig. 8.
Ramifying protrusions from basal layer into the underlying fibrous stroma. H&E

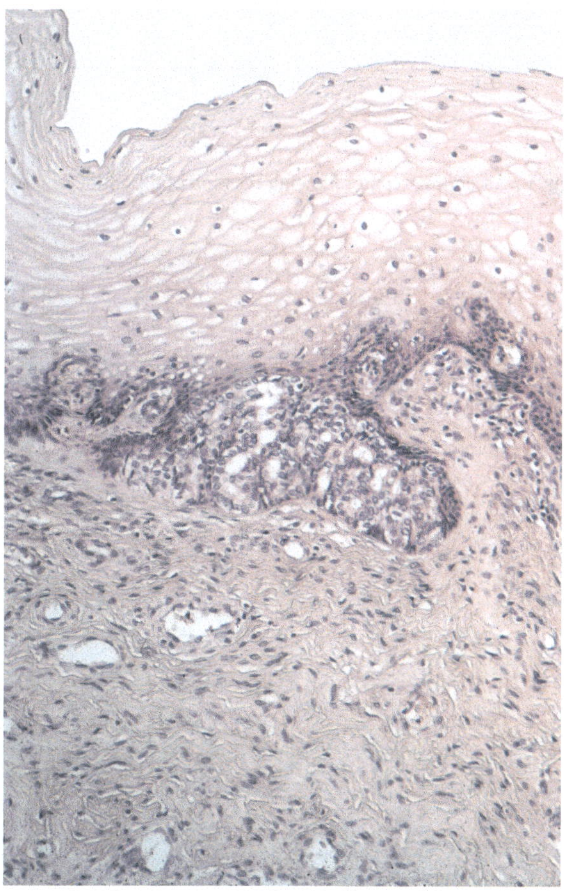

Fig. 9.
Formation of glands from the basal layer of the ectocervical epithelium. H&E

Ascending Repair (Figs. 10–13)

During reproductive life, and following eversion of the endocervical mucosa onto the portio, the ectocervical epithelium is capable of overgrowing the vulnerable endocervical epithelium by ascending repair (Figs. 10, 11), thereby often occluding the openings of

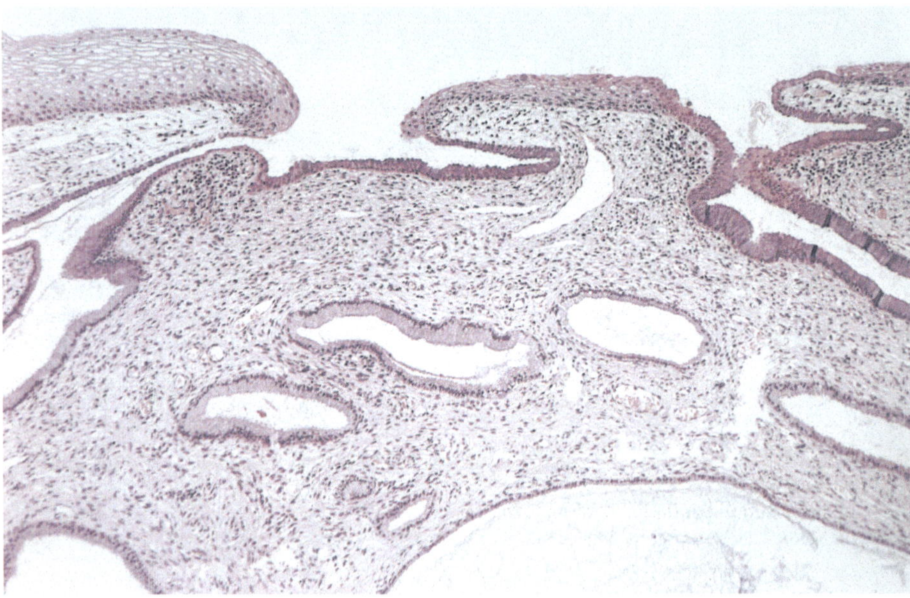

Fig. 10. Ascending repair following eversion of the endocervical mucosa onto the portio, early stage. H&E

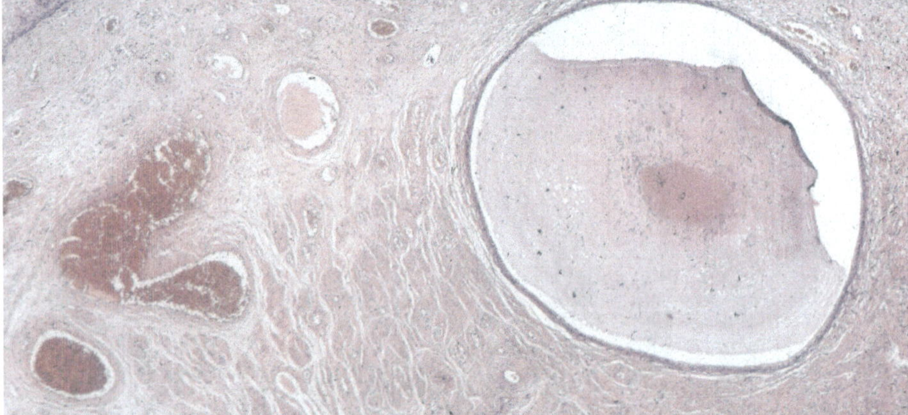

Fig. 11. Ascending repair following eversion of the endocervical mucosa onto the portio, advanced stage. H&E

endocervical glands, which may then become cystically dilated with inspissated mucus (Fig. 11).

In the early stages this regenerative epithelium consists of regular, but incompletely differentiated epithelial cells devoid of glycogen (Figs. 12, 13). Later, it cannot be distinguished from the original ectocervical epithelium (see p. 31, Fig. 31).

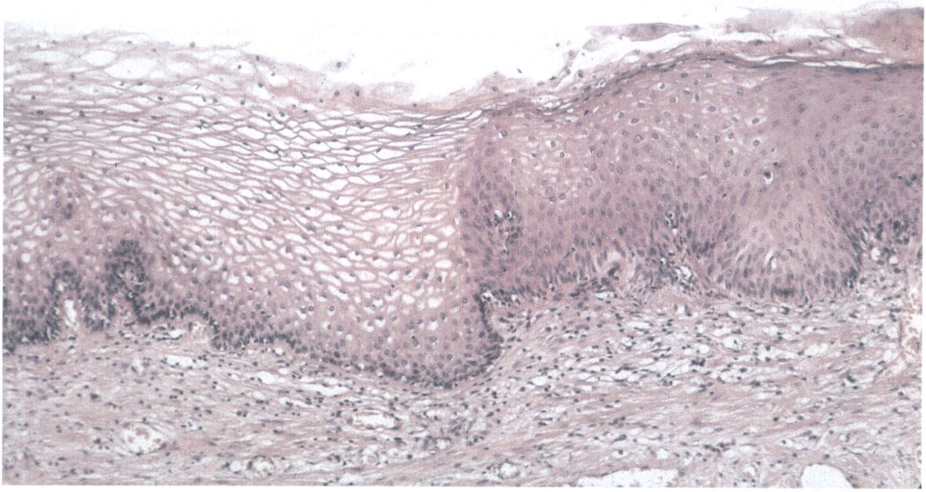

Fig. 12. Regenerative ectocervical epithelium sharply delineated from the original epithelium. H&E

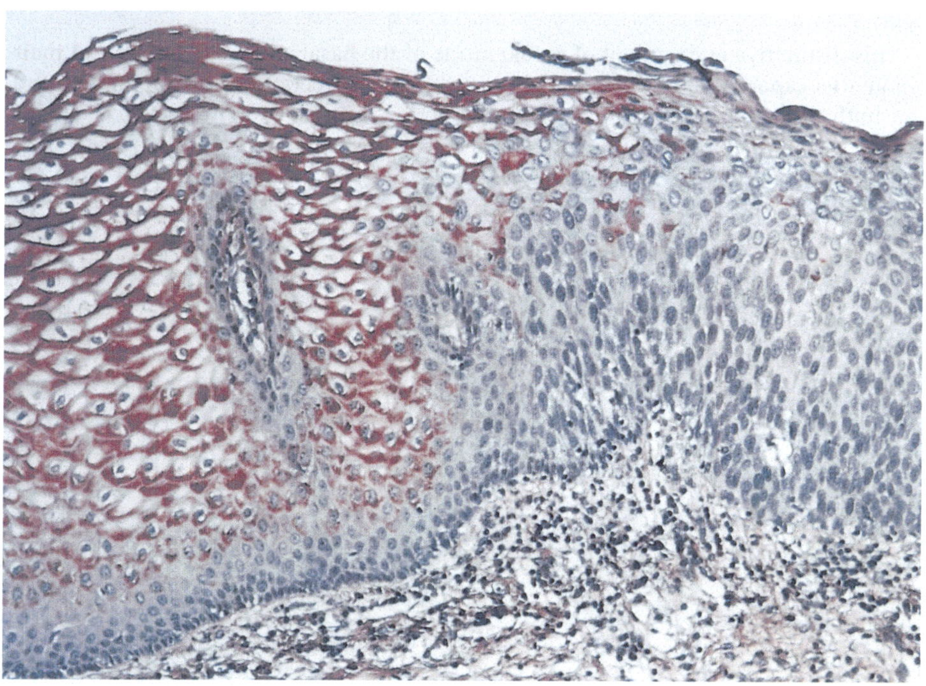

Fig. 13. Sharp line between original and regenerative epithelium. PAS reaction

Normal Endocervix (Figs. 14–18)

The normal endocervical mucosa consists of mucus-producing tubules and clefts (mucosal infoldings, usually called glands), loosely arranged in a fibrous stroma. A single layer of tall, columnar epithelial cells covers the mucosal surface and lines the intricate folds, clefts, and tubules. The small nuclei are basally placed during the early proliferative phase. The clear cytoplasm contains abundant mucus, especially in the late proliferative phase (Fig. 14). Where the endocervical mucosa merges with the isthmic mucosa, endometrial-type glands intermingle with endocervical glands (Figs. 15, 16).

Beneath the endocervical columnar epithelium a small single layer of reserve cells can often be detected (Figs. 17, 18). Immunohistochemically, these reserve cells differ in their cytoskeleton from the columnar cells. Although both cell types stain positively with broad-reacting cytokeratin antibodies, reserve cells remain unstained with antibodies against cytokeratin 18 (Fig. 17), but do react positively with antibodies against KA 1, detecting the complex of cytokeratin 5 with cytokeratin 14 (Gould et al. 1990), a reaction characteristic of squamous epithelium (Fig. 18). In contrast, the columnar cells stain with antibodies against cytokeratin 18 (Fig. 17), and 8, but not with antibodies against KA 1.

Consequently, the reserve cells of the endocervical epithelium differ immunohistochemically from the columnar cells covering them, much like the basal cells of the ectocervix differ from the cells overlying them, but in different ways. The basal layer of the ectocervix expresses cytokeratins characteristic for single (glandular) epithelial cells, yet is covered by squamous epithelium. The reserve cells of the endocervix contain cytokeratins characteristic for epithelial cells with squamous differentiation and are covered by a simple, glandular epithelium. Although the reserve cells are bipotential and capable of producing either keratin or mucin, they are not essentially precursors of the columnar cells, which can themselves proliferate by mitotic activity (Hiersche and Nagl 1980).

This distinctive endowment of cytokeratins of the basal and reserve cells and their bipotential capacities to differentiate in two different directions may explain how and why both epithelia at the squamocolumnar junction respond so characteristically to regenerative and metaplastic influences initiated by the eversion of the endocervix during the reproductive years.

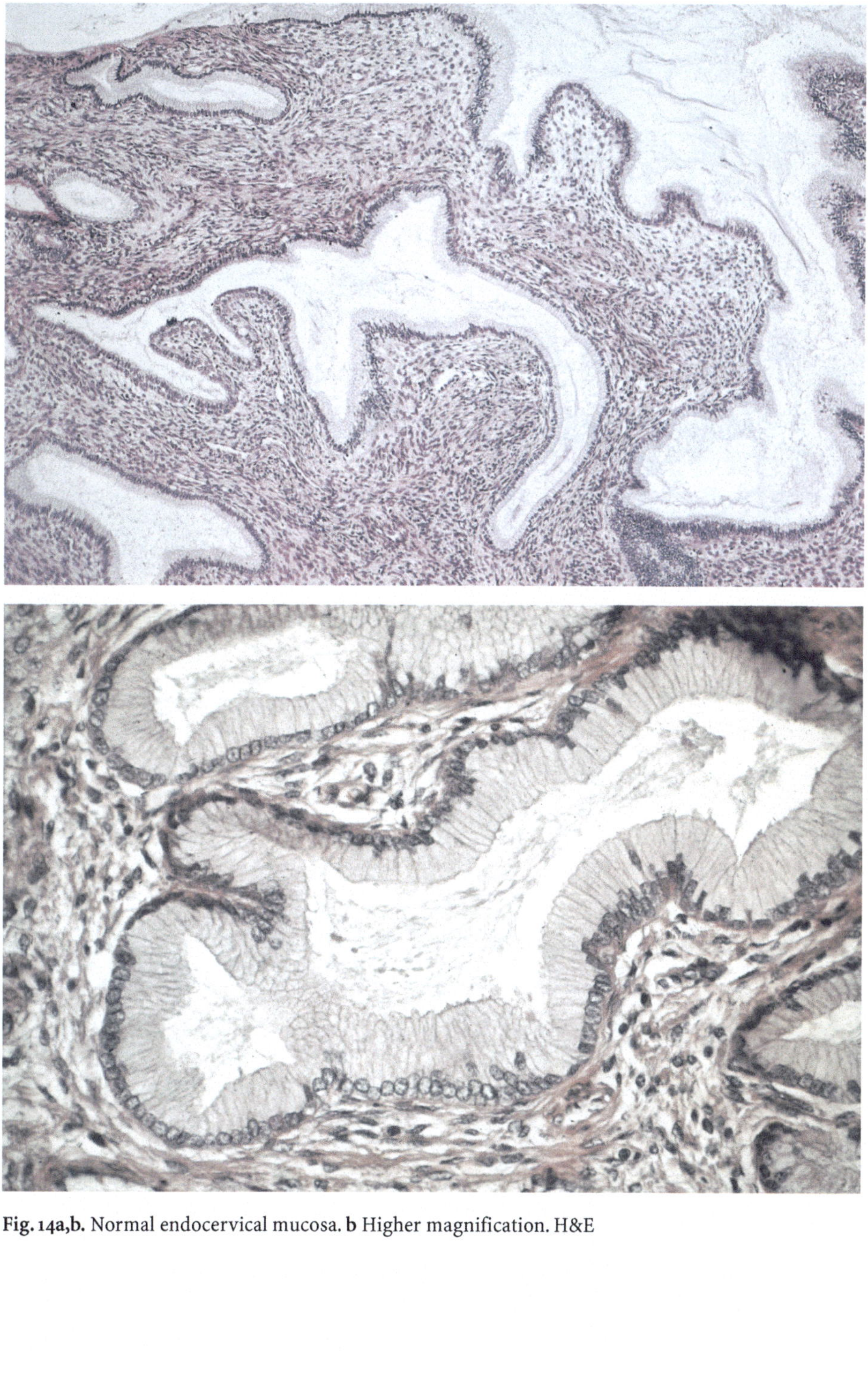

Fig. 14a,b. Normal endocervical mucosa. **b** Higher magnification. H&E

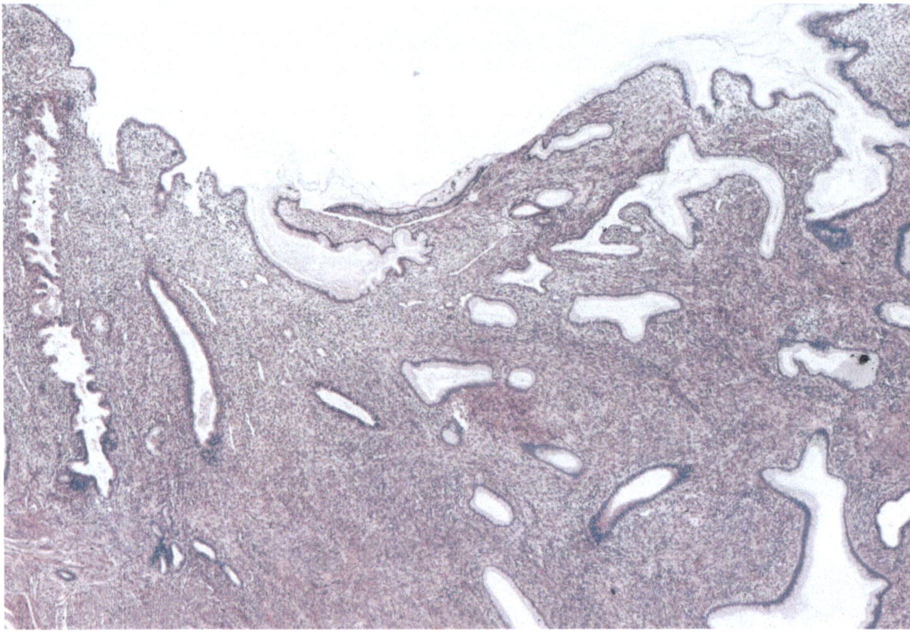

Fig. 15. Border between endocervical (*right*) and isthmic mucosa (*left*). H&E

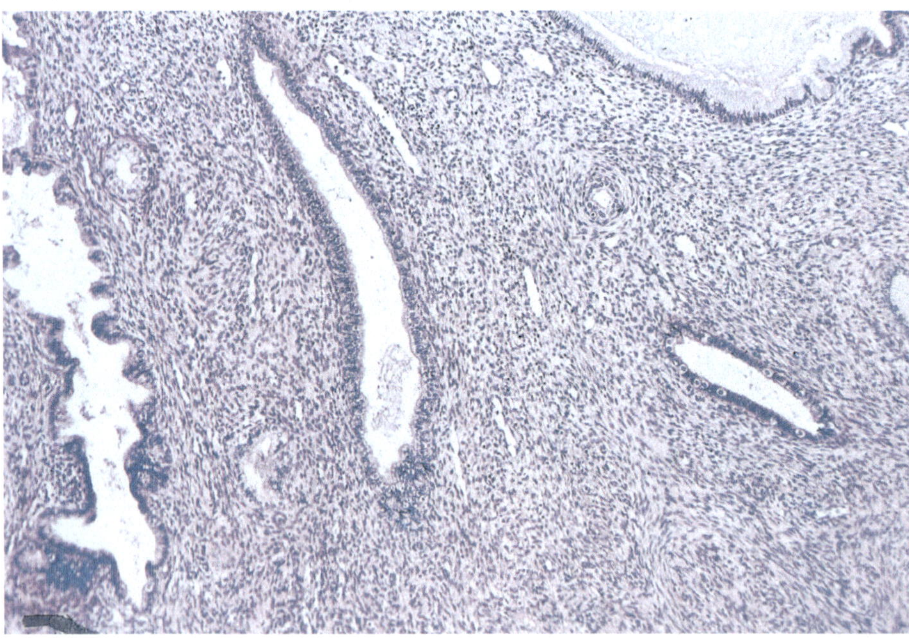

Fig. 16. Border between endocervical (*right*) and isthmic mucosa (*left*). H&E, higher magnification

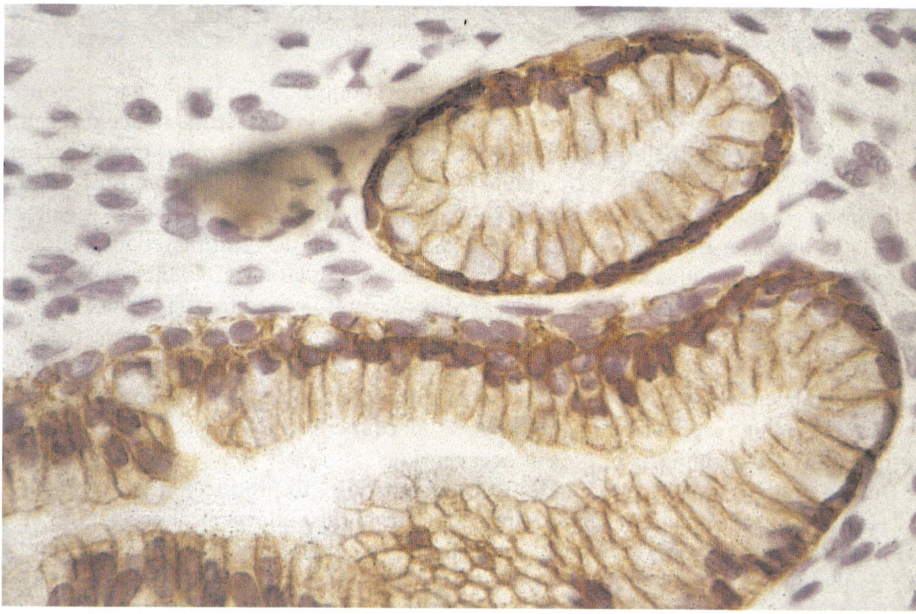

Fig. 17. Endocervical glands surrounded by a single layer of reserve cells. Immunohistochemical reaction with cytokeratin 18

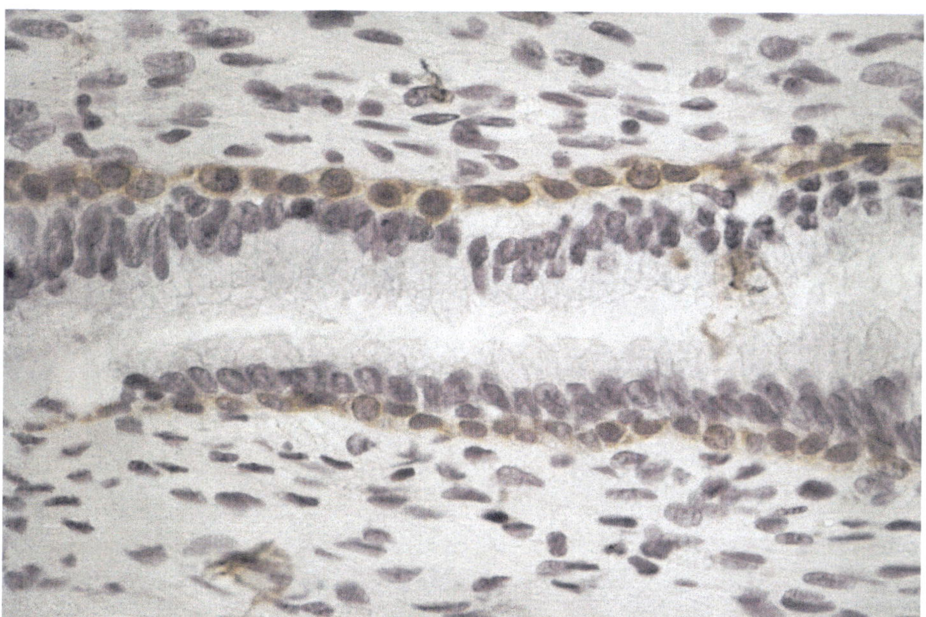

Fig. 18. Positive reaction of reserve cells with cytokeratin KA 1, columnar cells negative

Descending Repair (Figs. 19–27)

Endocervical mucosal surface epithelium that everts out onto the portio may become replaced by squamous epithelium in two ways: (1) by overgrowth from adjacent regenerative ectocervical epithelium, as in ascending repair (Figs. 10–13), or (2) by squamous metaplasia of the reserve cells of the endocervical epithelium, as in descending repair. Both processes may occur simultaneously or separately. In general, ascending repair is stimulated by endogenous or exogenous estrogens, whereas descending repair predominates under endogenous or exogenous gestagenic stimulation (Dallenbach-Hellweg 1981). Descending repair is preceded by a double- or multilayered hyperplasia of the reserve cells (Figs. 19, 20), which, in accordance with their cytokeratin endowment, undergo metaplastic change and differentiate into squamous epithelium (Figs. 21, 22). Some of these metaplastic cells, however, may retain their bipotential capacity and produce mucin, thereby being responsible for the monocellular mucin formation occasionally seen in squamous cell metaplasia of the endocervix (Figs. 23, 24).

During maturation to squamous cells, their capability to produce mucin is usually lost. In contrast, the squamous epithelium adjacent to the endocervical epithelium expresses cytokeratins of the squamous epithelium type in all layers, whereas the columnar epithelium neighboring it exhibits a positive reaction only in the underlying reserve cell layer (Fig. 25). With mucin stains, a faint positive reaction may be detected in the superficial cell layer, which may include the flattened atrophic remnants of columnar cells that originally covered the reserve cells (Figs. 26, 27).

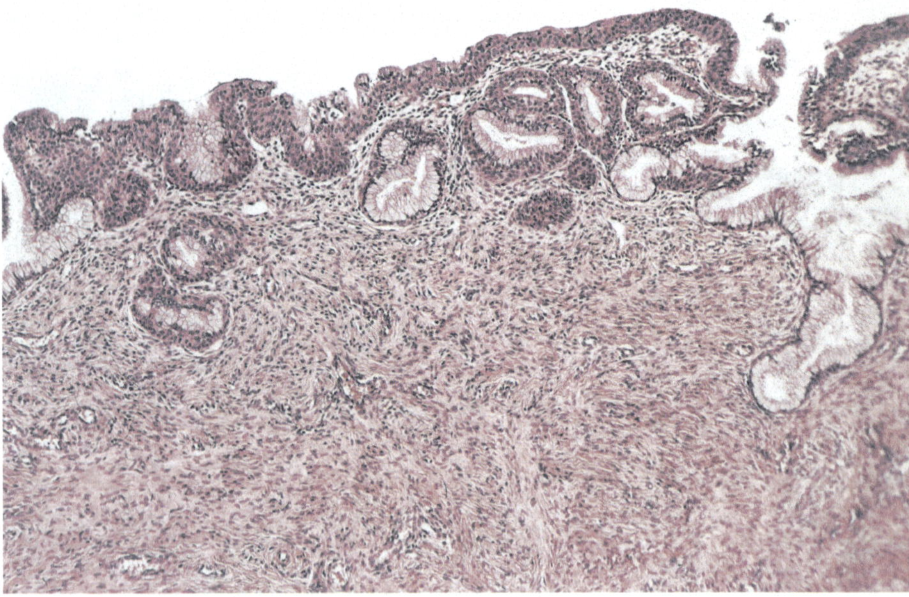

Fig. 19. Hyperplasia of reserve cells in descending repair. H&E

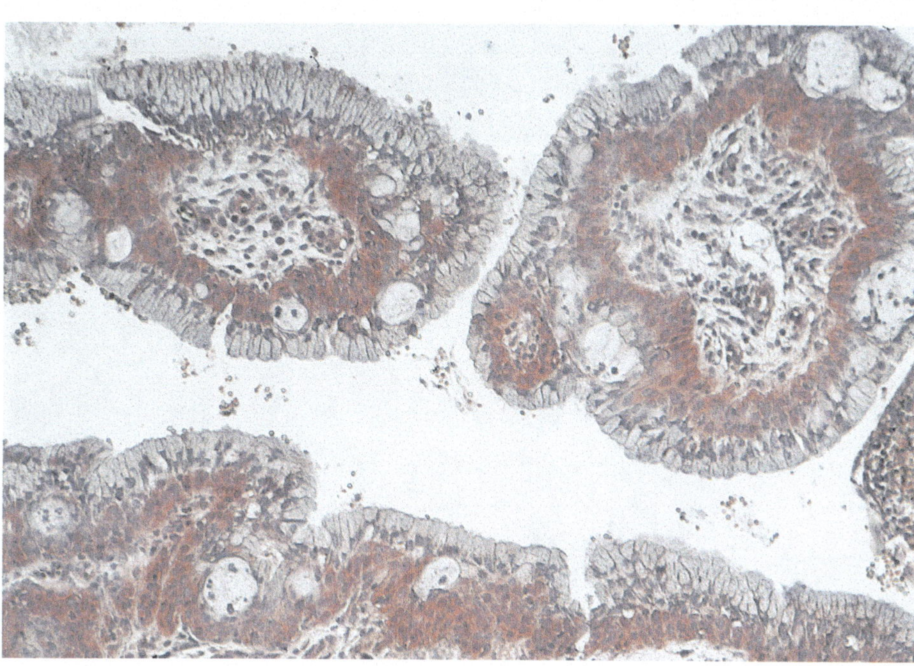

Fig. 20. Hyperplasia of reserve cells. Immunohistochemical reaction with cytokeratin 13

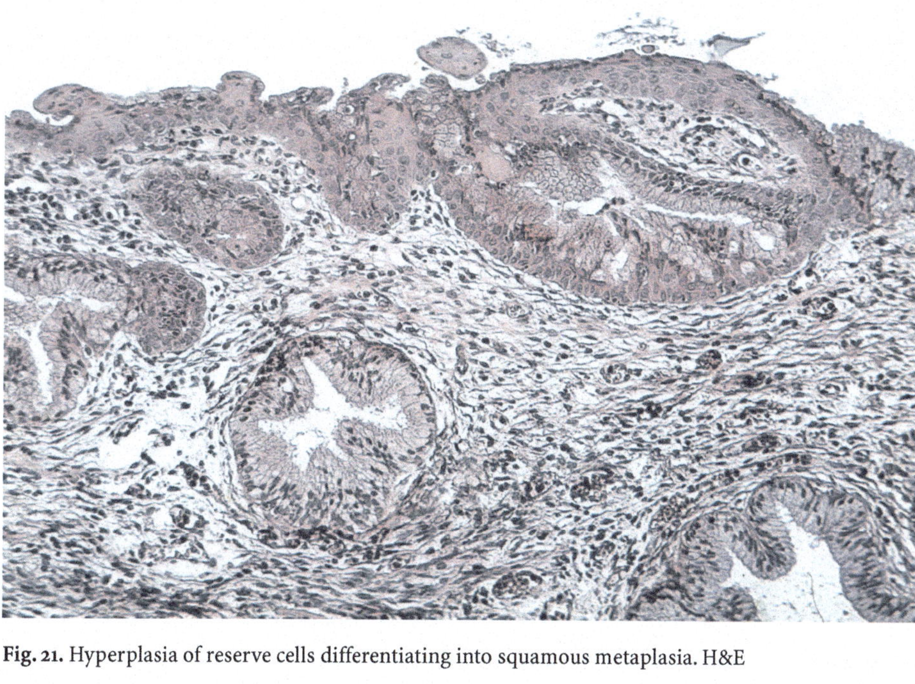

Fig. 21. Hyperplasia of reserve cells differentiating into squamous metaplasia. H&E

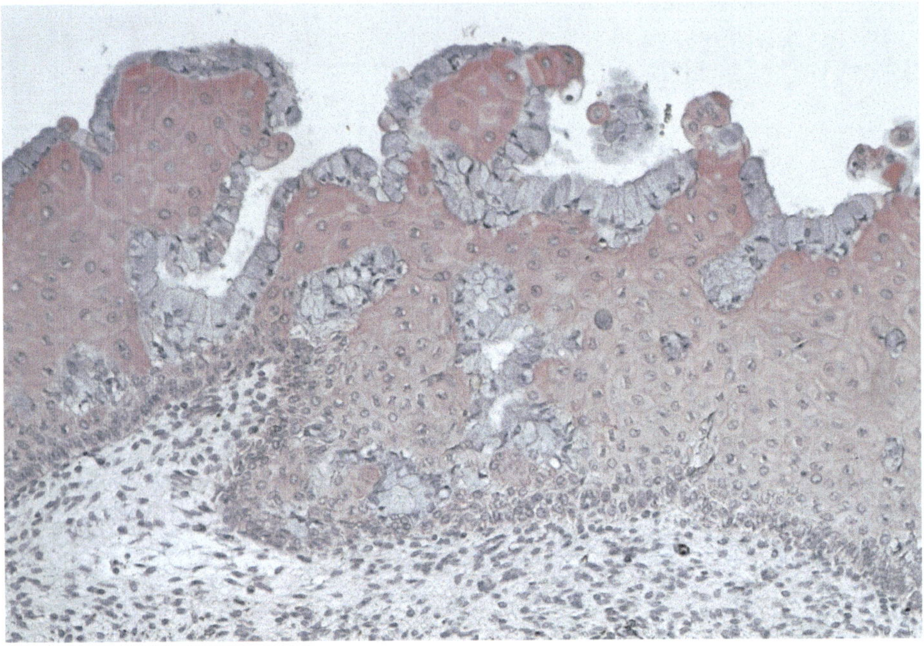

Fig. 22. Hyperplasia of reserve cells differentiating into squamous metaplasia. Immunohistochemical reaction with cytokeratin 13

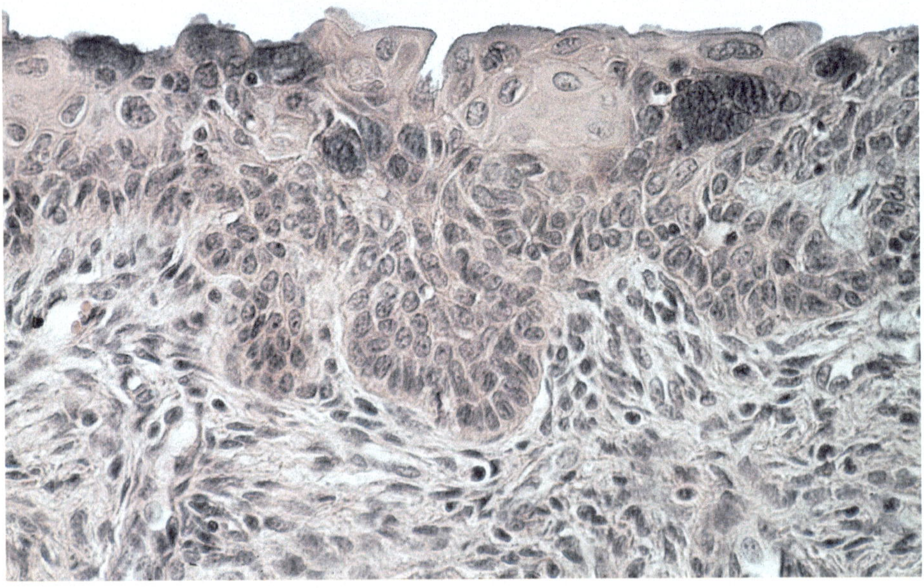

Fig. 23. Monocellular mucin formation in squamous metaplasia. H&E

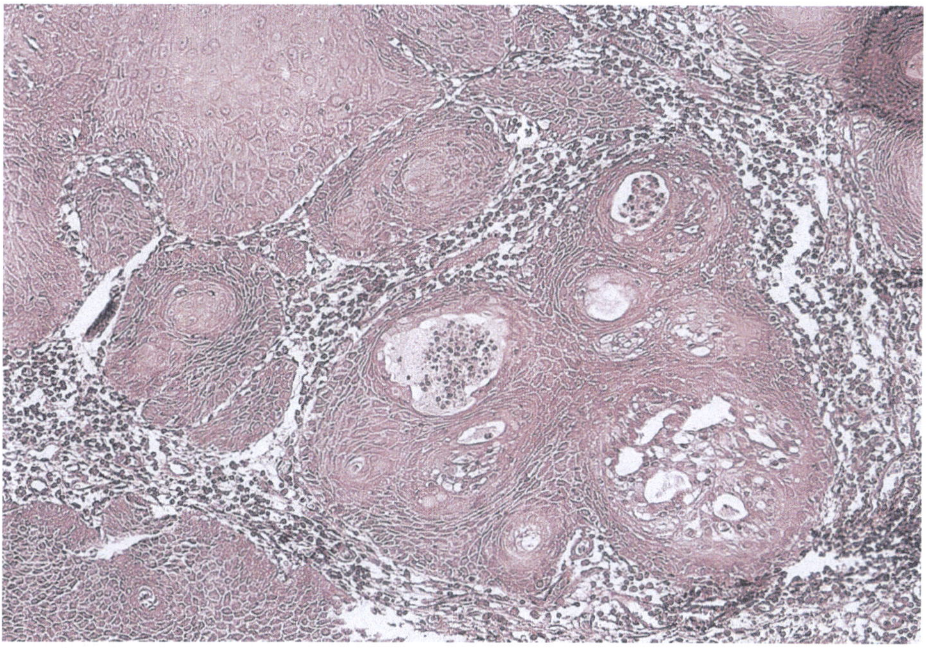

Fig. 24. Monocellular and multicystic mucin formation in squamous metaplasia. H&E

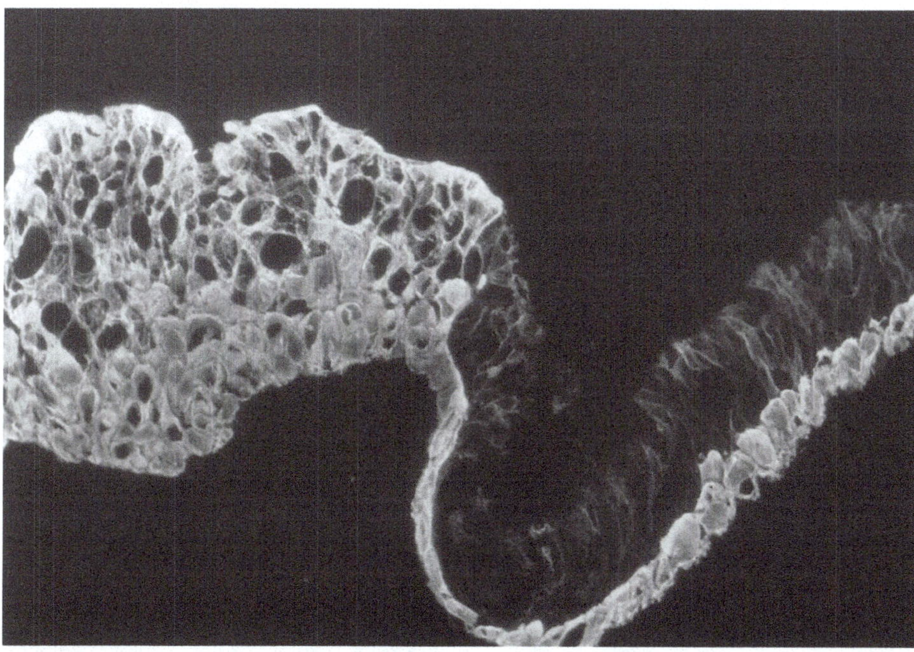

Fig. 25. Squamocolumnar junction with original squamous epithelium and adjacent reserve cell hyperplasia underneath the columnar epithelium. Immunohistochemical reaction with cytokeratin KA 1 (from Franke et al. 1986)

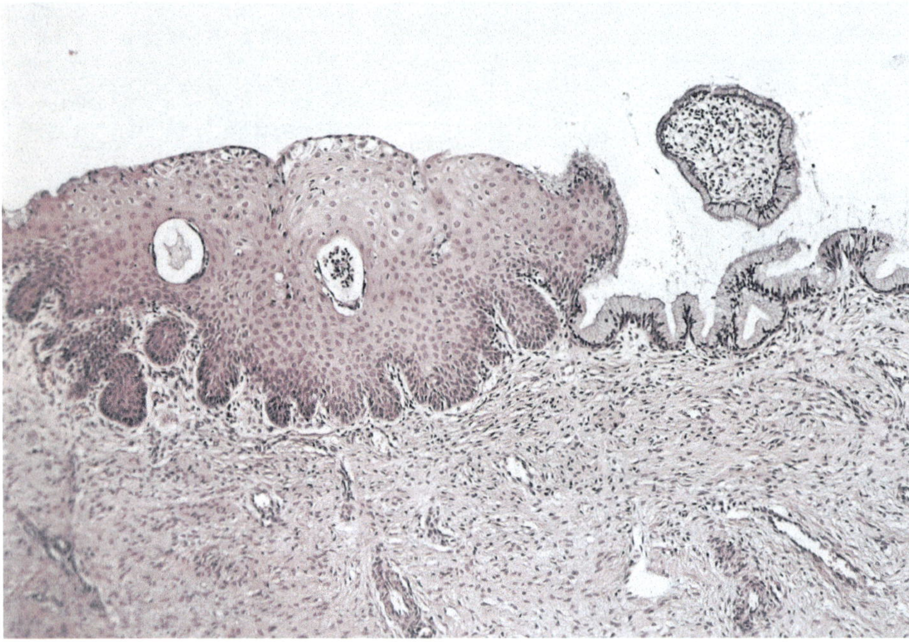

Fig. 26. Junction between squamous metaplasia and columnar epithelium. H&E

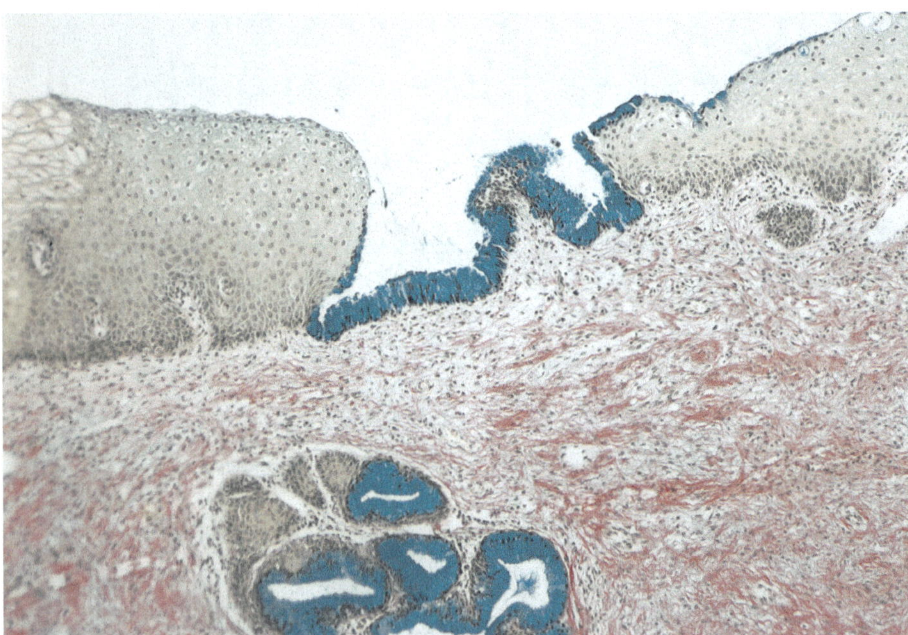

Fig. 27. Junction between squamous metaplasia and columnar epithelium. Alcian blue reaction

Transformation Zone (Figs. 28–31)

It is important to recognize and locate the transformation zone since most cervical neoplasias arise at or above this squamocolumnar junction. In their developmental stage they usually are limited to the transformation zone.

When the squamous epithelium that covers this repair zone (Figs. 28–30) does not undergo precancerous change, but, as in most instances, matures normally and completely, then at the end stage of repair it is impossible to distinguish the regenerative and metaplastic squamous epithelia from the adjacent primary ectocervical epithelium (Fig. 31). This "third mucosa" can only be recognized by the pinched off and often cystically dilated endocervical glands underlying the squamous epithelium. When these become large retention cysts, they may be recognized grossly as rounded protuberances (ovula Nabothi, Nabothian cysts; Fig. 11).

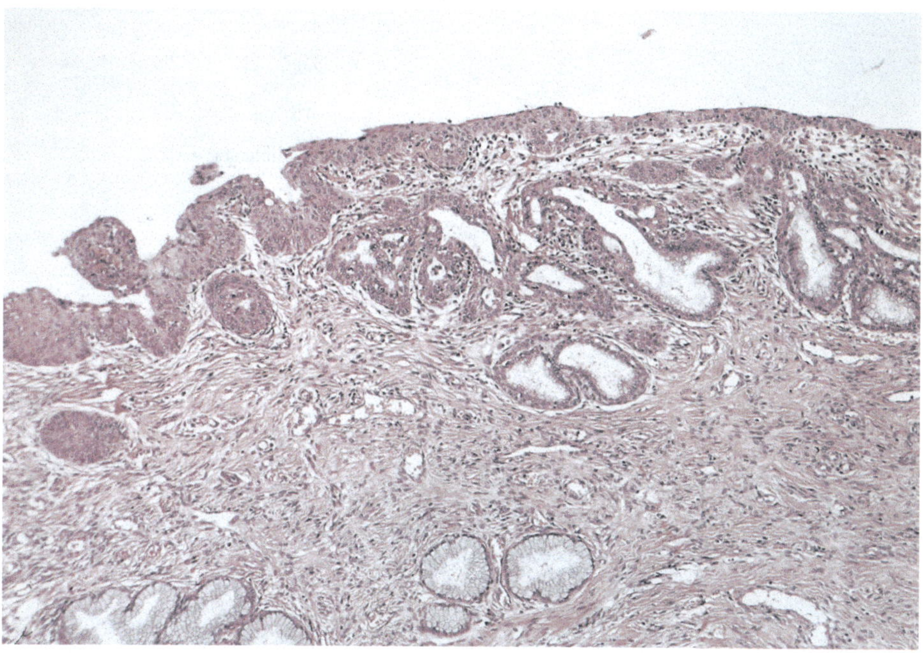

Fig. 28. Transformation zone covered by squamous metaplasia in descending repair, early stage. H&E

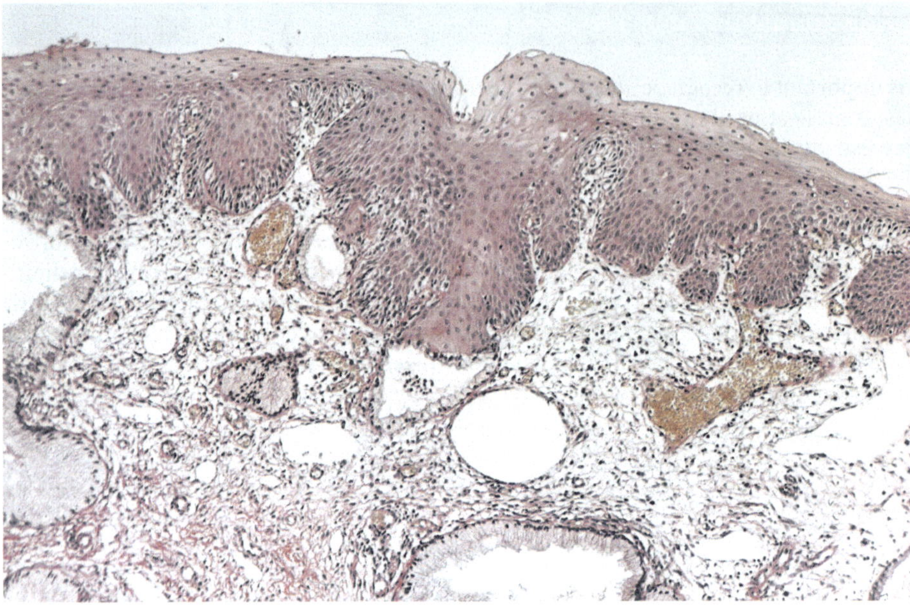

Fig. 29. Transformation zone covered by squamous metaplasia, intermediate stage. H&E

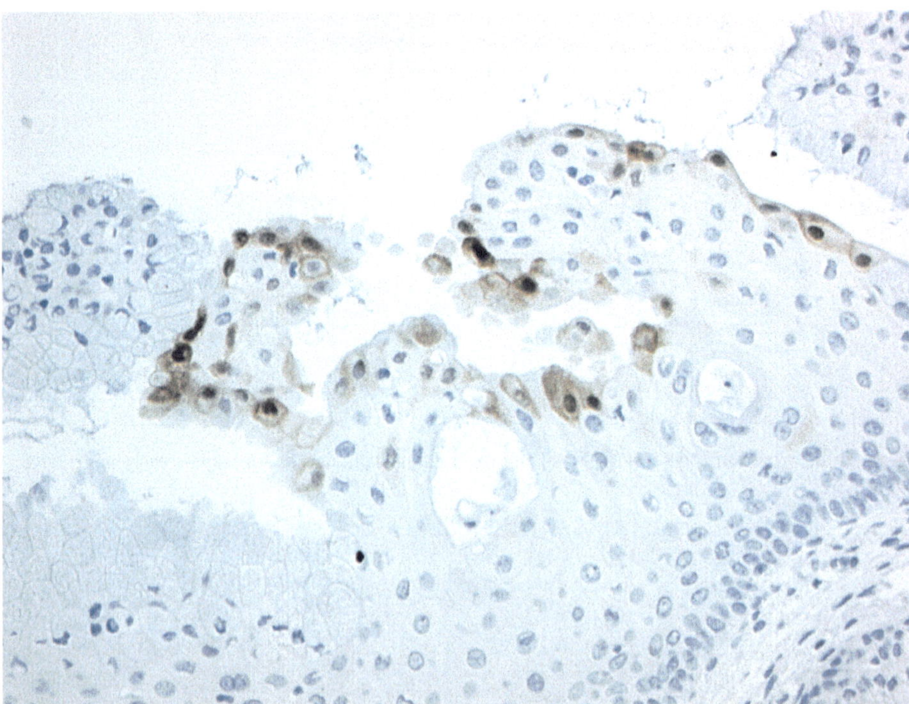

Fig. 30. Squamous metaplasia, physiologic p16^{INK4a}-expression in maturing epithelial cells. Focal staining pattern. p16^{INK4a} immunostain (see p. 9 f)

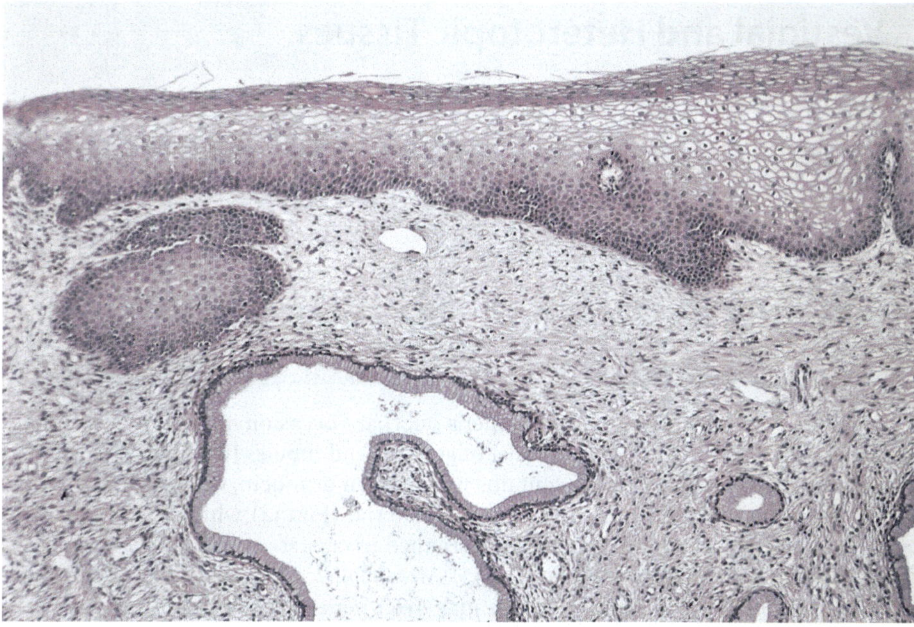

Fig. 31. Transformation zone covered by mature squamous epithelium, late stage. H&E

Vestigial and Heterotopic Tissues

Mesonephric Duct Remnants [2637/0] and Hyperplasia [7258/0] (Figs. 32–34)

Remnants of the mesonephric duct (Gartner's duct) are occasionally found deep in the lateral cervical wall (Fig. 32). They consist of small round tubules lined by a single layer of low cuboidal epithelium which contains no glycogen or mucin, whereas in the lumina one often finds eosinophilic homogenous material (Fig. 34) which is PAS-positive (compare Fig. 207). The tubules are often arranged in clusters, occasionally around an elongated remnant of a larger tubule (Fig. 33). *Mesonephric duct hyperplasia* consists of larger aggregates of such tubules, which may even penetrate the entire cervical wall (florid type) (Fig. 209).

Differential Diagnosis. Hyperplasia must be carefully distinguished from: (a) mesonephric adenocarcinoma, which shows hobnail cells with cytological atypia, intraglandular epithelial papillae, and frank stromal invasion; and (b) minimal deviation adenocarcinoma of the endocervix, which shows intracellular mucin formation, a positive re-

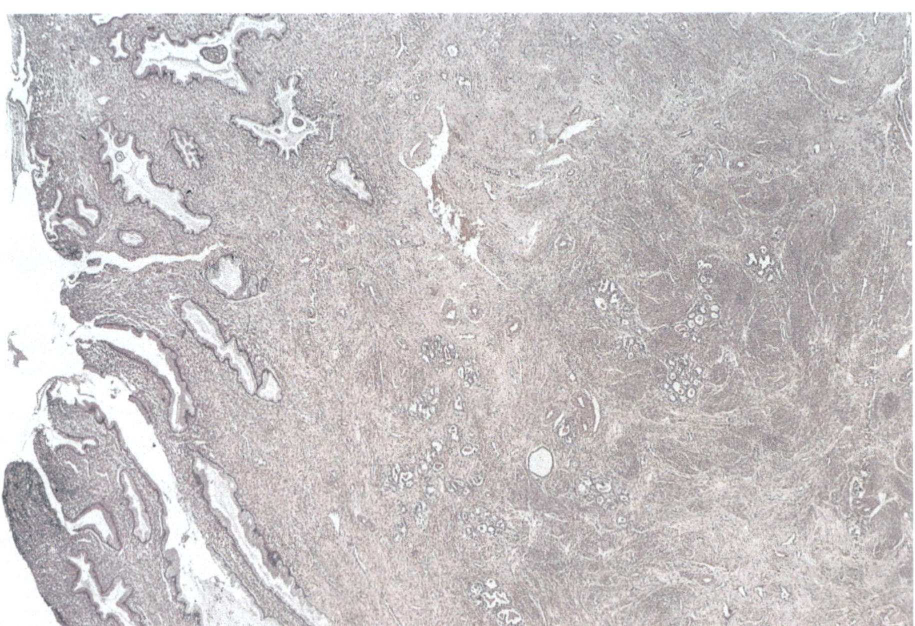

Fig. 32. Remnants of mesonephric duct in the cervical wall. H&E

action with CEA, periglandular edema with mucin pools, a desmoplastic stromal reaction around the invading tubules, and a histological transition between normal endocervical glands and the carcinomatous tubules (Shah et al. 1980; Ayroud et al. 1985).

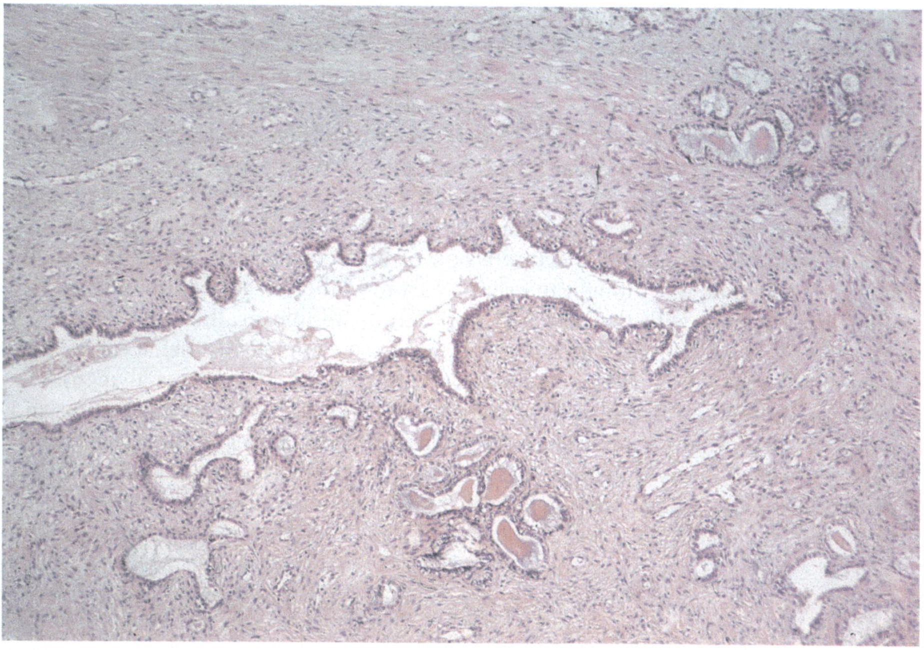

Fig. 33. Remnants of mesonephric duct in the cervical wall. H&E

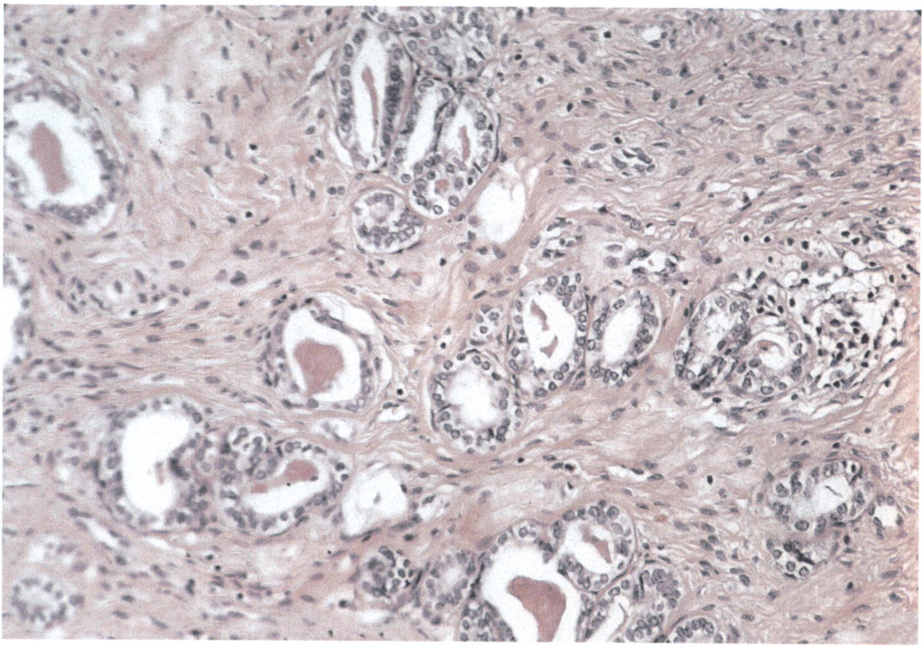

Fig. 34. Remnants of mesonephric duct in the cervical wall. H&E, higher magnification

Müllerian Duct Remnants and Metaplasia (Figs. 35–42)

Foci of ectocervical *endometriosis* [7650/0] may be located beneath the ectocervical epithelium and bulge forth as nodules (Fig. 35), grossly recognizable by the old and fresh hemorrhages in and around them (Figs. 35, 36), or be located deep in the cervical wall (Figs. 37, 38). These deep foci correspond in their location and structure to adenomyosis of the myometrium. The glands are characteristically surrounded by an endometrial-type stroma. In some instances, endocervical glands may be lined by columnar ciliated cells resulting from a *ciliated cell (tubal) metaplasia* (Figs. 39–42). Such glands are devoid of surrounding endometrial-type stroma and correspond to the foci of *endosalpingiosis* occasionally found scattered about the small pelvis (Wells and Brown 1986). Foci of *intestinal metaplasia* [7332/0] may also be observed within endocervical glands.

Transitional cell metaplasia is a rare lesion of the ectocervical epithelium usually seen in older women. It is thought to originate from Müllerian epithelium of the early genitourinary system with the potential to differentiate into urothelium (Weir et al. 1997). Since the reaction to CK 20 is negative, however, complete urothelial differentiation cannot be verified on immunohistological examination (Harnden et al. 1999). The ectocervical epithelium is replaced by transitional cells with lack of maturation and spindled nuclei with longitudinal nuclear grooves and perinuclear halos. Transitional cell metaplasia may be overdiagnosed as dysplasia, from which it can be differentiated by its regular nuclear shape and the lack of mitoses. Squamous cell metaplasia can be distinguished by its round nuclear shape.

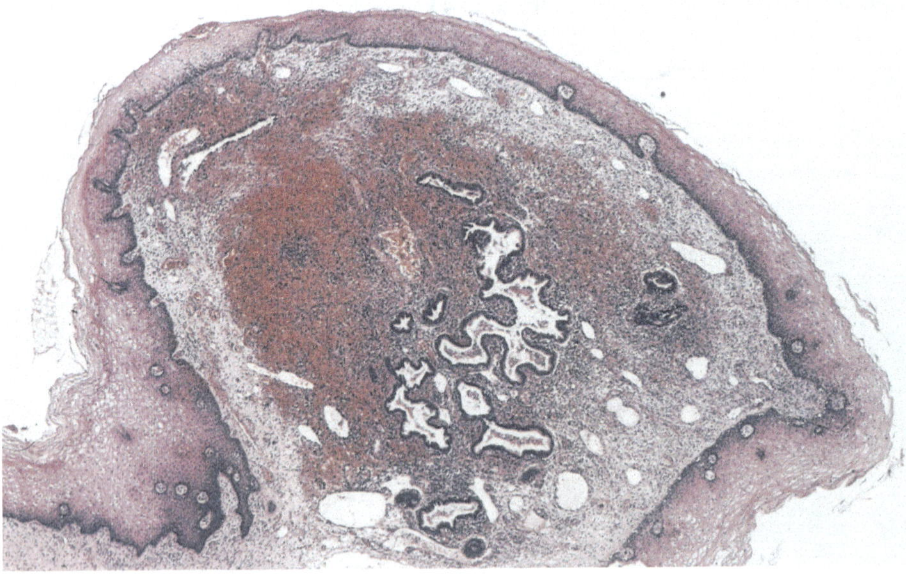

Fig. 35. Focus of endometriosis underneath ectocervical epithelium. H&E

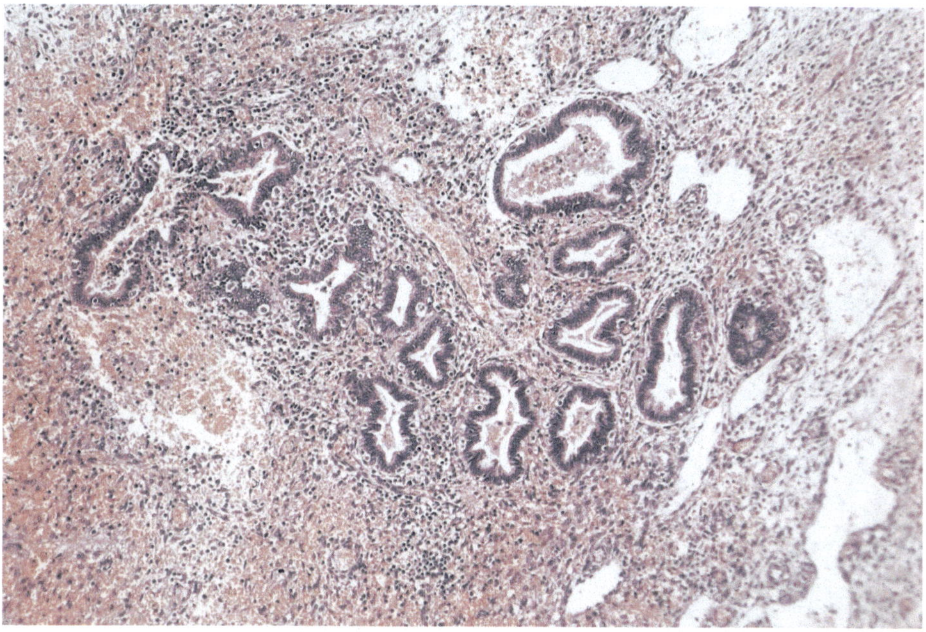

Fig. 36. Focus of endometriosis underneath ectocervical epithelium. H&E, higher magnification

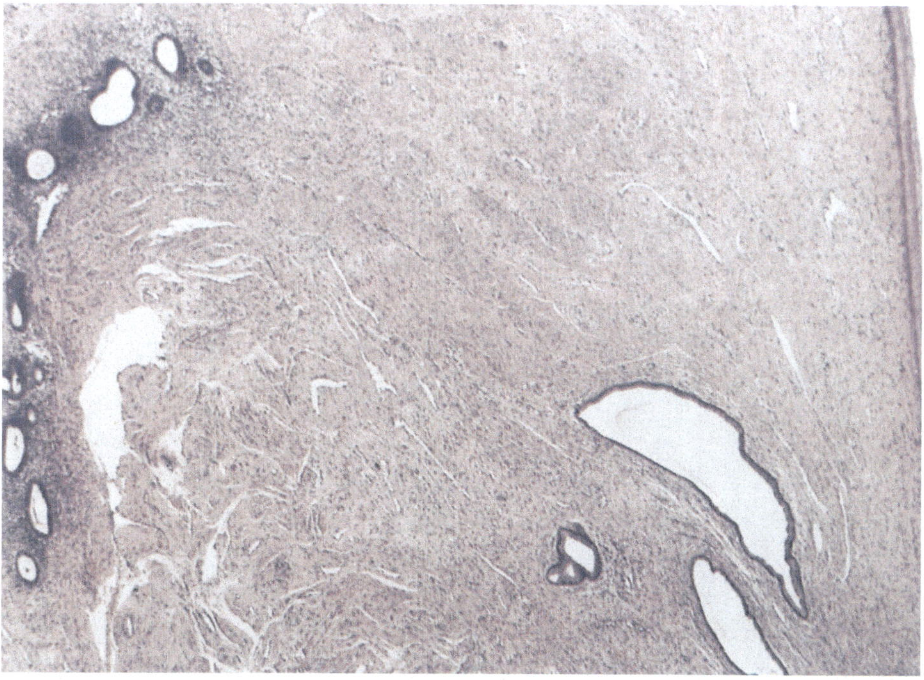

Fig. 37. Focus of endometriosis in the cervical wall. H&E

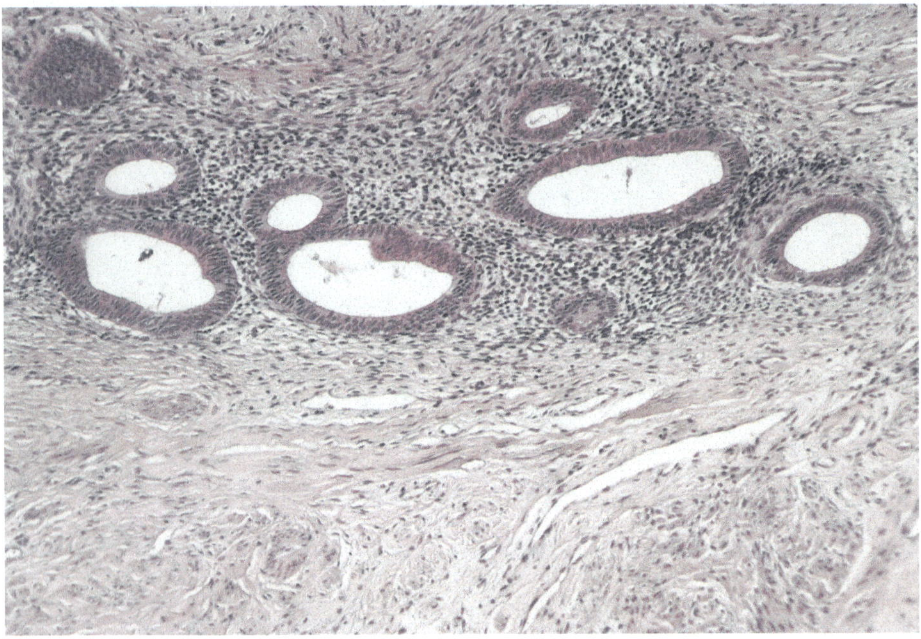

Fig. 38. Focus of endometriosis in the cervical wall. H&E higher magnification

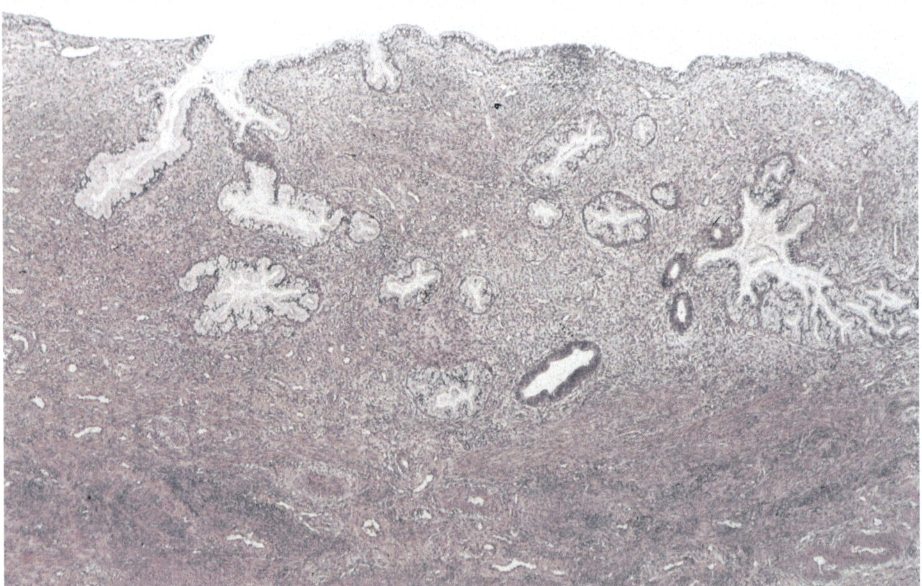

Fig. 39. Ciliated cell (tubal) metaplasia of endocervical glands. H&E

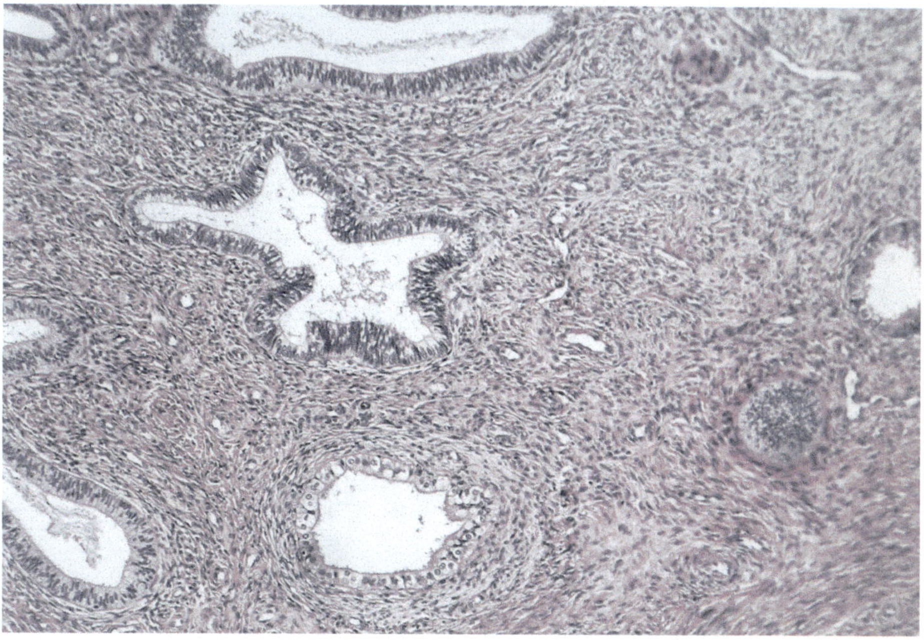

Fig. 40. Ciliated cell (tubal) metaplasia of endocervical glands. H&E, higher magnification

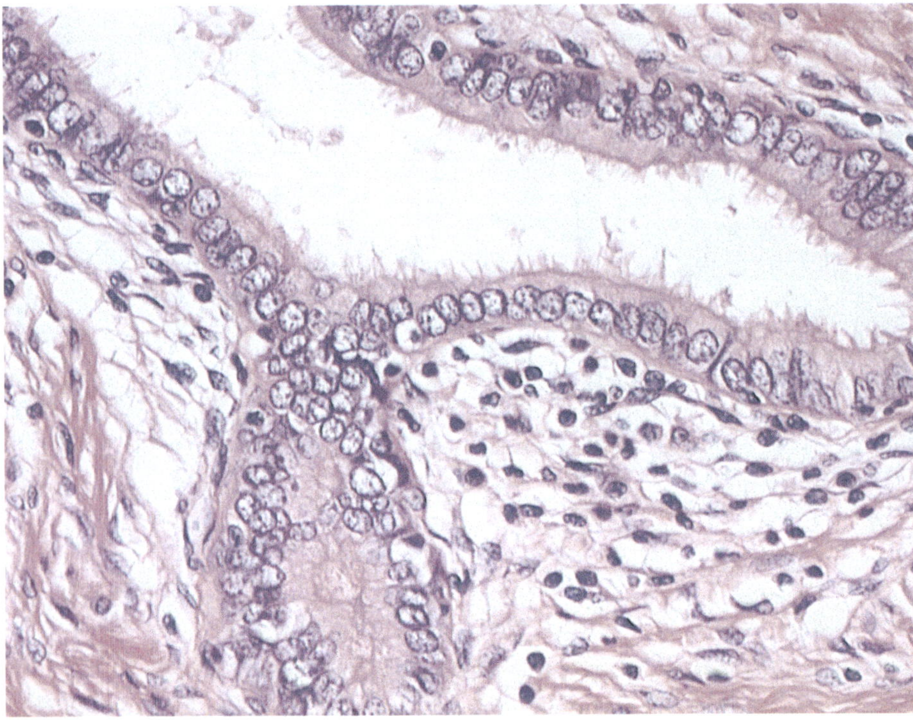

Fig. 41. Ciliated cell (tubal) metaplasia of endocervical glands. H&E

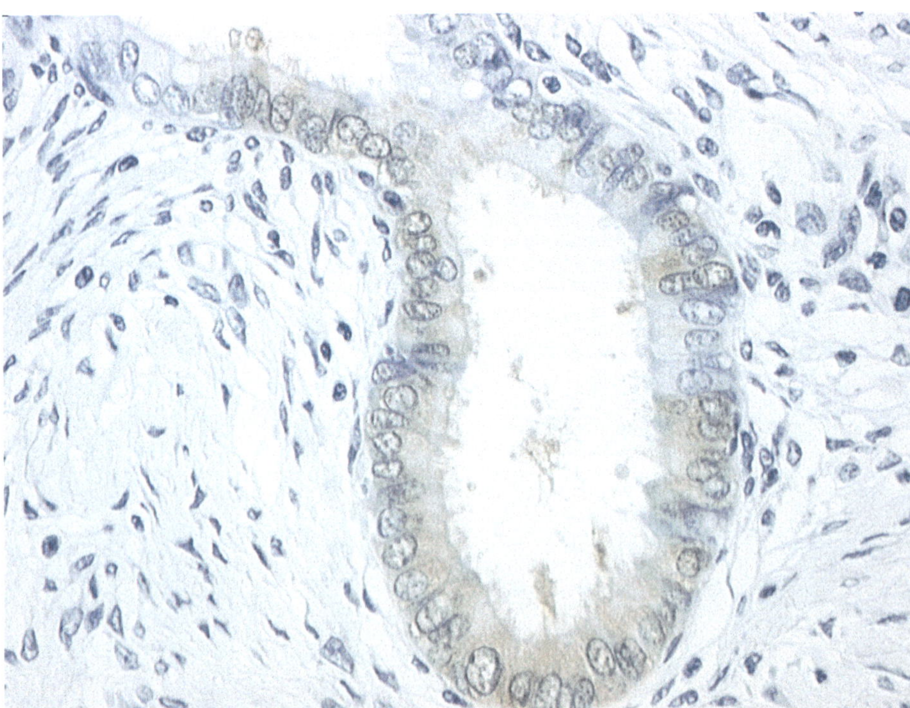

Heterotopic Ectodermal and Mesodermal Structures (Figs. 43–47)

Rarely, heterotopic "neometaplasia" (Young et al. 1981) may result in the formation of *epidermoid or dermoid cysts* [9084/0] (Figs. 43–45) or give rise to sebaceous or sweat gland formations beneath the ectocervical epithelium (Figs. 46, 47; Dougherty et al. 1962). These structures have no clinical significance.

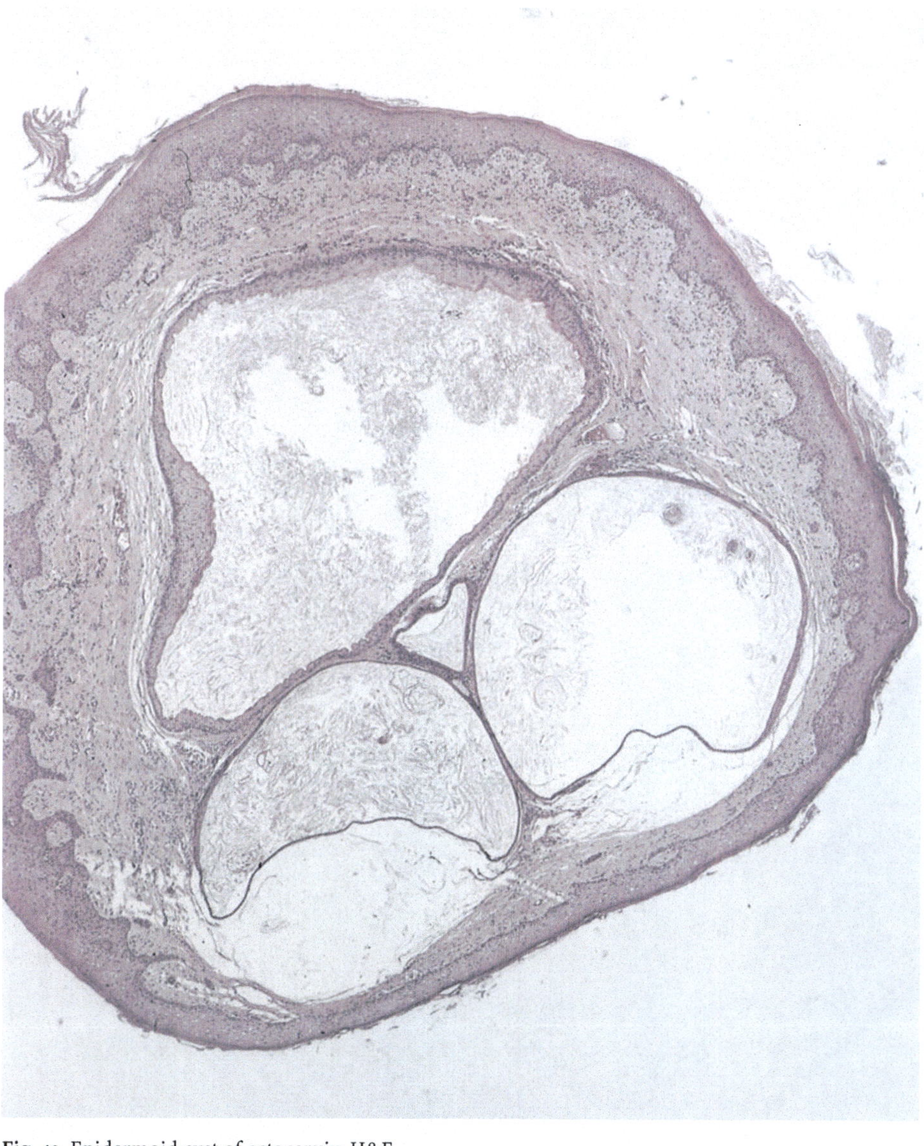

Fig. 43. Epidermoid cyst of ectocervix. H&E

Fig. 42. Ciliated cell (tubal) metaplasia of endocervical glands. Same case as in Fig. 41. Focal, noncontinuous positivity for $p16^{INK4a}$. $p16^{INK4a}$ immunostain

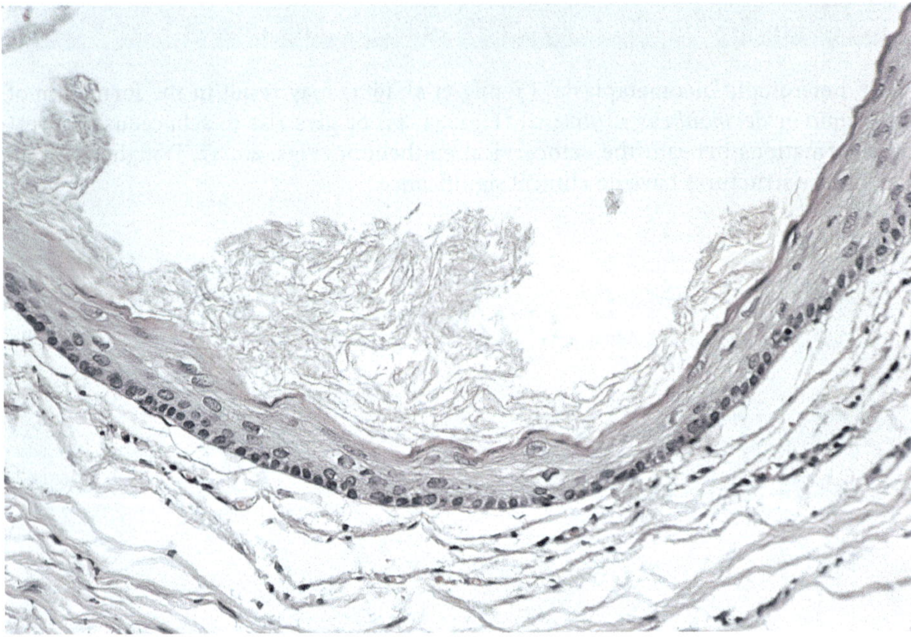

Fig. 44. Epidermoid cyst of ectocervix. H&E, higher magnification

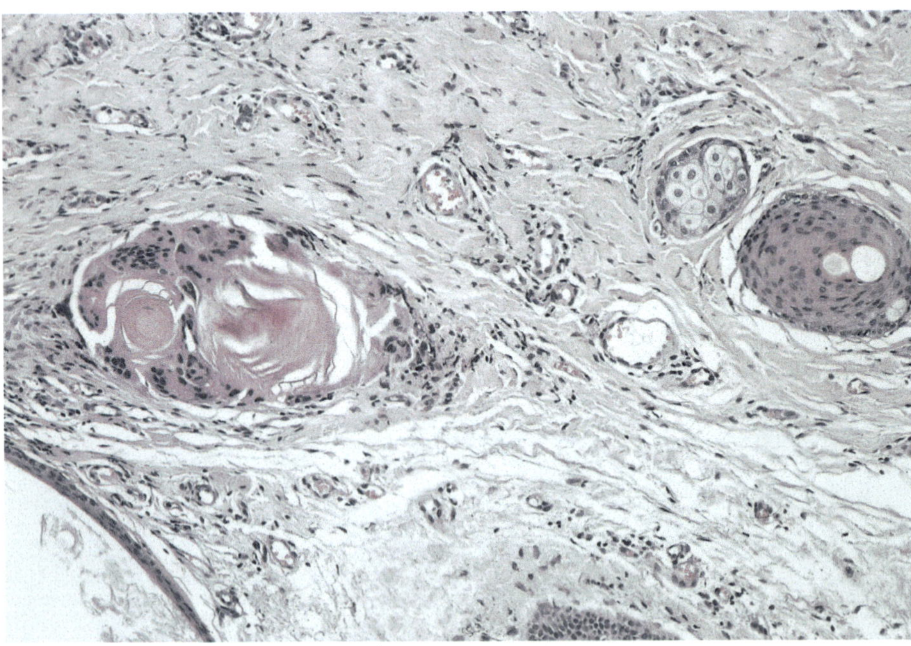

Fig. 45. Epidermoid cyst of ectocervix. Foreign body reaction around squamous cells. H&E

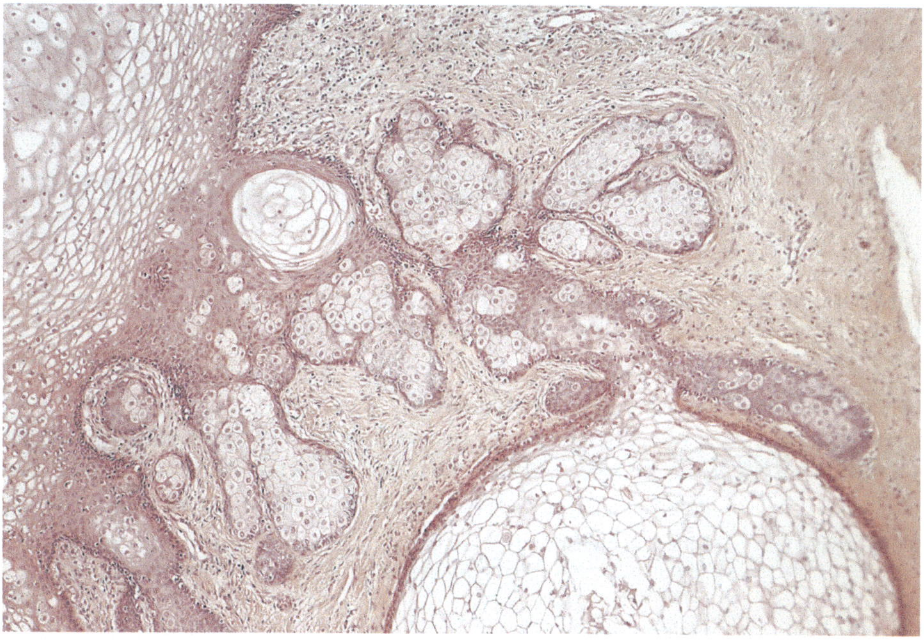

Fig. 46. Formation of sebaceous glands beneath ectocervical epithelium. H&E

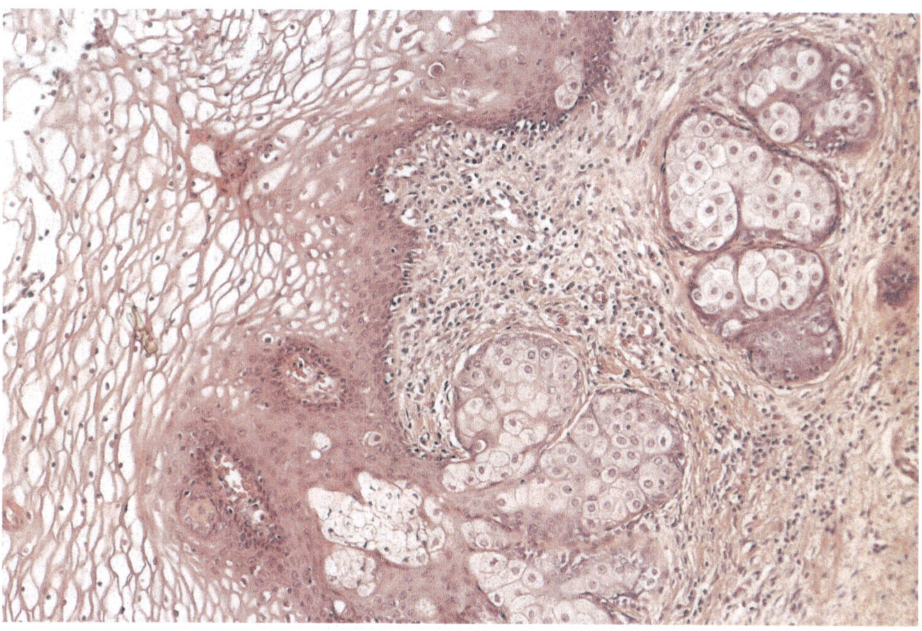

Fig. 47. Formation of sebaceous glands beneath ectocervical epithelium. H&E, higher magnification

Hormonally Induced Changes

Estrogens and gestagens act as antagonists not only on the endometrium but also on the ecto- and endocervix (Dallenbach-Hellweg 1981; Table 2).

Table 2. The effects of ovarian hormones on the uterus

	Estrogen	Progesterone
Ectocervix	Proliferation, para- and hyperkeratosis	Differentiation, desquamation
Endocervix	Differentiation: glands: secretion of mucin; reserve cells: squamous metaplasia	Proliferation (regeneration), glandular and reserve cell hyperplasia
Endometrium	Proliferation	Differentiation: glands: secretion of glycogen; stroma: decidualization

Effects of Estrogen (Figs. 48–54)

Parakeratosis and Hyperkeratosis of the Ectocervix

Estrogens stimulate proliferation of the squamous epithelium of the ectocervix, resulting in a well-developed superficial cell layer often covered by a fairly thick layer of parakeratotic cells (Figs. 48, 49), which become keratinized prematurely. In endogenous or exogenous hyperestrogenism, the keratinization may become exaggerated, whereby a thin (Fig. 50) or thick (Fig. 51) layer of hyperkeratosis is devoid of nuclei.

The proliferative effect of estrogens, furthermore, promotes ascending repair of columnar epithelium or epithelial defects, which are overgrown by regenerative epithelium of ectocervical origin (see p. 19. Similar hyperkeratinization follows the stimulatory effects induced by chronic trauma, as in uterine prolapse.

Cystic Hyperplasia of the Endocervix [3340/0]

Under estrogenic stimulation, the epithelial cells of the endocervical glands differentiate and produce mucin, which may become excessive with long-standing unopposed estrogen. Consequently, the glands become cystically dilated with inspissated mucin (Figs. 52–54). Thereby they become closely clustered, and the glandular region enlarges by extending down into the cervical wall. Reserve cells or areas of preceding reserve cell hyperplasia may differentiate and undergo squamous cell metaplasia (see p. 24).

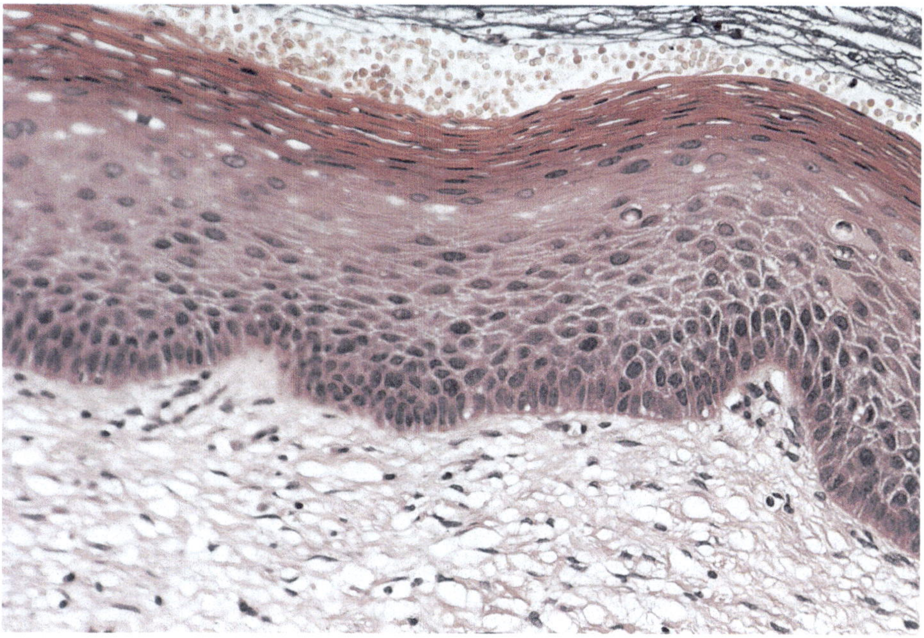

Fig. 48. Parakeratosis of ectocervical epithelium. H&E

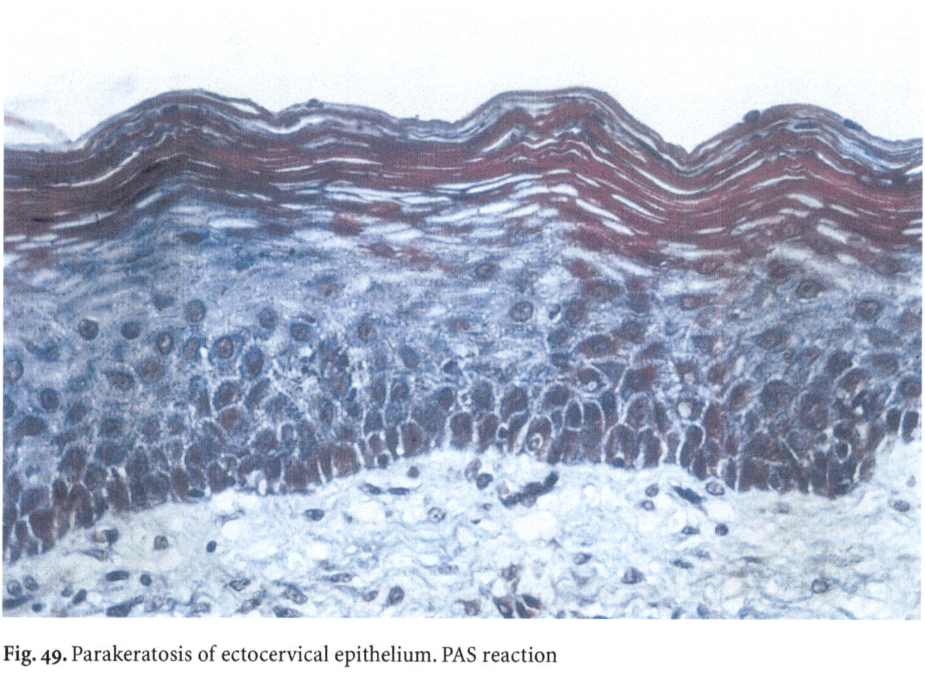

Fig. 49. Parakeratosis of ectocervical epithelium. PAS reaction

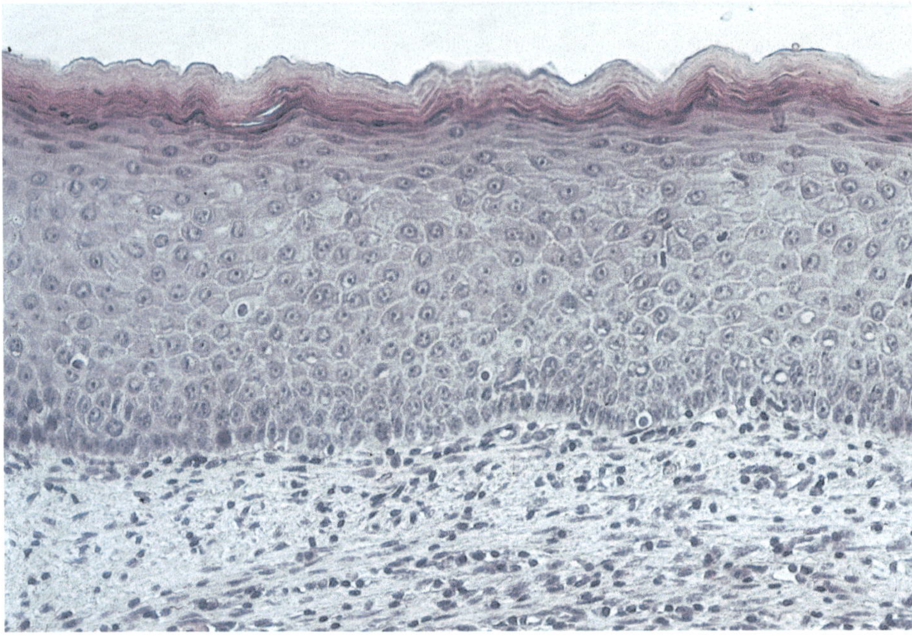

Fig. 50. Hyperkeratosis of ectocervical epithelium, mild. H&E

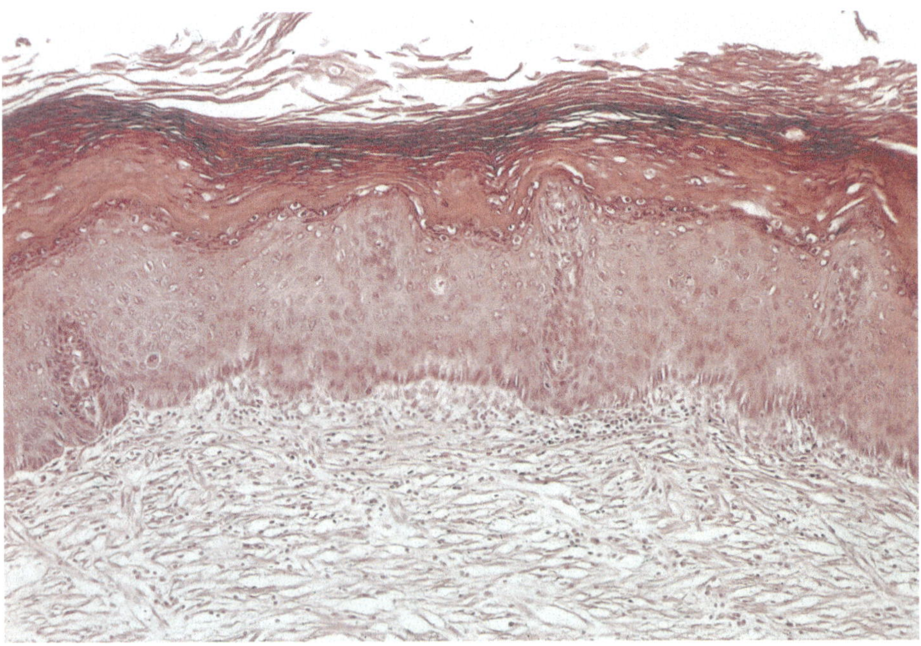

Fig. 51. Hyperkeratosis of ectocervical epithelium, extensive. H&E

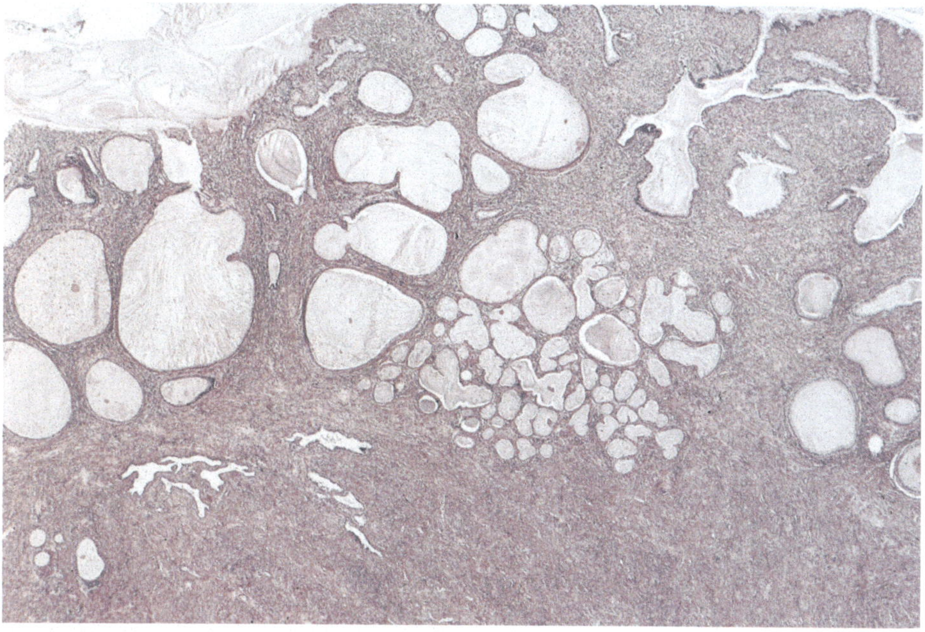

Fig. 52. Cystic hyperplasia of endocervix, mild, with focal formation of tunnel clusters (*middle right*). H&E

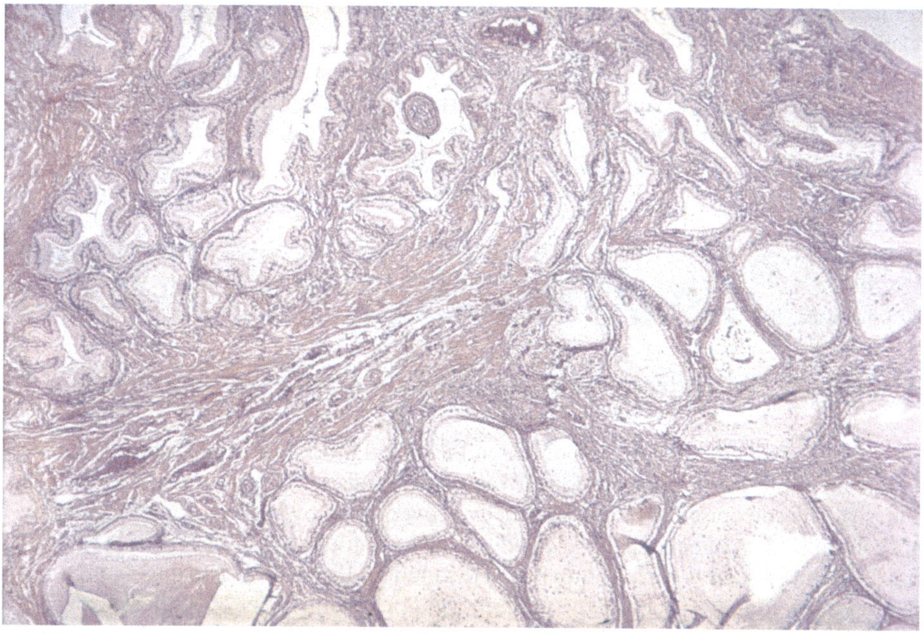

Fig. 53. Cystic hyperplasia of endocervix, extensive. H&E

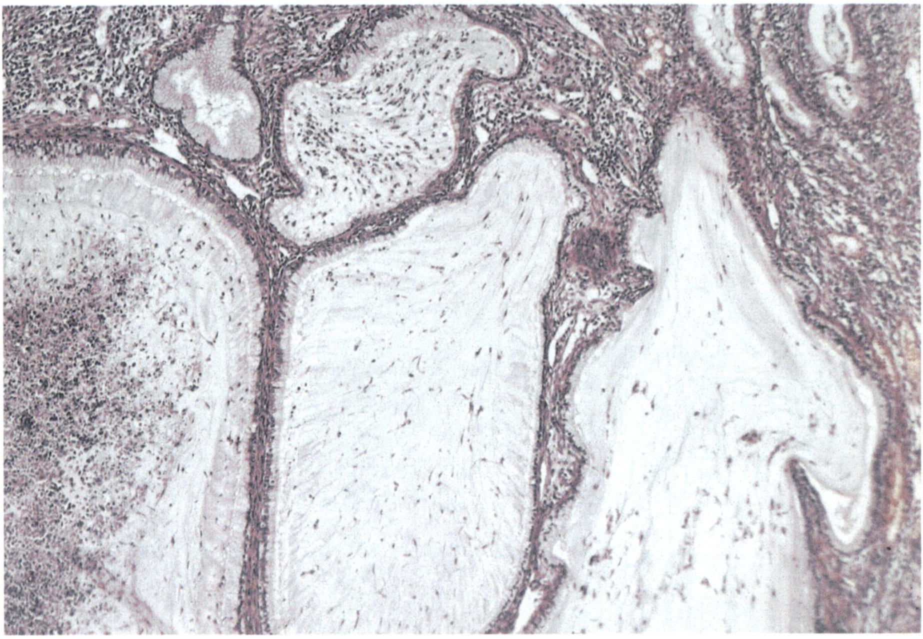

Fig. 54. Cystic hyperplasia of endocervix, extensive. H&E, higher magnification

Subinvolution of previously cystic hyperplastic glands may result in the formation of *tunnel clusters* (Fig. 52), consisting of multifocal areas of closely packed, dilated endocervical glands with inspissated mucus. The glandular epithelium is mostly flat, nonatypical. Occasional foci may contain noncystic, closely packed glands lined by slightly irregular epithelium and may falsely be interpreted as adenocarcinoma with minimal deviation. Distinction from carcinoma is possible by their lack of invasion and the negative reaction for CEA (Segal and Hart 1990; Gilks at al. 1989).

Effects of Endogenous Progesterone under Hypersecretion (Figs. 55–58)

Glandular and Cystic Hyperplasia of the Endocervix [3340/0]

The physiologic hyperstimulation of the endocervical mucosa during gestation induces a mild or moderate hypersecretion of the glands and a proliferation of reserve cells (Fig. 56). The ectropionized mucosa usually is overgrown by an ascending regenerative epithelium (Fig. 55). Foci of *ectopic decidua* may be found in the endocervix and appear much like those seen at various other sites throughout the small pelvis during pregnancy. They show that they possess the inherent genetic potentialities of Müllerian-derived cells. In like manner, an *Arias-Stella reaction* [7943/0] (see Figs. 57, 58) is also occasionally observed in endocervical glands.

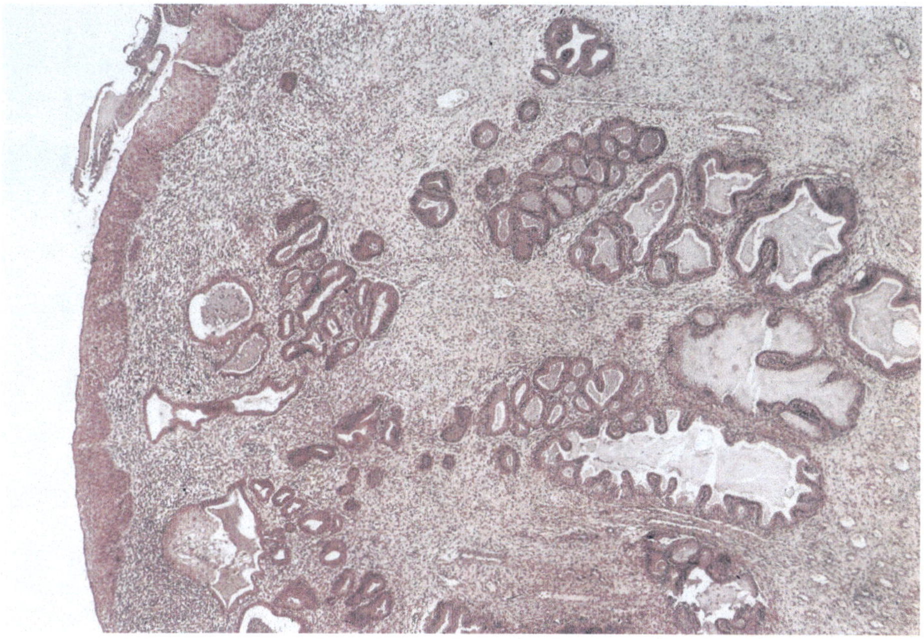

Fig. 55. Glandular (and cystic) hyperplasia of endocervix during pregnancy, with proliferation of reserve cells. H&E

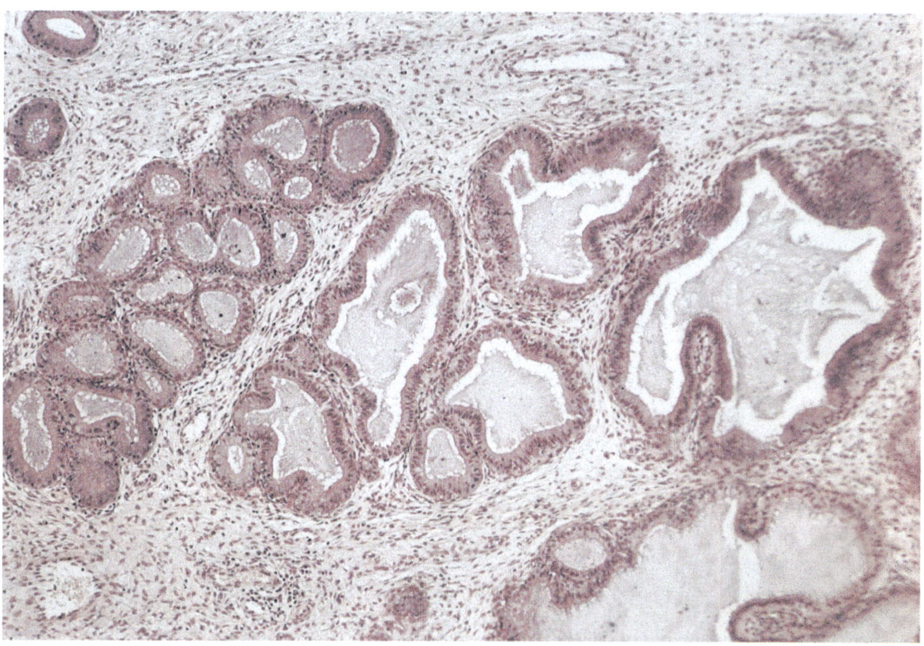

Fig. 56. Glandular (and cystic) hyperplasia of endocervix during pregnancy, with proliferation of reserve cells. H&E, higher magnification

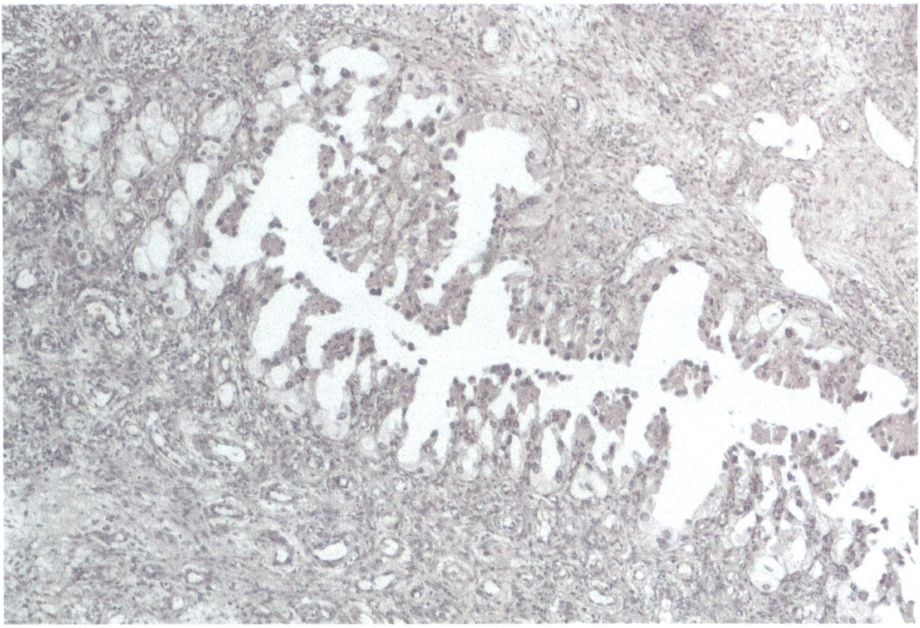

Fig. 57. Arias-Stella reaction of endocervical glandular epithelia during pregnancy. H&E

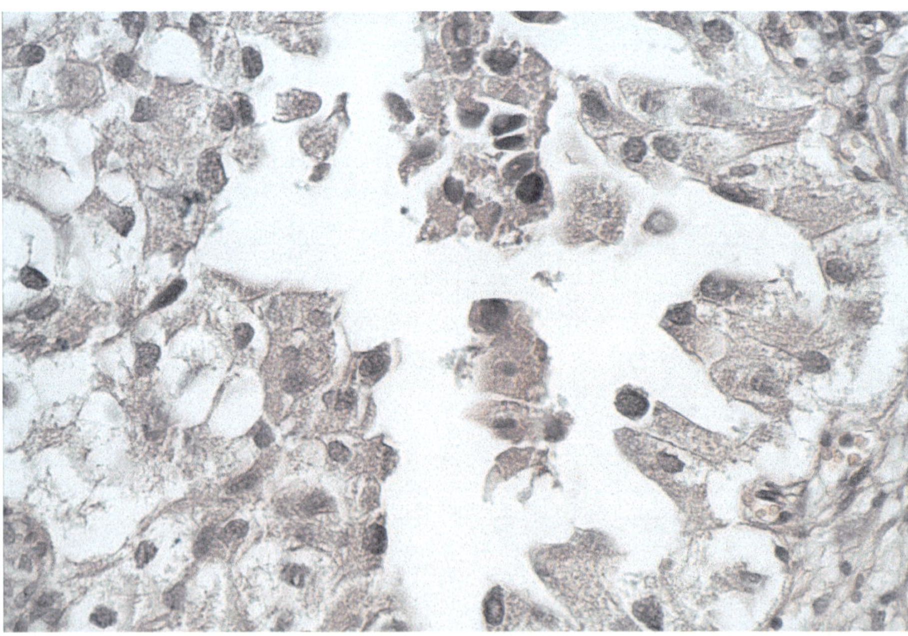

Fig. 58. Arias-Stella reaction of endocervical glandular epithelia during pregnancy. Hyperplastic endocervical epithelia with hobnail nuclei. H&E, higher magnification of Fig. 57

Effects of Exogenous Gestagens (Figs. 59–65)

Under the influence of synthetic gestagens, the maturation of the ectocervical stratified squamous epithelium ceases at the intermediate stage, and desquamation is enhanced. In contrast, under the same hormonal stimulation, the endocervix shows proliferative changes, the intensity and histological appearance of which vary depending on the length of administration, dose, potency, and chemical structure of the gestagen given (Moltz and Becker 1977). Glandular proliferation may be either predominantly adenomatous or microglandular, the immature glandular epithelium either single- or multilayered. The proliferation of the glandular epithelium is often accompanied by a multilayered hyperplasia of underlying reserve cells.

Glandular (Adenomatous) Hyperplasia of the Endocervix

New glands form and the glandular epithelial cells become pseudostratified (Fig. 62), containing elongated hyperchromatic nuclei in a less well-differentiated cytoplasm. The glands may ramify (Fig. 59) or become crowded (Fig. 60), occasionally resulting in a diffuse laminar glandular pattern (Jones et al. 1991; Nucci 2002). The production of mucin is reduced or absent and occurs irregularly from one gland to another (Fig. 61) or within the same gland (Fig. 62). Cells with mucin and those without may lie together. In addition, the chemical composition of the mucus is often changed (Gaton et al. 1982).

The reserve cells underneath the glandular and superficial epithelium may undergo hyperplasia to form several layers. That hyperplasia is stimulated by the gestagens. Such hyperplastic reserve cells may appear quite immature and contain depolarized hyperchromatic nuclei (Gall et al. 1969).

■ **Differential Diagnosis.** These adenomatous proliferations have to be distinguished from a well-differentiated adenocarcinoma of the endocervix. The invading carcinomatous glands induce, in most instances, a stromal reaction as they grow into the cervical wall. A large biopsy of the cervical wall may be required to make the distinction with H & E sections. If only a small portion of tissue is available, the immunohistochemical reaction for CEA is of great help – an adenomatous hyperplasia is negative for CEA, whereas an invasive adenocarcinoma reacts positively in most cases. An ACIS can be distinguished from adenomatous hyperplasia by its cytological atypias, cellular stratification, densely arranged hyperchromatic nuclei, and by its positive immunostaining reaction for CEA (Fig. 140a). $p16^{INK4a}$ is diffusely positive in adenocarcinoma and ACIS, whereas it is negative or focally positive in adenomatous hyperplasia.

It is well known that milder degrees of epithelial atypia may develop in some or parts of glands in cases of ACIS and invasive adenocarcinoma of the cervix. Similar epithelial atypia may also occur alone. For these changes the term cervical glandular atypia has been proposed; they probably represent a continuum from low-grade atypia to ACIS (Wells and Brown 1986). In the current WHO classification these changes are termed *glandular dysplasia* (Zaino 2002; Tavassoli and Devilee 2003).

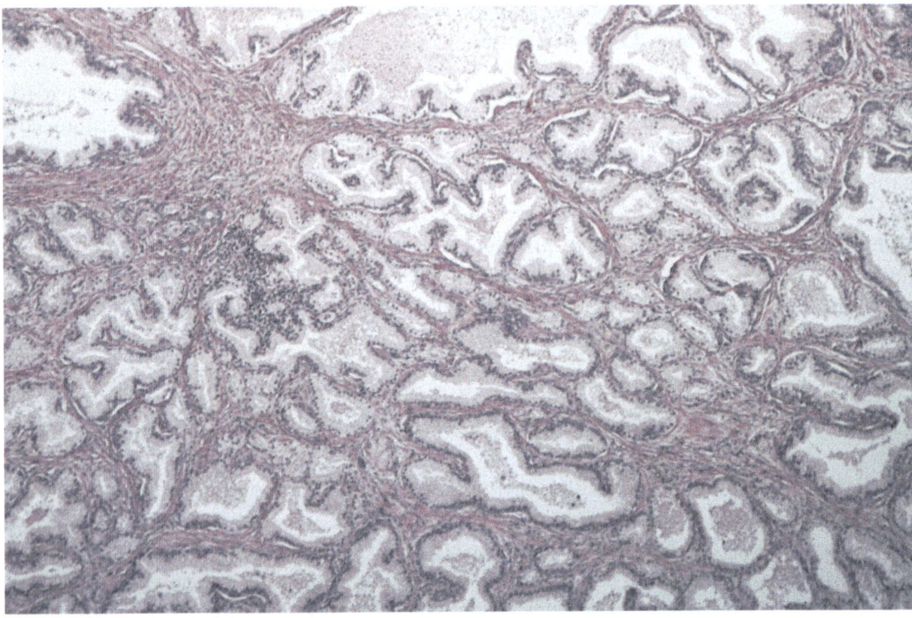

Fig. 59. Glandular (adenomatous) hyperplasia of endocervix. H&E

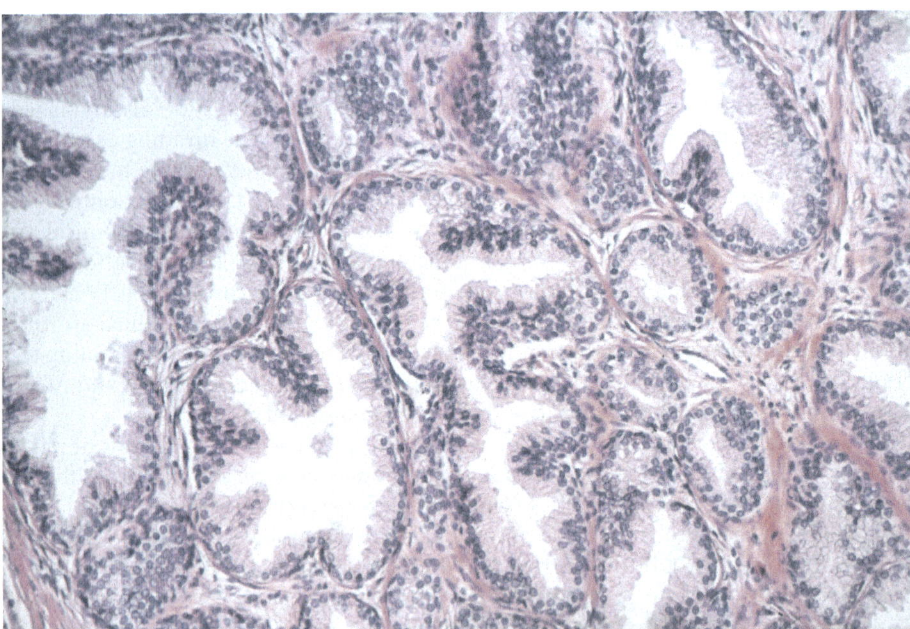

Fig. 60. Glandular (adenomatous) hyperplasia of endocervix with crowding of glands. H&E

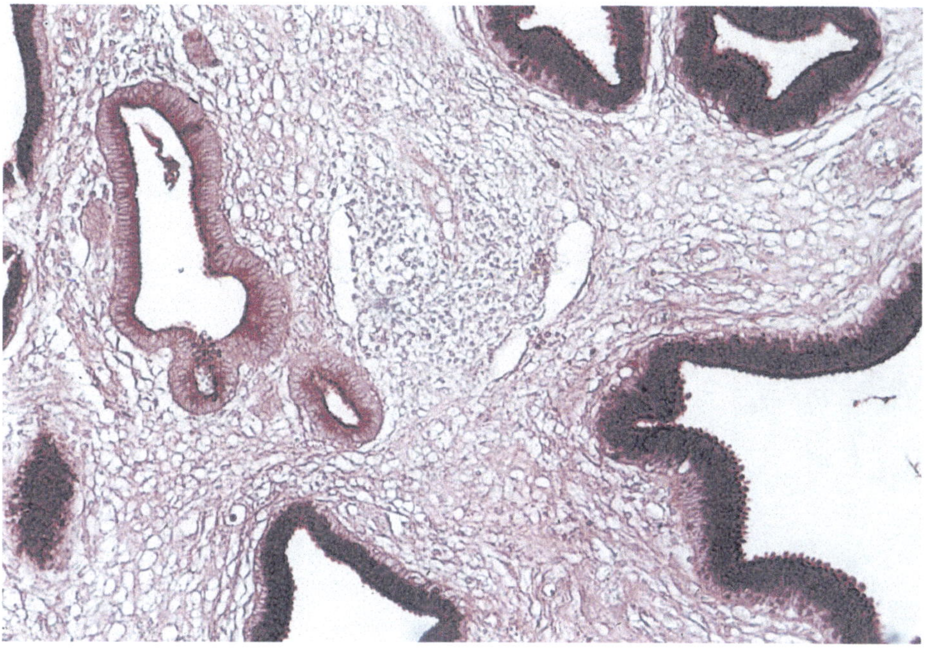

Fig. 61. Glandular (adenomatous) hyperplasia of endocervix, variable content of mucin from one gland to another. PAS reaction

Microglandular Hyperplasia of the Endocervix [7248/0] (Figs. 63–65)

With increasing potency of the gestagen used, endocervical glandular proliferation is more likely to develop into microalveolar changes with disappearance of the intervening stroma (Figs. 63–65). The low cuboidal, undifferentiated, glandular epithelial cells can hardly be distinguished from the surrounding hyperplastic reserve cells. Occasionally a solid sheetlike proliferation of reserve cells, signet-ring cells or hobnail cells may be observed. These changes, too, may be misdiagnosed as invasive adenocarcinoma or clear cell carcinoma (Taylor et al. 1967; Candy and Abell 1968; Kyriakos et al. 1968; Talbert and Shery 1969; Helmerhorst et al. 1984; Wells and Brown 1986; Young and Scully 1989).

Differential Diagnosis. Several features may help to differentiate a microglandular hyperplasia from an invasive carcinoma. The cells of microglandular hyperplasia show less nuclear atypia, they have a low proliferation index (MIB-1) and their cytoplasm contains mucin, not glycogen. In contrast to invasive adenocarcinoma, microglandular hyperplasia reacts negatively for CEA and for $p16^{INK4a}$.

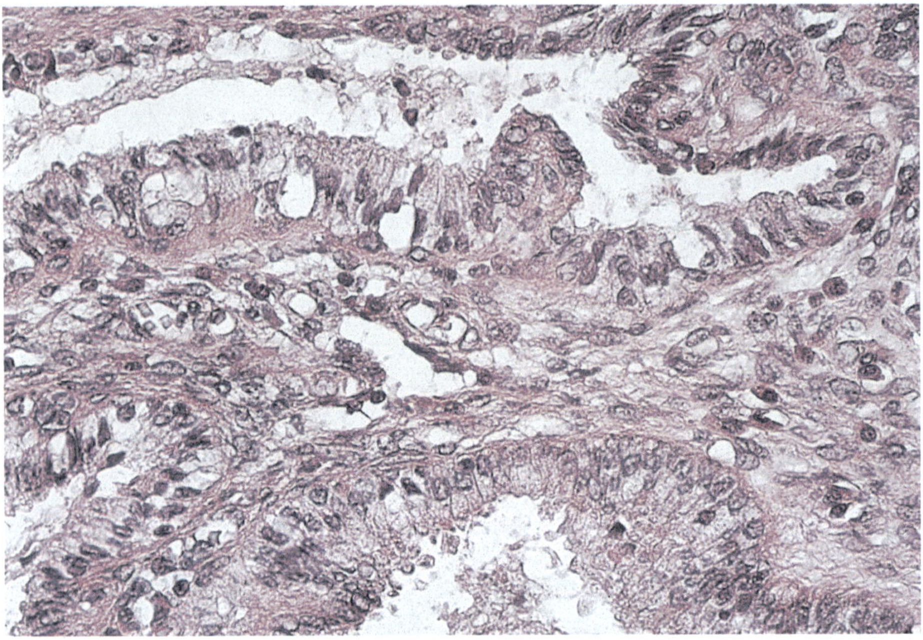

Fig. 62. Glandular (adenomatous) hyperplasia of endocervix with pseudostratified nuclei. H&E

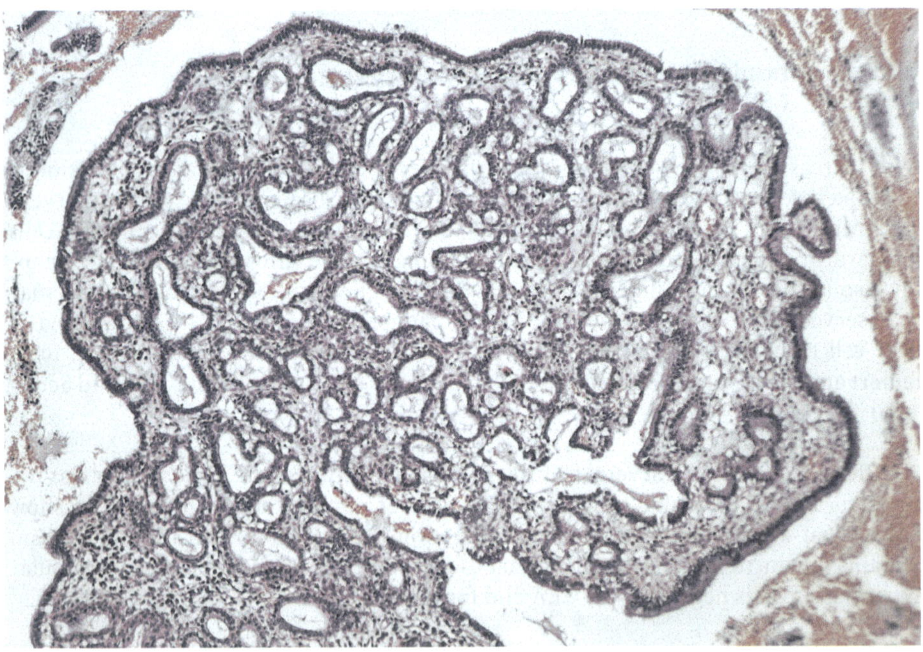

Fig. 63. Microglandular hyperplasia of endocervix. H&E

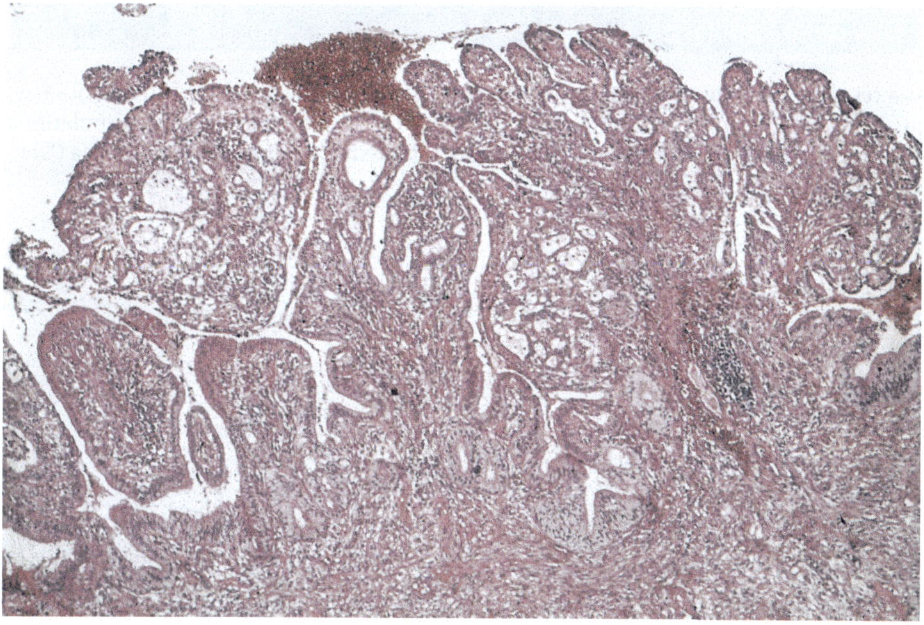

Fig. 64. Microglandular hyperplasia of endocervix, with reserve cell hyperplasia. H&E

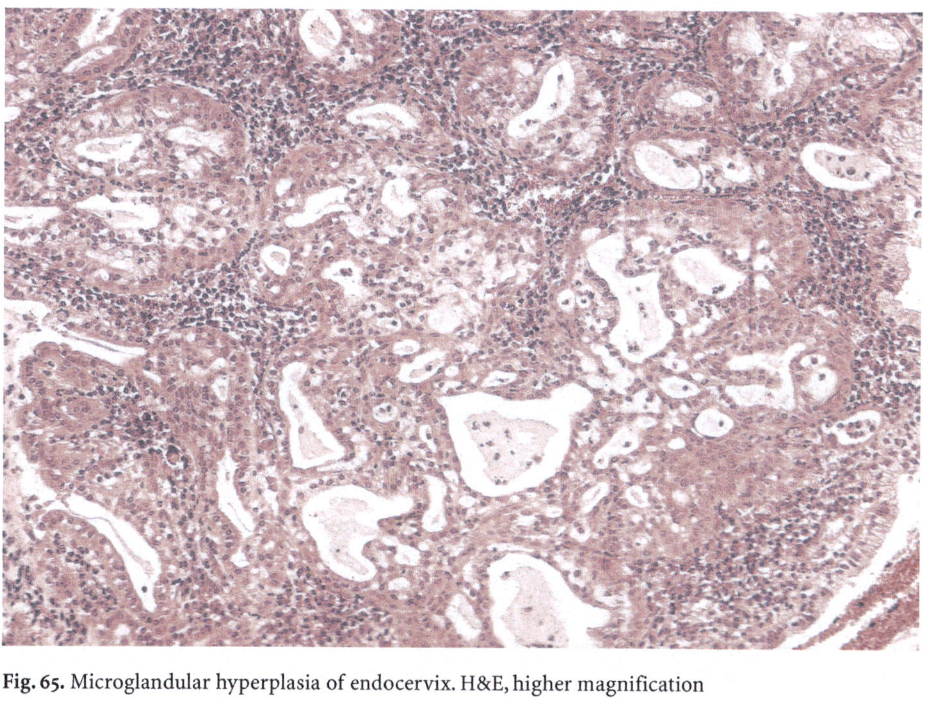

Fig. 65. Microglandular hyperplasia of endocervix. H&E, higher magnification

Glandular Papillary Ectropion (Fig. 66)

As a result of excessive proliferation and growth pressure, the endocervical mucosa frequently protrudes onto the ectocervical surface (Fig. 66). Under gestagenic stimulation, epidermization of such an ectropion is usually initiated by reserve cell hyperplasia ("descending repair," p. 24).

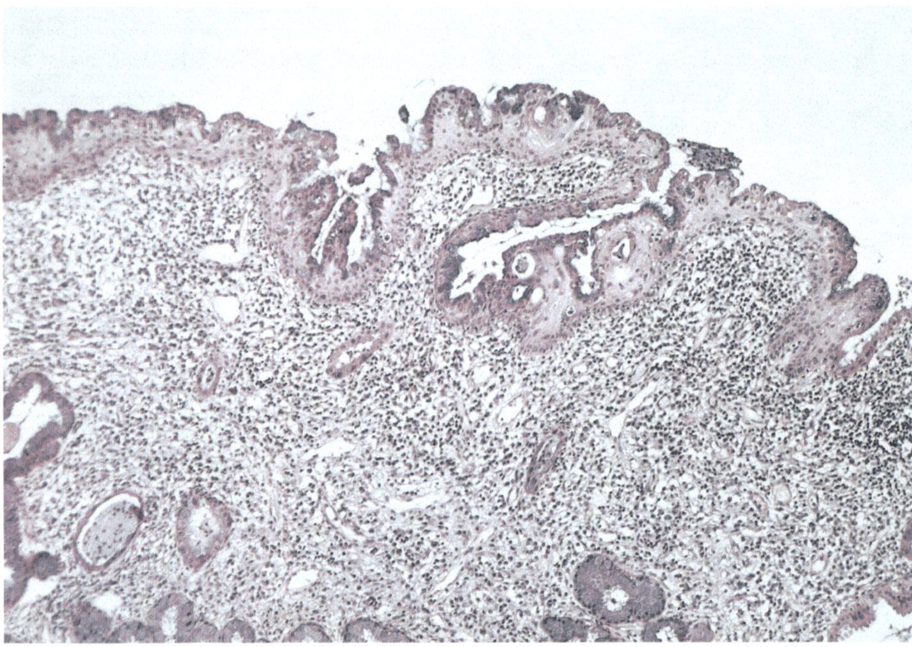

Fig. 66. Eversion (protrusion) of hyperplastic endocervical mucosa onto the ectocervical surface with epidermization (descending repair). H&E

Polyps of the Ecto- and Endocervix (Figs. 67–69)

Focal proliferation of the endocervical mucosa leads to polyp formation. Depending upon their glands, they may be either cystic (Fig. 67), adenomatous, or microglandular; depending upon their stromal content, they may be either fibrous, angiomatous (Fig. 68), edematous (Fig. 67), or cellular (Fig. 68). Their surface may be papillary (Fig. 67) or smooth (Fig. 68). When these polyps protrude through the external os, the surface epithelium may be replaced by reserve cell hyperplasia (Fig. 68), which can differentiate to squamous metaplasia and finally to mature stratified squamous epithelium. When such polyps are completely overgrown by squamous epithelium, they are then classified as ectocervical polyps (Fig. 69).

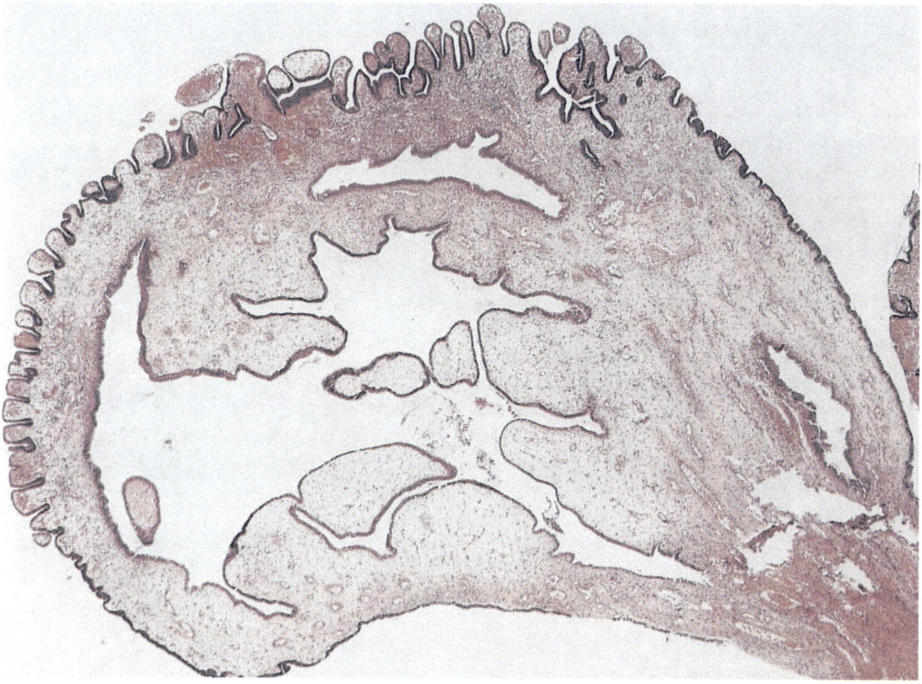

Fig. 67. Papillary endocervical polyp. H&E

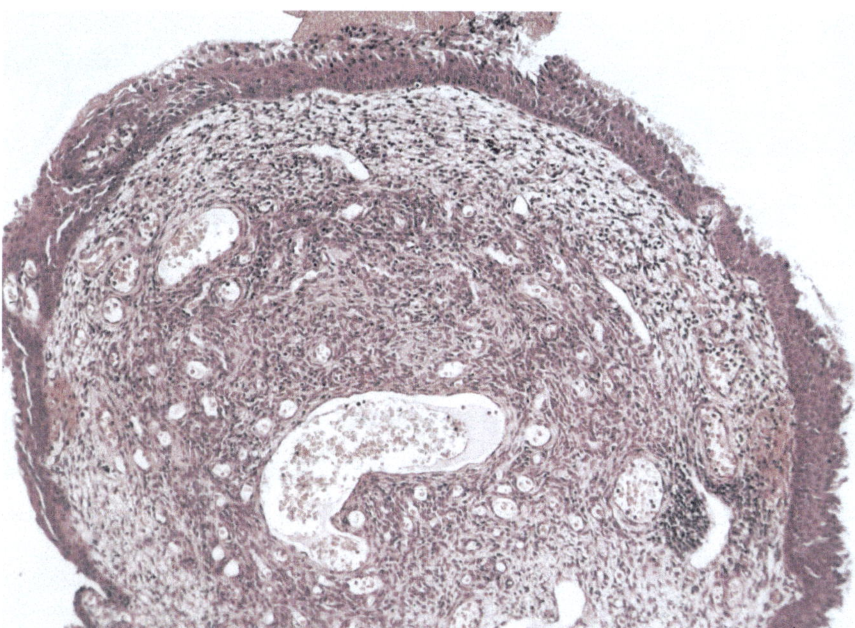

Fig. 68. Endocervical polyp with angiomatous, cellular stroma, covered by reserve cell hyperplasia. H&E

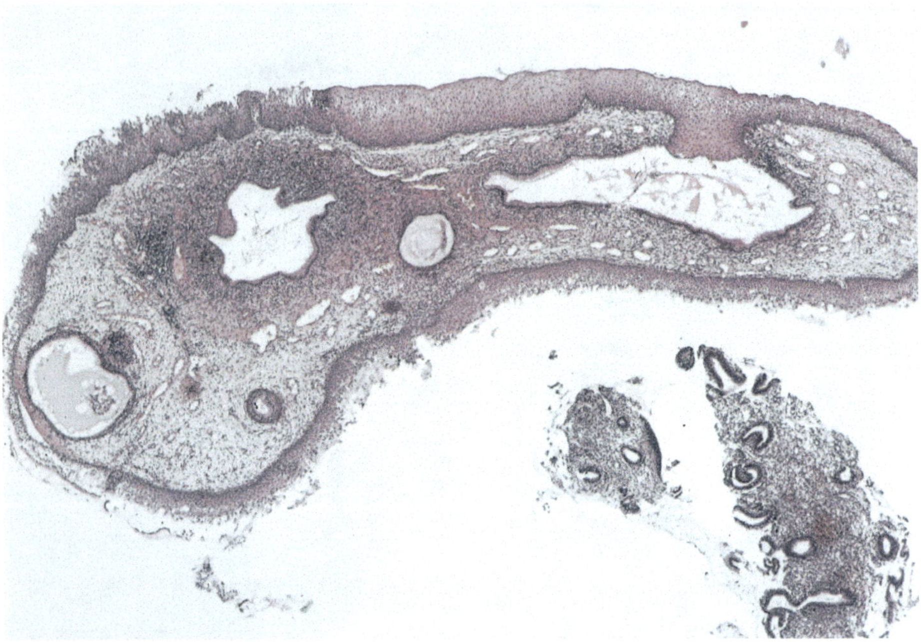

Fig. 69. Ectocervical polyp. H&E

Inflammatory Lesions

Nonspecific Ecto- and Endocervicitis (Figs. 70–76)

Nonspecific cervicitis may be chemically induced or caused by trauma in the presence of a "locus minoris resistentiae," such as postmenopausal atrophy of the ectocervical epithelium, or eversion of the vulnerable endocervical mucosa onto the ectocervix (ectropion) during the reproductive age.

Acute and *subacute ectocervicitis* (Figs. 70–72) is characterized by vascular congestion, edema, and infiltration of inflammatory cells, mainly neutrophilic granulocytes. When the inflammation is mild, the overlying epithelium remains intact (Fig. 70). With more severe inflammation, the epithelium is destroyed, sloughed off, leading to an erosive or ulcerative ectocervicitis (Fig. 71, 72).

Acute and *subacute endocervicitis* (Figs. 73–75) presents similar signs of inflammation (Figs. 73, 74) and occasionally ulceration (Fig. 75).

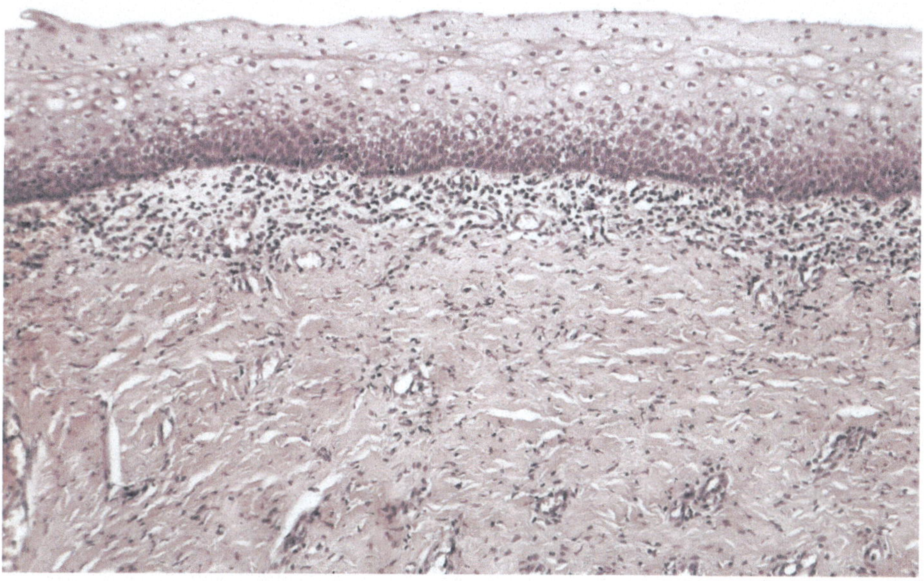

Fig. 70. Chronic ectocervicitis, mild. H&E

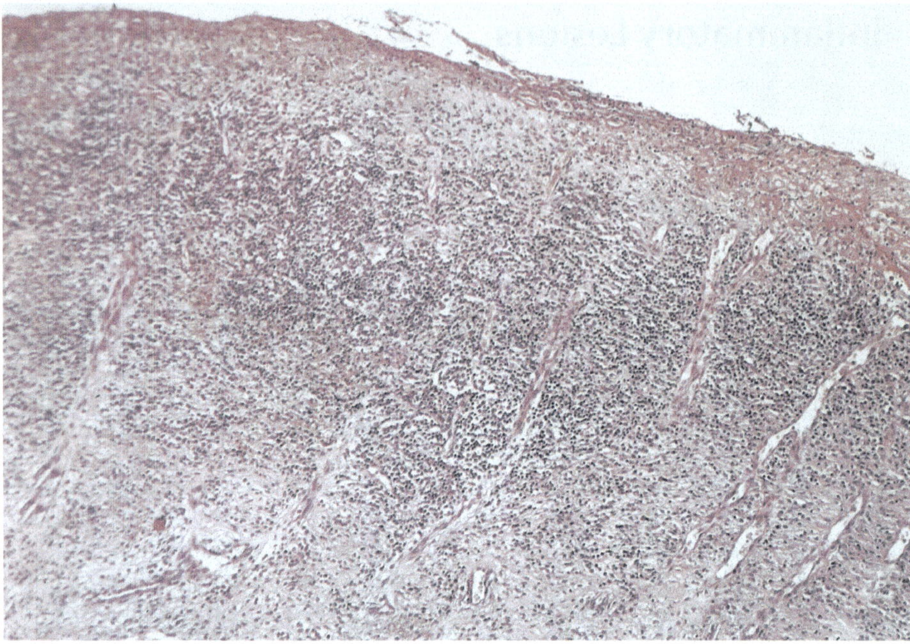

Fig. 71. Subacute ulcerative ectocervicitis. H&E

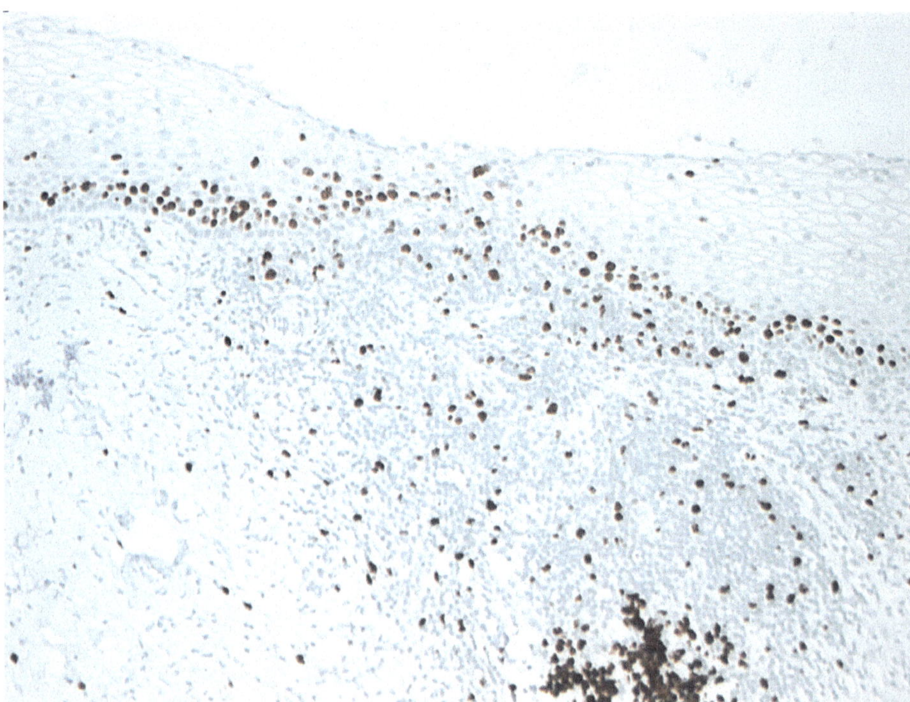

Fig. 72. Subacute ulcerative ectocervicitis. Positivity for MIB-1 in parabasal cell layer of squamous epithelium and in lymphocytic infiltrate in stroma. MIB-1 immunostain

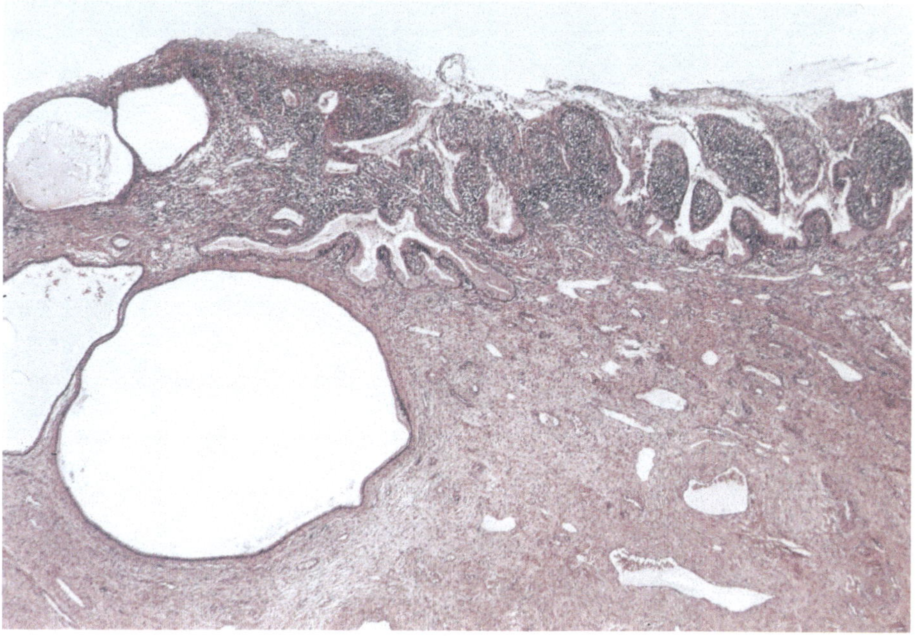

Fig. 73. Subacute endocervicitis. H&E

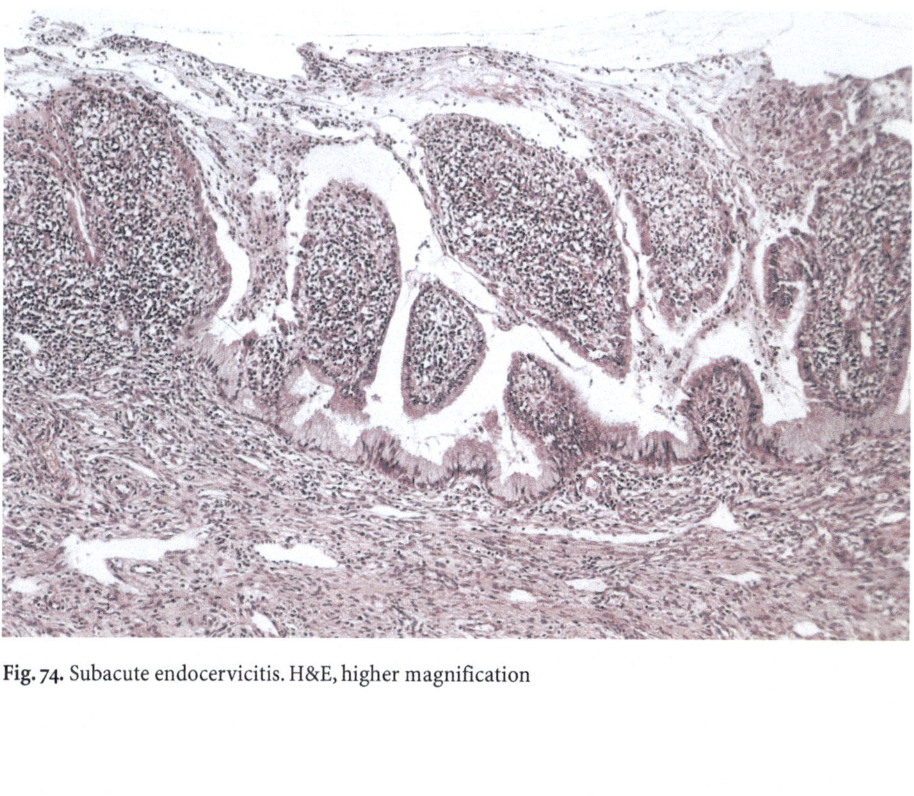

Fig. 74. Subacute endocervicitis. H&E, higher magnification

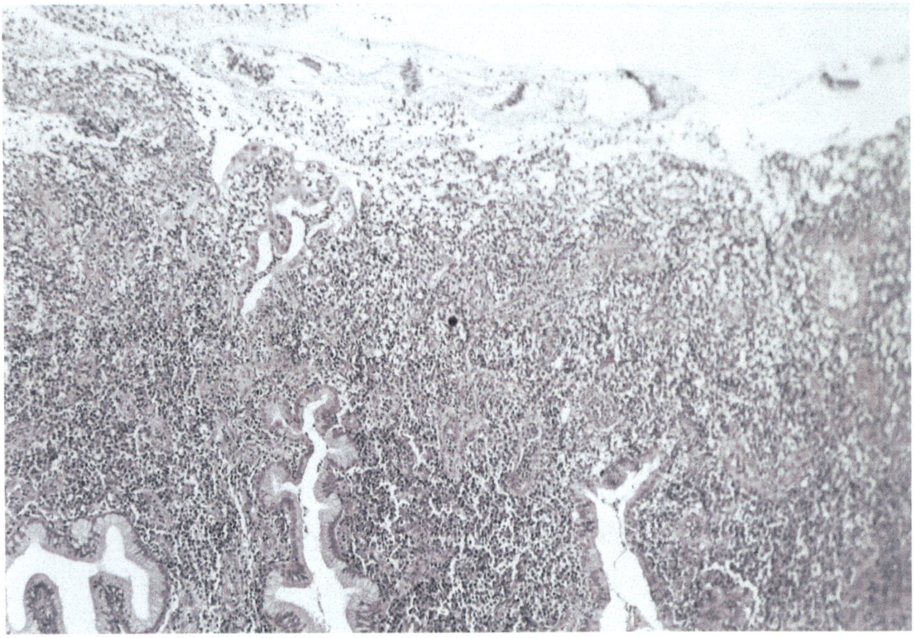

Fig. 75. Subacute ulcerative endocervicitis. H&E

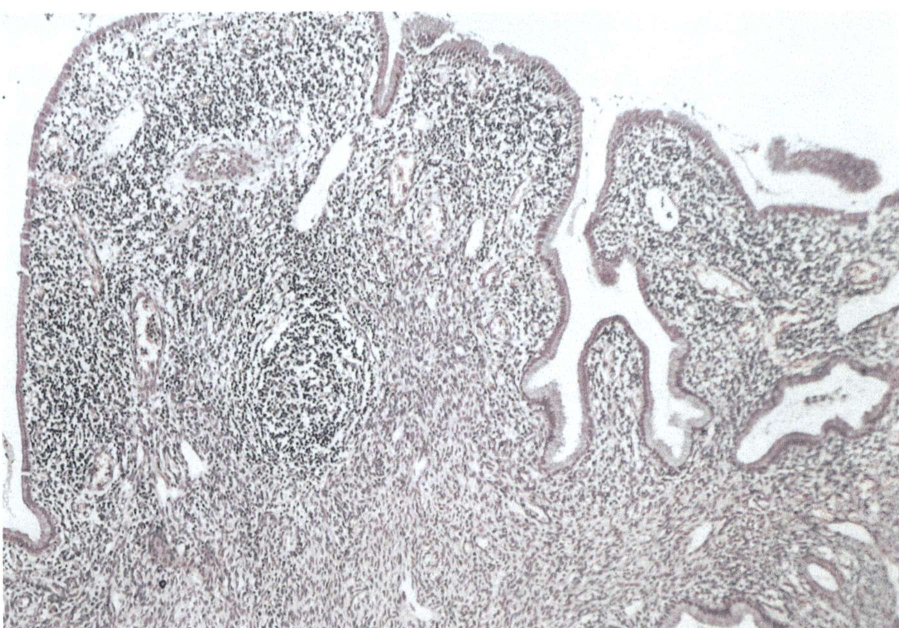

Fig. 76. Follicular endocervicitis. H&E

In *chronic ecto-* and *endocervicitis*, rather dense subepithelial infiltrates of predominantly lymphocytes and plasma cells are found, often accompanied by proliferating capillaries and fibroblasts. The overlying epithelium is usually intact. In prolonged or severe chronic endocervicitis, lymphoid follicles may develop (*follicular endocervicitis*, Fig. 76), and the overlying columnar epithelium may show polymorphic, hyperchromatic, and depolarized nuclei. When detected in cervical smears, such reactive nuclear changes may be misinterpreted by the screening cytologist and lead to false-positive readings.

■ **Differential Diagnosis.** Severe subacute and chronic follicular and ulcerative cervicitis may be misdiagnosed as lymphoma when large lymphoid cells, immunoblasts, and mitoses are found. However, surface ulceration and a polymorphic inflammatory infiltrate with neutrophils and plasma cells are rarely seen in lymphomas, which show instead an extensive, monomorphic infiltrate of lymphoid cells (Fig. 235; Young et al. 1985).

Specific Inflammations (Figs. 77–89)

Viral Infections

Viral infections of the ecto- and endocervix can cause characteristic morphological changes, by which they can be recognized. The accompanying inflammatory infiltrate may be scant (as with HPV infection) or extensive (as with herpes virus infection).

Infection with HPV usually starts at the basal or parabasal cells and may initiate here a latent infection that remains morphologically inapparent. If the infection changes to the productive phase, strong viral gene expression and production of new virus particles are observed in the intermediate and superficial layers of the epithelium, resulting in characteristic morphological changes that are typical for HPV infections (Middleton et al. 2003). These include koilocytosis of the ectocervical (Fig. 77, 78) and endocervical epithelia (Fig. 121), and may also lead to less specific changes such as acanthosis, papillomatosis, giant nuclei, multinucleated cells, monocellular keratinization, hypergranulation, and superficial ortho- and/or parakeratosis. Because of these cellular and nuclear alterations, they have to be classified as mild (reversible) dysplasia (CIN 1, see p. 87).

A *koilocyte* is a dyskaryotic epithelial cell with a deformed, often angulated, hyperchromatic nucleus surrounded by a swollen cytoplasm, which shows a clear perinuclear halo and a thickened cytoplasmic membrane (Fig. 78). Both signs, the atypical degenerating nucleus and the clear, blown-up cytoplasm, are essential features of a true koilocyte. Sometimes other agents may cause similar but nonspecific koilocyte-like cellular changes. For example, clear cells with ballooned cytoplasm and a normal nucleus may be seen after a gestagen-predominant hormonal stimulation, whereby glycogen accumulates in the cytoplasm (Fig. 79). In contrast, the cytoplasm of true koilocytes is devoid of glycogen. A degenerative vacuolation of the cytoplasm may occur in other nonspecific inflammatory lesions. Koilocytes can also be observed in columnar epithelial cells (Fig. 121) of the endocervix. Viral DNA is reproduced in the nuclei of koilocytes, and in the cytoplasm viral particles are accumulated.

Persisting infection with HR-HPV (see Table 4, p. 83) may in some cases result in dysplastic transformation of the epithelium that is reflected by higher-grade cervical intraepithelial neoplasia (CIN 2/3) or even progression to invasive cancer. HR-HPV infection resulting in carcinogenesis is discussed therefore at greater length in "Premalignant Lesions" (p. 82 ff). Infections with LR-HPV types, however, in almost all cases regress spontaneously within several months (Ho et al. 1998; Wang and Hildesheim 2003).

It is important to note that not all HPV infections result in detectable morphological changes (Fuchs et al. 1988). Samples taken from women between 15 and 50 years of age with normal cytologic smears harbor HR-HPV DNA in about 10% (de Villiers et al. 1987). The percentage of HPV-positive women with normal cytologic smears depends significantly on the women's age. In general the percentage of younger women with a HR-HPV-positive test result is significantly greater than that of older women (Schiffman and Kjaer 2003). For a detailed description of the taxonomy and the epidemiological distribution of HPV infection, the reader is referred to de Villiers et al. (2004) and Munoz et al. (2003).

Infection with herpes virus (Figs. 80–83) involves chiefly herpes simplex virus (HSV) type 2. In the acute stage, the infection can be easily recognized cytologically by the large multinucleated epithelial cells with characteristic intranuclear, ground-glass, viral inclusions (Fig. 80). On histological examination, small or larger vesicles may be found within the ectocervical epithelium containing such giant cells with intranuclear viral inclusions (Fig. 81). These vesicles ultimately burst, forming confluent ulcers surrounded by cellular debris and dense inflammatory infiltrates (Figs. 82, 83). During pregnancy, infection of the fetus or placenta may cause spontaneous abortion (Corey 1984).

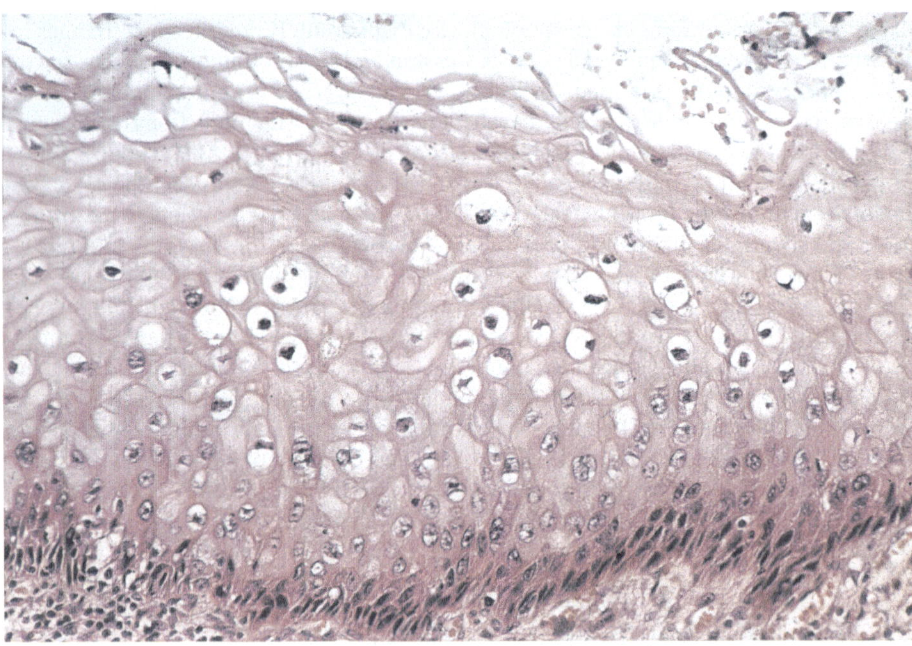

Fig. 77. Infection of ectocervical epithelium with human papillomavirus. H&E

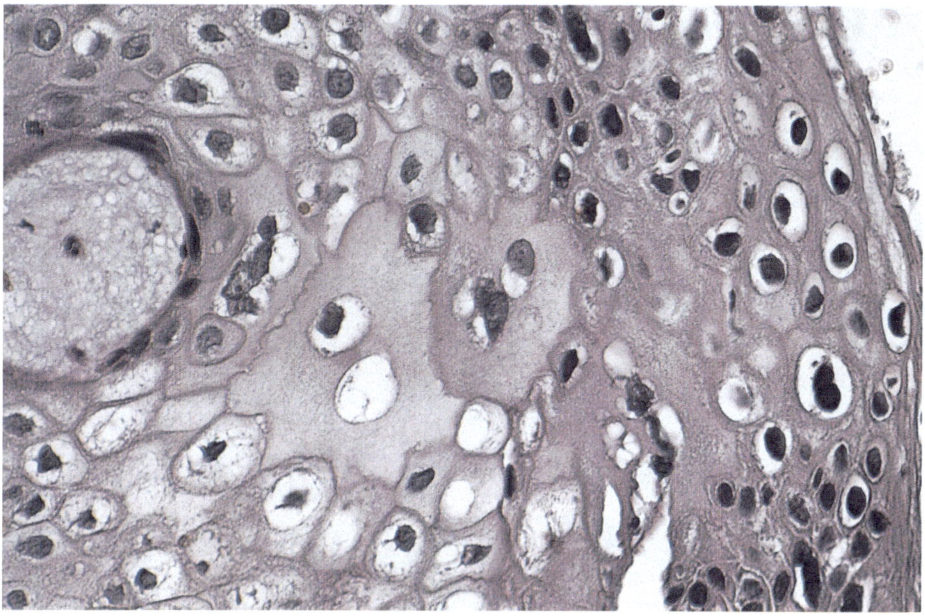

Fig. 78. Dysplastic squamous epithelium with true koilocytes. H&E

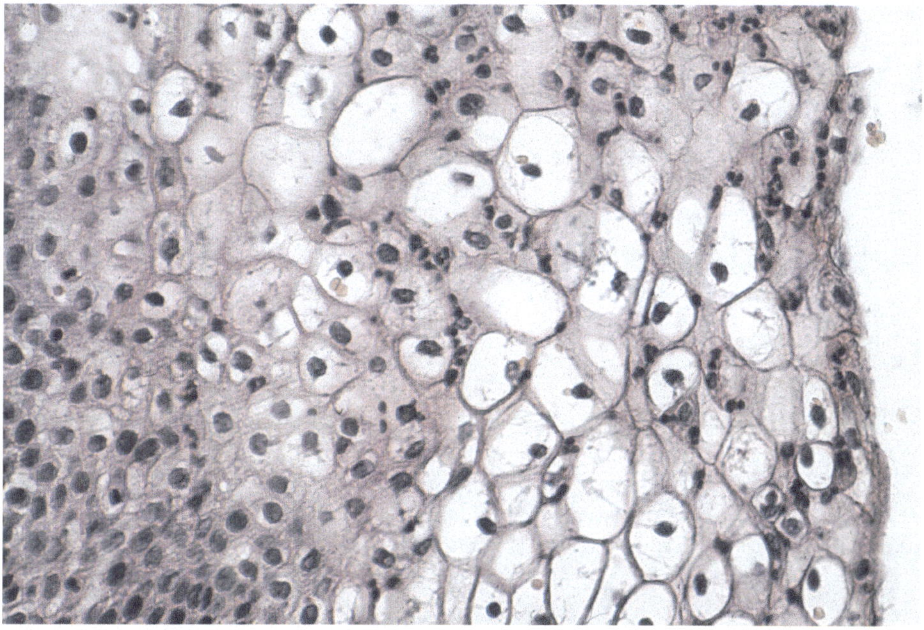

Fig. 79. Squamous epithelium with "false" koilocytes. H&E

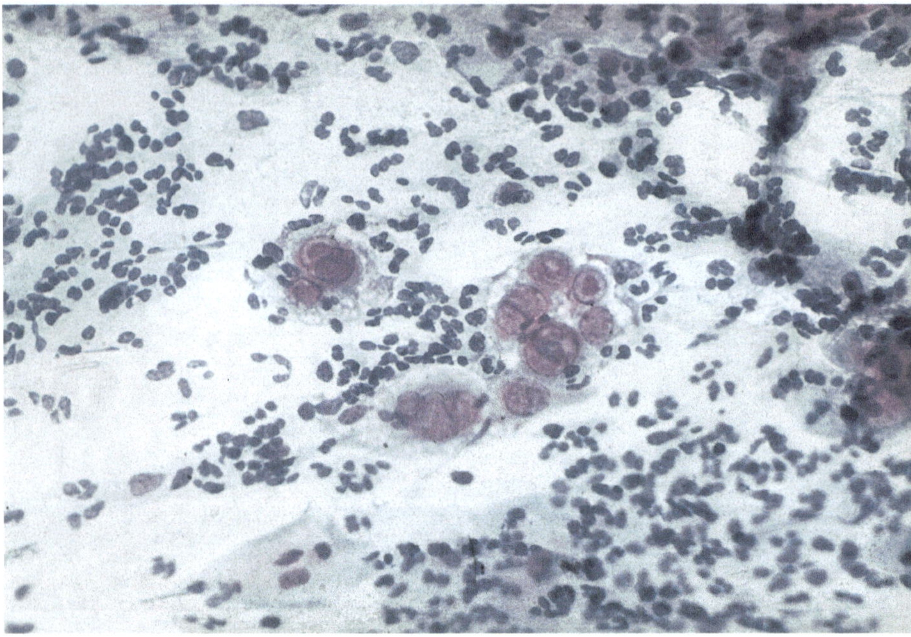

Fig. 80. Vaginal cytological smear with intranuclear inclusions of herpes virus. Papanicolaou

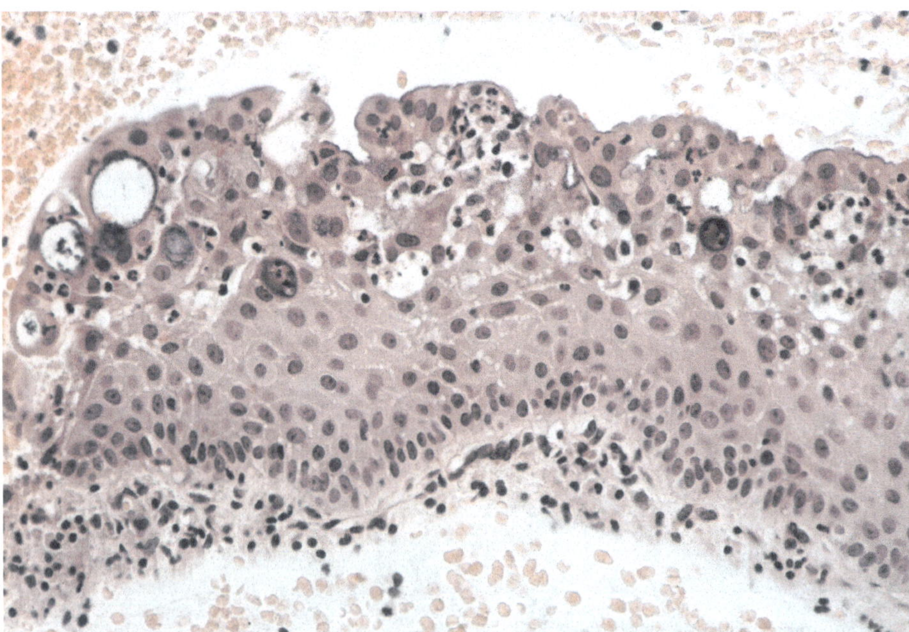

Fig. 81. Ectocervical epithelium with intranuclear inclusions of herpes virus. H&E

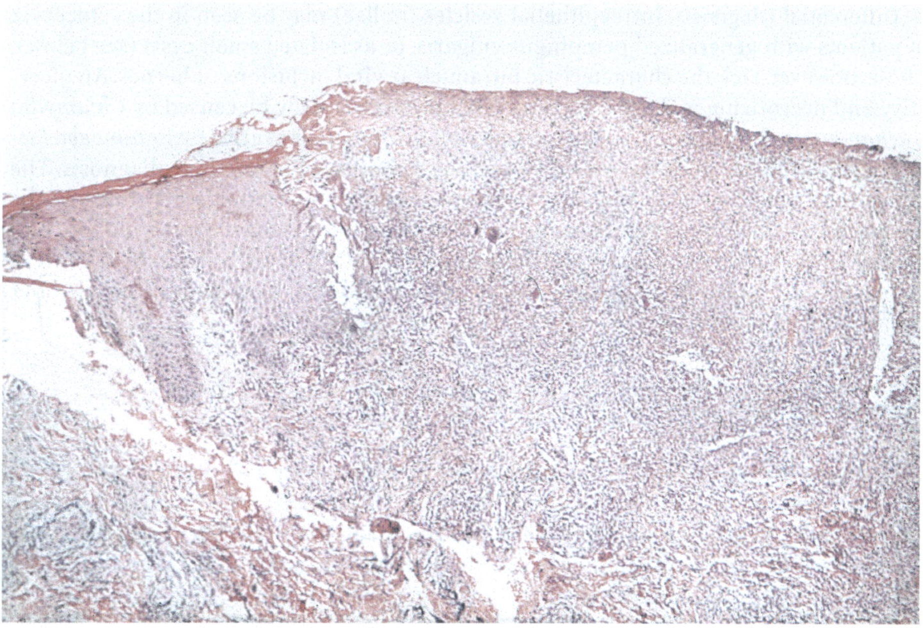

Fig. 82. Florid ulcerative ectocervicitis caused by herpes virus. H&E

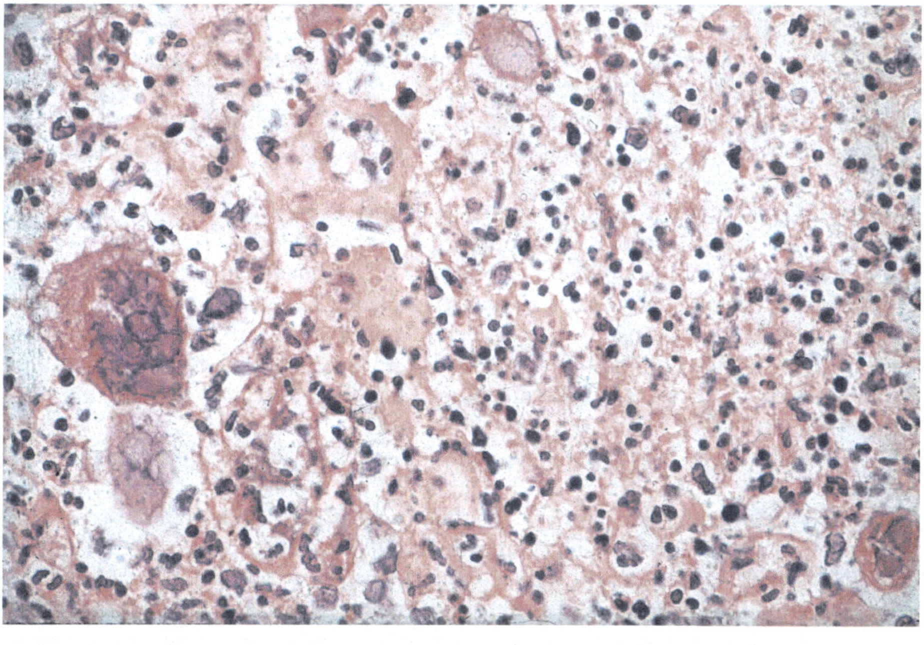

Fig. 83. Florid ulcerative ectocervicitis caused by herpes virus. H&E, higher magnification

■ **Differential Diagnosis.** Intraepithelial vesicles (bullae) may be seen in the ectocervix in patients with generalized pemphigus vulgaris, or as isolated small cysts (see below). These, however, lack the characteristic intranuclear viral inclusions of herpes. An ulcerative and necrotizing infection of the cervix may occasionally be caused by *Chlamydia trachomatis*, or by protozoa, such as *Trichomonas vaginalis*, or rarely by *Entamoeba histolytica*. Identification of the causative agent is essential for a definitive diagnosis. The cytoplasmic chlamydial inclusions can best be detected immunohistochemically; the most sensitive method to assess the presence of *Chlamydia* is the examination for chlamydial DNA, either by polymerase chain reaction (PCR) or with the hybrid capture technique. The motile protozoa are most readily identified in fresh native smears under phase-contrast microscopy.

Bacterial Infections

Tuberculous cervicitis (Fig. 84) almost always develops from an infection descending from tuberculous salpingitis or endometritis. The tuberculous granulomas can be recognized by aggregates of epitheloid cells and Langhans giant cells surrounded by lymphocytes. Caseation is rare in the cervix. Since similar granulomatous lesions of other causes may occur here, and some of them are even more common, the diagnosis of tuberculosis has to be verified by the demonstration of acid-fast mycobacteria (tuberculosis), with the Ziehl-Neelsen stain, or a modification of it.

■ **Differential Diagnosis.** Under low microscopic magnification, foreign body granulomas may appear very similar. They can often be distinguished from tuberculous granulomas by identifying intracytoplasmic inclusions of foreign material in multinucleated giant cells under polarized light. Most of these inclusions are double refractile under polarized light (such as talcum crystals or suture material). Infectious granulomas such as *lues*, *lymphogranuloma venereum*, *granuloma inguinale*, *schistosomiasis*, and *sarcoidosis* must be distinguished from tuberculosis by using special stains or bacteriological and immunological methods, since individual morphological features are often lacking.

Chlamydial cervicitis is being observed with increasing frequency (Winkler and Crum 1986) and is now the most common sexually transmitted infection in the Western world (Stamm and Holmes 1984). It is considered a cofactor to HPV in the etiology of cervical cancer (Smith et al. 2002). The causative agent, *Chlamydia trachomatis*, is sexually transmitted and has an affinity for cervical columnar cells or basal (reserve) cells. Concomitant infection of other tissues leads to urethritis, endometritis, salpingitis, and proctitis, which are common. Other infections, such as gonorrhea, often occur at the same time.

Histologically, severe nonspecific inflammation is typical, but in some cases chronic follicular endocervicitis is observed (Winkler and Crum 1986). Slight atypia of both columnar and metaplastic cells has been described. Only in a small number of cases can cytoplasmic inclusions, comprising aggregates of *Chlamydia trachomatis* organisms, be found in columnar or metaplastic basal cells of smears or sections (Fig. 85a, b). Recognition in vaginal PAP smears is difficult, since many degenerative cytoplasmic inclusions occurring in metaplastic epithelial cells closely resemble the various developmental stages of chlamydial inclusions. These consist of cytoplasmic vacuoles containing

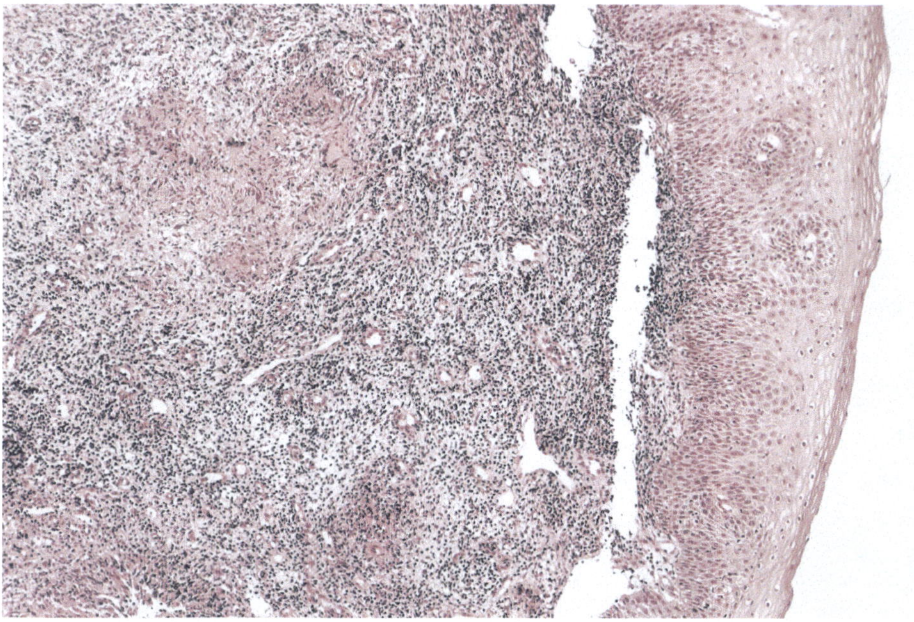

Fig. 84. Tuberculous cervicitis. H&E

few or numerous tiny particles. The most sensitive method to assess the presence of *Chlamydia* is the examination for chlamydial DNA, either by PCR or with the hybrid capture technique.

It is important to treat the patients as well as their male partners since chlamydial urethritis may be asymptomatic.

■ **Differential Diagnosis.** Distinction from severe subacute or chronic nonspecific cervicitis is virtually impossible on histological grounds alone. Many of these so-called nonspecific infections actually are unrecognized chlamydial cervicitis, as Paavonen et al. (1982) could show for follicular endocervicitis. Distinction from gonorrhea is possible bacteriologically, from trichomonal infection by vital cytology under phase-contrast microscopy (see below).

Parasitic Infections

Trichomonas cervicitis (Fig. 86) is caused by an ascending infection with *Trichomonas vaginalis*, a flagellated protozoon most easily recognized in a fresh vaginal smear under phase-contrast microscopy (Stoll 1969). In histological preparations an inflammatory infiltrate is seen, whereby the desquamating epithelial cells reveal nuclear swelling and chromatin clumping.

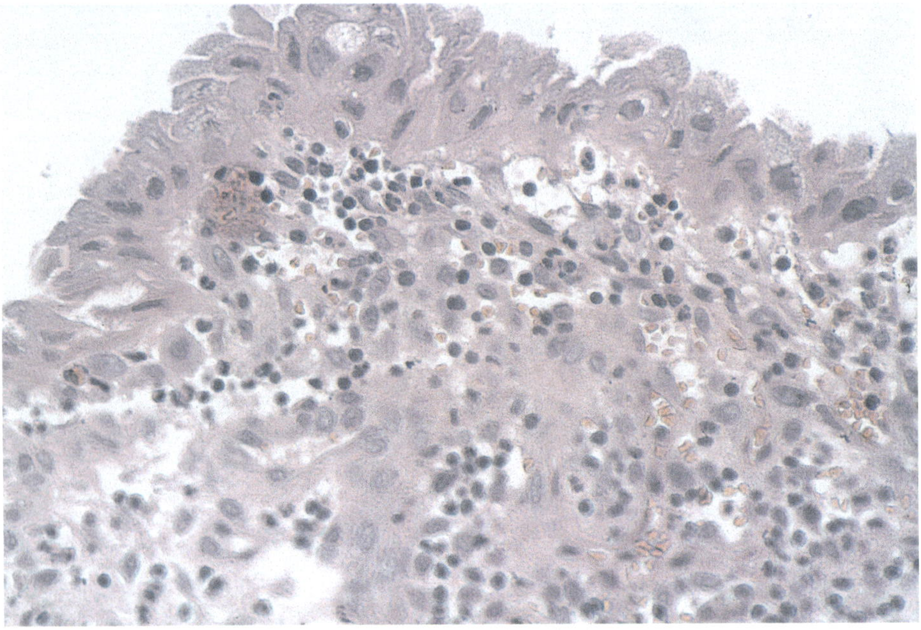

Fig. 85a. Subacute endocervicitis with intracytoplasmic inclusions of *Chlamydia trachomatis* in metaplastic epithelial cells. H&E

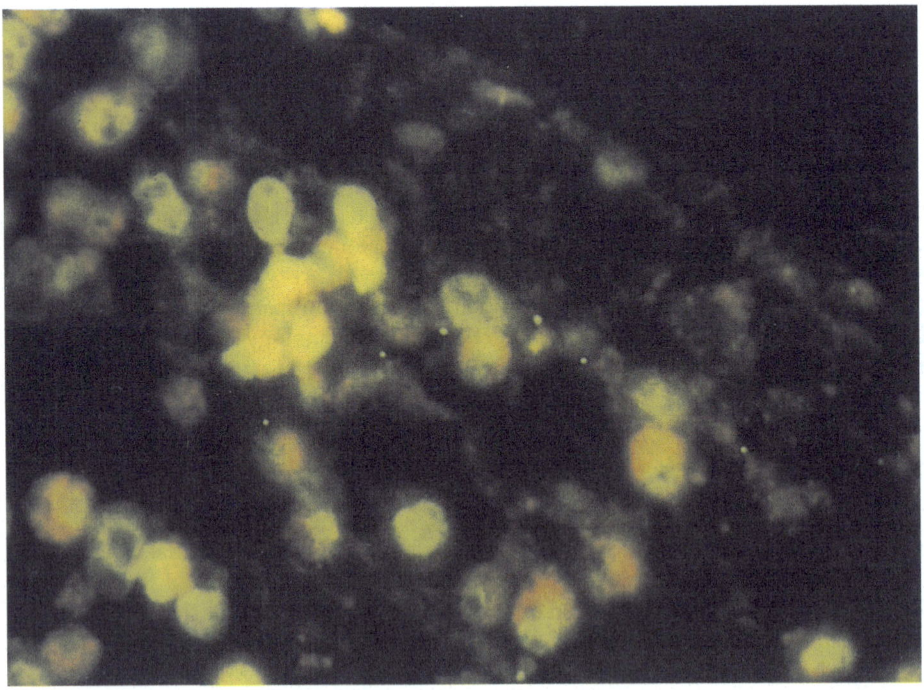

Fig. 85b. Intracytoplasmic inclusions of *Chlamydia trachomatis* showing uniform green fluorescence. Immunohistochemistry with specific antibodies

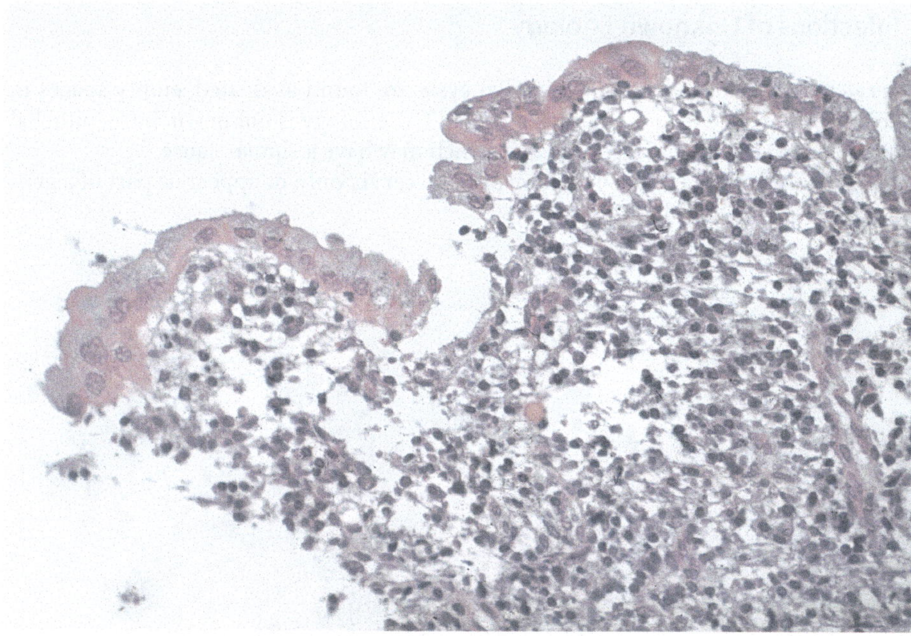

Fig. 86. Endocervicitis caused by ascending infection with *Trichomonas vaginalis*. H&E

■ **Differential Diagnosis.** Nonspecific acute and subacute purulent cervicitis, follicular (chlamydial) cervicitis, granuloma inguinale, and lymphogranuloma can be distinguished by detecting the causing agent. Rare parasitic infections involving the cervix are: schistosomiasis (endemic in Africa), echinococcosis, and infections with *Entamoeba histolytica*.

Fungal Infections

Actinomycosis of the cervix (Fig. 87) may result from infectious trauma from an intrauterine device or surgical procedures (Burkman and Damewood 1985). Microscopically, a dense inflammatory infiltrate with abscess formation is seen, consisting mainly of neutrophils and histiocytes. Characteristic gram-positive rods arranged in a radial fashion, and located in the center of the abscess, are diagnostic.

■ **Differential Diagnosis.** Inspissated mucus or groups of autolytic, swollen, endocervical epithelial cells arranged in a radial position may have a very similar appearance. Distinction is possible by immunohistochemical detection of *Actinomyces* organisms (Pine et al. 1985).

Infection with *Candida albicans* rarely involves the cervix and is secondary to involvement of vulva and vagina.

Infections of Unknown Etiology

In *cervicitis emphysematosa*, subepithelial cysts are found as dilated, empty spaces in the connective tissue without epithelial lining. The etiology is unknown. Intraepithelial cysts are occasionally observed (Fig. 88), which may have a similar cause.

Polyarteriitis nodosa (Fig. 89) can involve the cervix only, or appear as part of a generalized (autoimmune) disease.

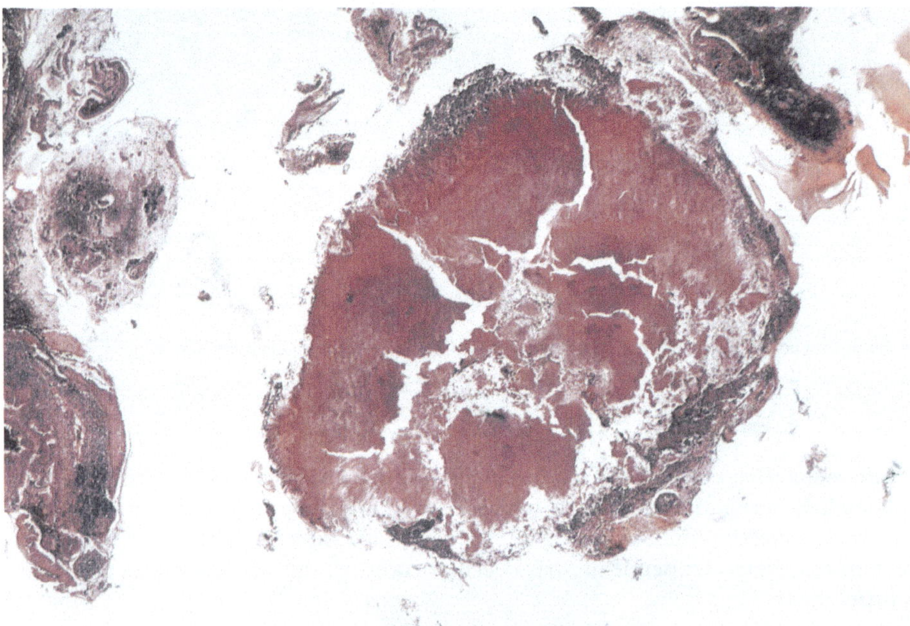

Fig. 87. Actinomycosis of the cervix. H&E

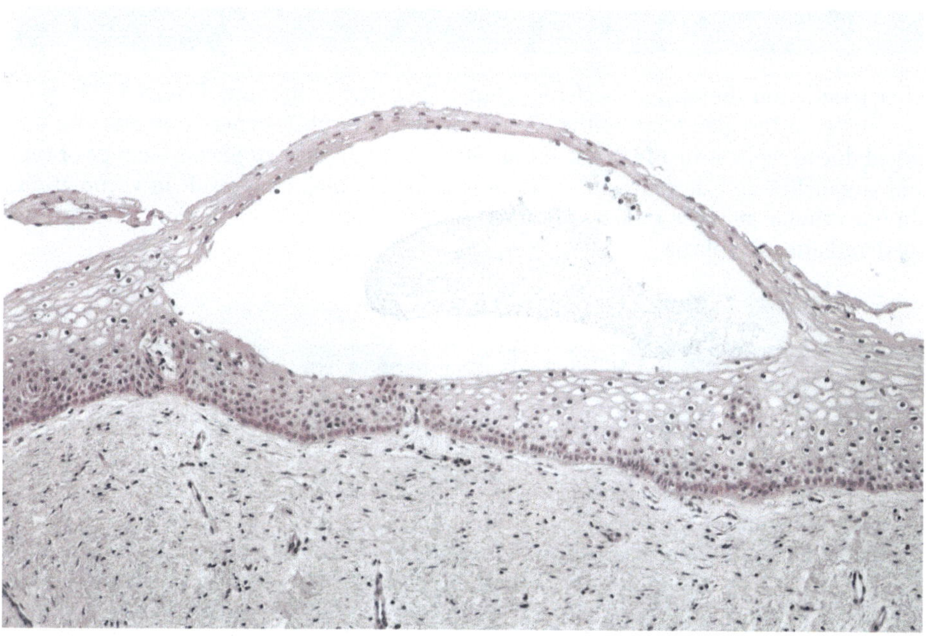

Fig. 88. Cervicitis emphysematosa. H&E

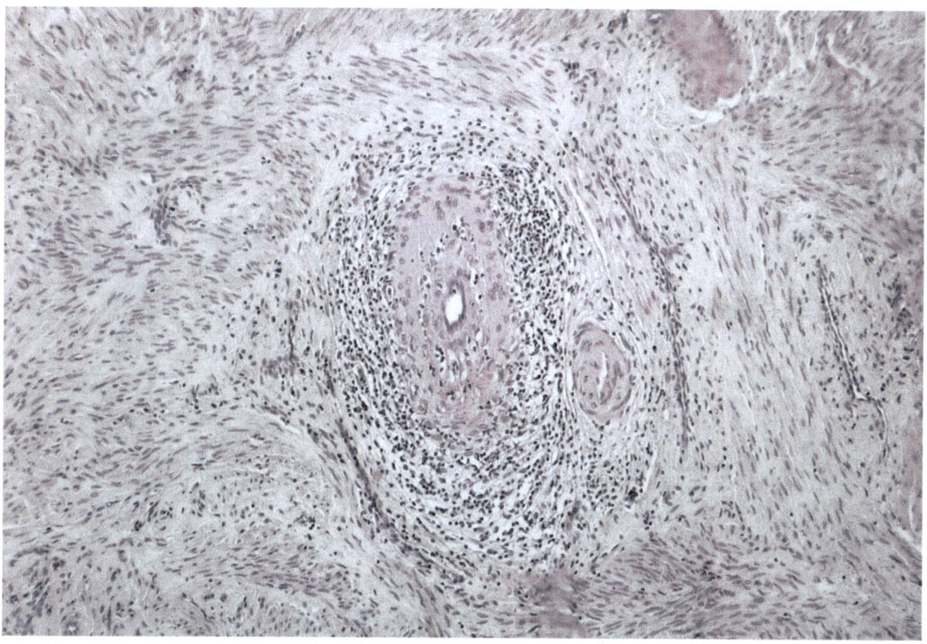

Fig. 89. Polyarteritis nodosa of the cervix. H&E

Irradiation Changes (Fig. 90)

After irradiation therapy, pre-existing glandular patterns become distorted (Fig. 90). The nuclei of the glandular epithelial cells are pleomorphic, hyperchromatic and enlarged due to replication of DNA without cell division. In the cytoplasm, damage of various organelles and destruction of lysosomal membranes may result in vacuolation. Similar cellular changes may be observed in the ectocervical epithelium resulting in postirradiation dysplasia.

Postoperative Spindle Cell Nodule

This reactive benign lesion develops at the site of a recent operation and consists of densely packed proliferating mesenchymal spindle cells, capillaries and inflammatory cells. Distinction from leiomyosarcoma is clinically important and will be facilitated by the clinical history of a previous operation at the site of the nodule (Nielsen and Young 2001). Rarely, a non-neoplastic *traumatic neuroma* [4977/0] may develop postoperatively at the site of cervical amputation. *Retention of fetal glial tissue* may follow a previous abortion.

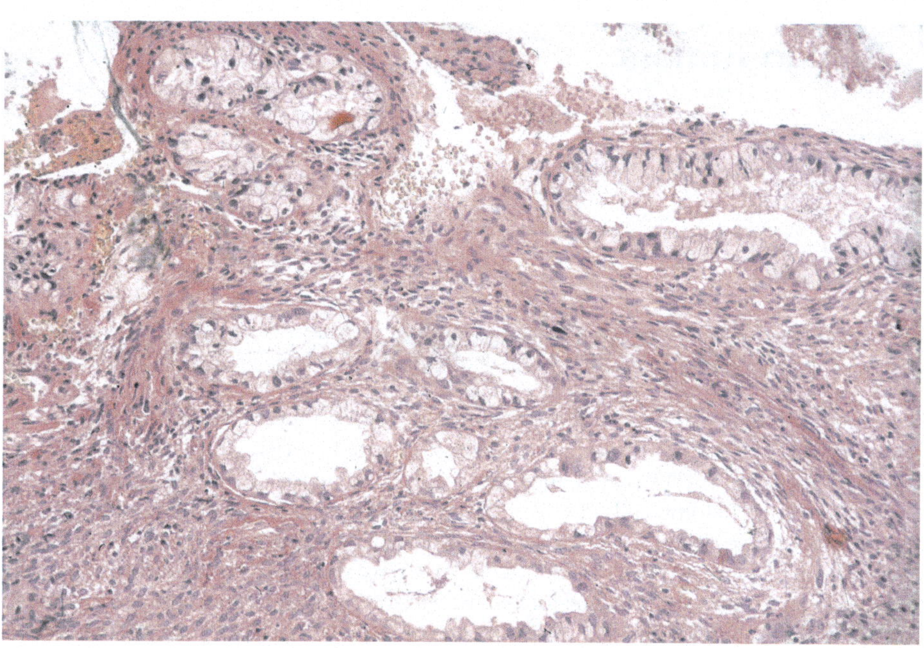

Fig. 90a. Endocervical glands after irradiation therapy with periglandular fibrosis. H&E

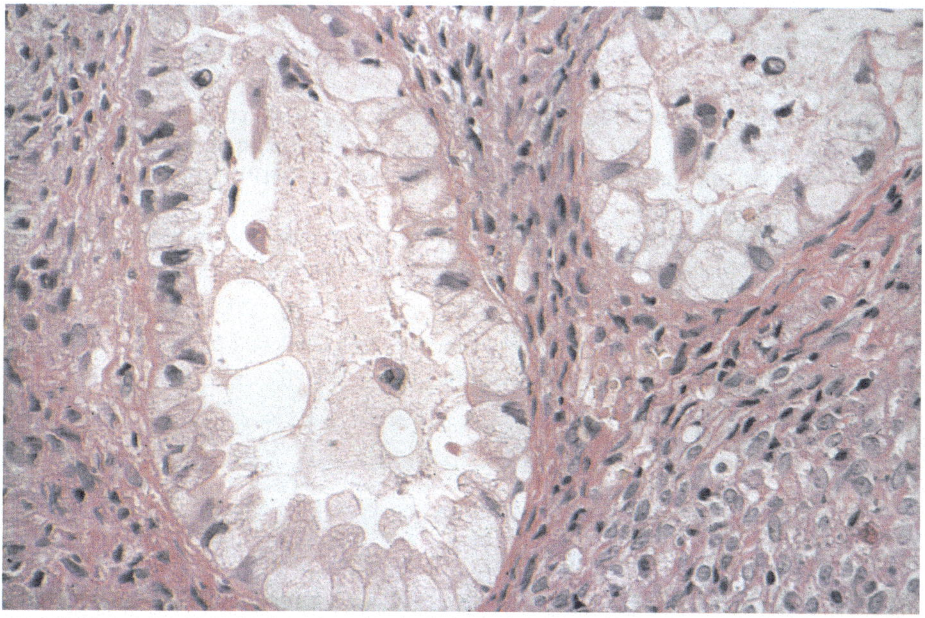

Fig. 90b. Same as Fig. 90a. Pleomorphic nuclei and vacuolated cytoplasm of glandular epithelium. H&E

Benign Tumors

Epithelial Tumors (Figs. 91–94)

Squamous papillomas [8052/0] of the ectocervix (Figs. 91–94) occur predominantly in young women and are mainly caused by infection with low-risk HPV (LR-HPV) types, such as types 6 and 11 (Ward et al. 1992; see Table 3). Some may be inverted, hence their surfaces are flat. Histologically they consist of thick layers of stratified squamous epithelium with elongated rete pegs that extend deeply into the lamina propria (Fig. 91). The basal membrane is intact, the epithelial layers are well differentiated, and acanthosis is usually pronounced. Some lesions may also contain koilocytes in the upper layers. Mitoses are rare. Besides the flat, inverted type of papilloma, others may present as *exophytic condylomatous lesions* [7672/0] and closely resemble the condylomata of the vulva and vagina (Fig. 92) or form verrucae covered by parakeratosis or hyperkeratosis (Fig. 93). These papillomas may be sessile or pedunculated. Since these lesions reflect acute virus-producing infections of low-risk type, they may display all morphological features of active papillomavirus replication (see HPV infection, p. 61).

Differential Diagnosis. On gross examination the condylomatous papillomas may resemble an invasive carcinoma. Histologically, they can be distinguished by lack of cellular atypia, absence of mitoses, and the intact basal membranes. Ectocervical papilloma, depending on the type of HPV causing it, may later become malignant, whereas condylomas of the vulva and vagina usually due to infection by LR-HPV types almost invariably remain benign (Willett et al. 1989).

The previously introduced term "flat condyloma" for inverted papilloma should be avoided, as it may mislead the clinician. These lesions may represent infection with LR-

Table 3. Classification systems of HPV-associated intraepithelial lesions of the cervix

Term	HPV risk category	Three-tiered CIN	Two-tiered CIN	SIL (Bethesda like)
Exophytic condyloma	Low risk	–	–	LGSIL
Squamous papilloma	Low risk	–	–	LGSIL
Flat condyloma	Low and high risk	–	–	LGSIL
Mild dysplasia	Low and high risk	CIN 1	Low-grade CIN	LGSIL
Moderate dysplasia	High risk	CIN 2	High-grade CIN	HGSIL
Severe dysplasia	High risk	CIN 3	High-grade CIN	HGSIL
Carcinoma in situ	High risk	CIN 3	High-grade CIN	HGSIL

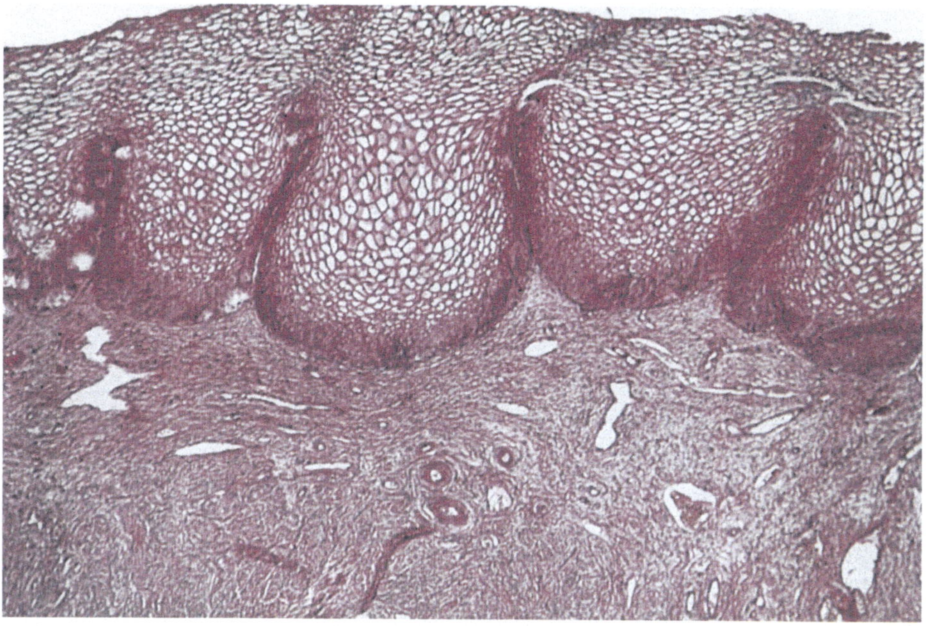

Fig. 91a. Papilloma of the ectocervix, early stage. H&E

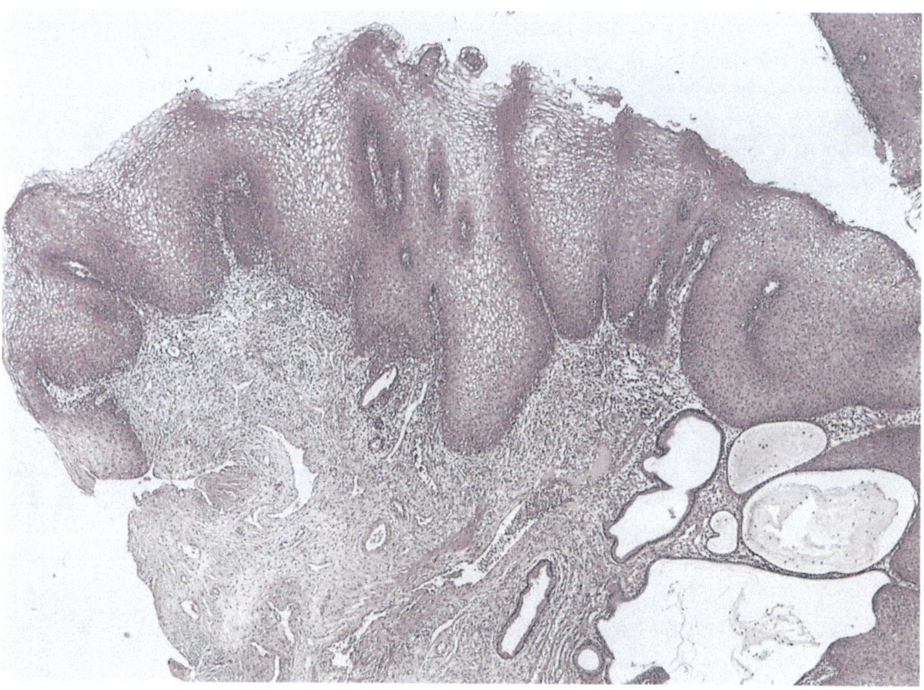

Fig. 91b. Papilloma of the ectocervix, advanced stage. H&E

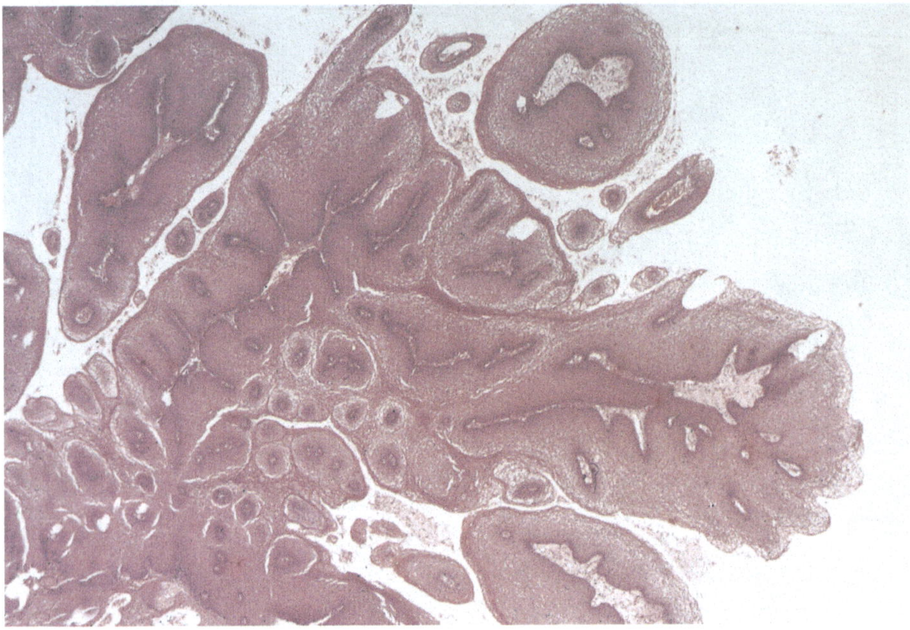

Fig. 92. Papilloma of the ectocervix, condylomatous. H&E

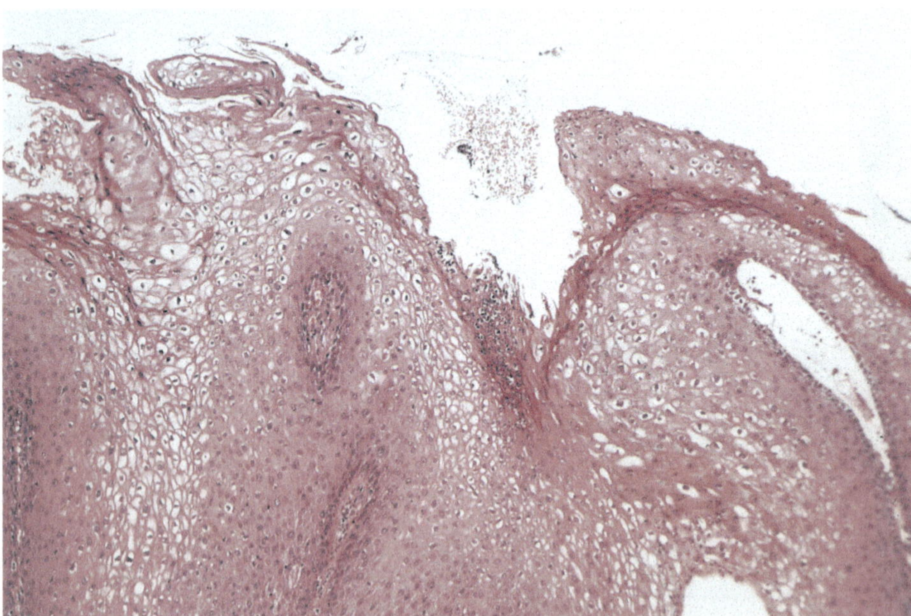

Fig. 93. Papilloma of the ectocervix, verrucous surface. H&E

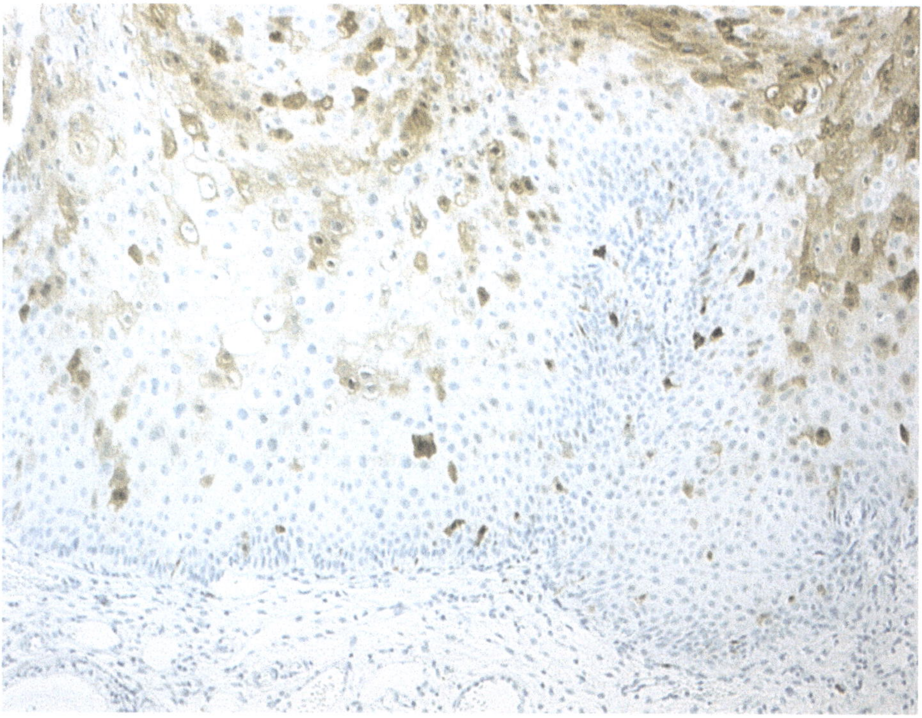

Fig. 94. Focal staining pattern of p16^{INK4a} in papilloma of the ectocervix. p16^{INK4a} immunostain

HPV types (e.g., HPV 6 and 11) that cause koilocytic alterations histologically classified as CIN 1. They may, however, also be induced by high-risk HPV types (see Table 3), representing the acute stage of the infection and eventually persist or progress to high-grade dysplasia or carcinoma.

In unclear cases it is important to determine the type of the underlying HPV infection. If HR-HPV types were identified, high-grade dysplasia may be present or may develop, whereas lesions that only harbor LR-HPV types do not progress to invasive carcinoma. The use of p16^{INK4a} as a dysplasia-associated antigen is very useful in the differentiation of benign condylomas and premalignant lesions induced by persistent papillomavirus infections (Fig 94). Strong diffuse expression of p16^{INK4a} in the basal and parabasal cell layers is restricted to lesions induced by HR-HPV (see Figs. 110, 111), whereas the condylomatous lesions induced by LR-HPV types may display focal p16^{INK4a} staining in the intermediate or superficial cell layers, but never show a diffuse staining in the basal or parabasal cell layers (see Fig. 94). p16^{INK4a} immunostaining is the simplest way to distinguish benign condylomatous lesions from true dysplastic lesions induced by HR-HPV types (Sano et al. 1998; Klaes et al. 2001; von Knebel Doeberitz 2002; Negri et al. 2004).

In many cases, however, both groups of HPV types are found concomitantly in one lesion. Here surveillance of the patients is particularly mandatory.

Besides diffuse or focal adenomatous hyperplasia (see p. 49), circumscribed benign *adenomas* may rarely develop from metaplastic foci. A *villous adenoma* (*Müllerian papilloma*) (Michael et al. 1986) derived from intestinal metaplasia of the endocervical epithelium occurs almost exclusively in young children (Smith et al. 1998).

Mesenchymal Tumors (Fig. 95–97)

Leiomyomas [8890/0] (Fig. 95) consist of smooth muscle cells more or less intermingled with fibroblasts and abundant blood vessels of various sizes. These leiomyomas resemble in most respects those of the myometrium (Tiltman 1998).

Hemangiomas (Fig. 96) of the cervix are rare (Gusdon 1965). They consist of compact tangles of venules (Fig. 96) or capillaries that through their growth often cause a bulging of the surface.

Blue nevi [8780/0] (Fig. 97) very rarely occur in the endocervix (Patel and Bhagavan 1985). They are composed of slender, wavy dermal melanocytes with long dendritic processes. These cells, either grouped or dispersed among variable numbers of melanophages, fibroblasts, and collagenous fibers, are usually laden with fine granules of melanin.

Other benign mesenchymal tumors, such as *rhabdomyoma*, *neurinoma*, *neurofibroma*, and *lipoma* are rare, compared with their counterparts in other tissues (Nielsen and Young 2001).

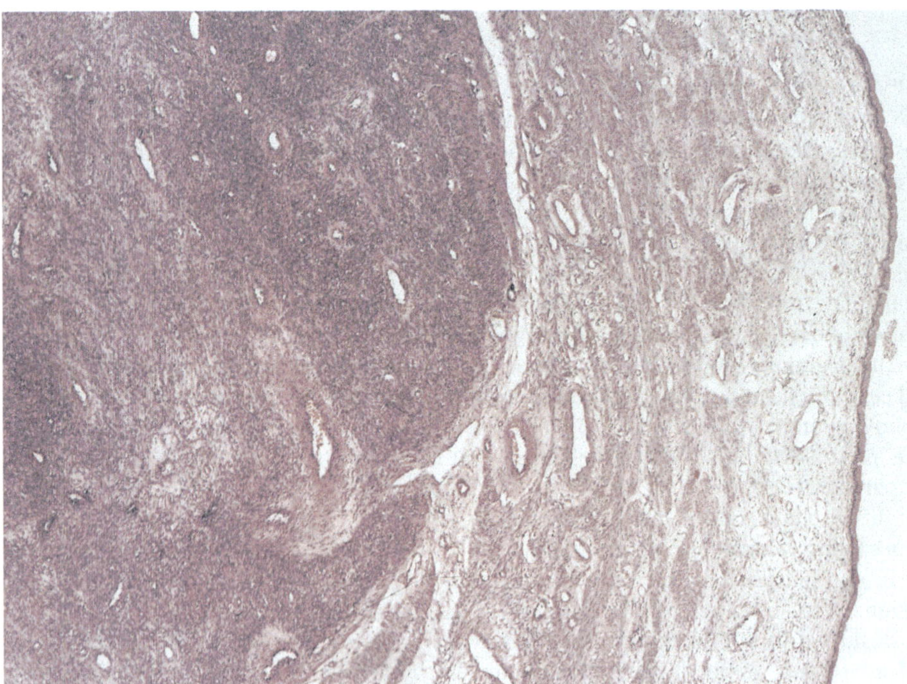

Fig. 95. Leiomyoma of the cervix. H&E

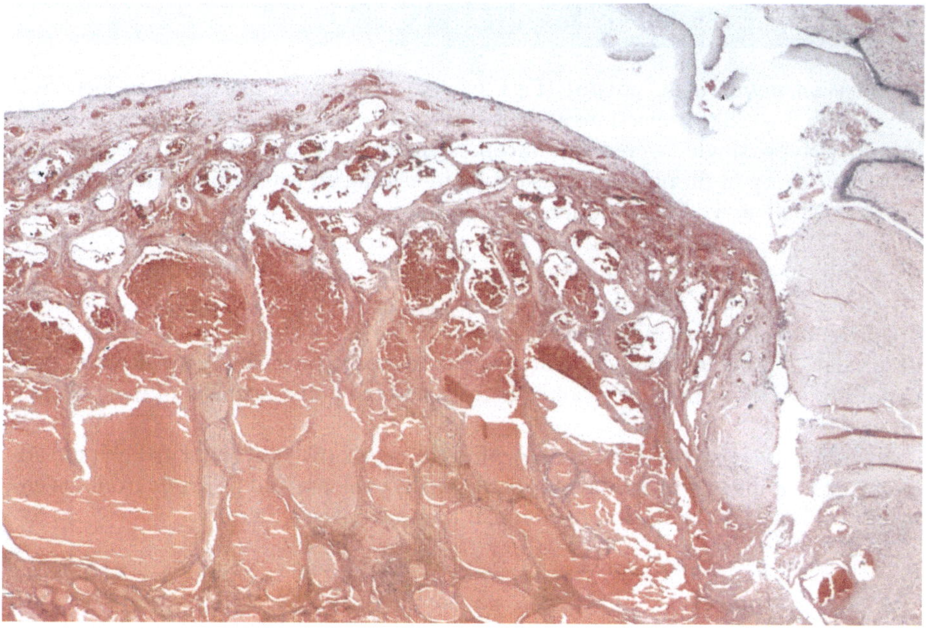

Fig. 96. Hemangioma of the cervix. H&E

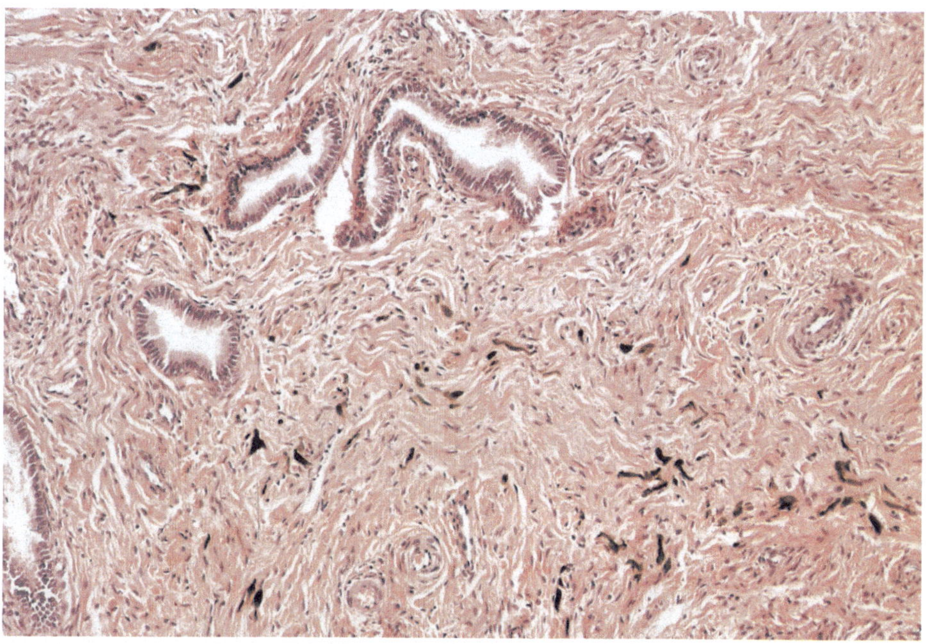

Fig. 97. Blue nevus of the cervix. H&E

Mixed Tumors (Figs. 98, 99)

Papillary adenofibromas [9013/0] (Figs. 98, 99) are shaped like large endocervical polyps with fingerlike projections at their surface. The covering epithelium is of the endocervical type, single layered, and inconspicuous. Their stroma is very cellular and dense, consisting of fibroblasts, occasionally intermingled with leiomyoblasts. Mitoses are rare (Abell 1971). These tumors are seen almost exclusively in postmenopausal women. They recur frequently, and after several recurrences, their stroma may undergo malignant change to become an adenosarcoma (see Figs. 231, 232).

■ **Differential Diagnosis.** Endocervical polyps can be distinguished by their either loose, edematous or fibrous, acellular stroma. Adenosarcomas are recognized by their high mitotic activity, their periglandular cuffs, and the polymorphism of their stromal cell nuclei.

Adenomyomas [8932/0] rarely arise within the cervix (Gilks at al. 1989). Polypoid adenomyomas of the endometrium may occasionally prolapse and protrude from the endocervical canal, giving the impression that they have arisen there.

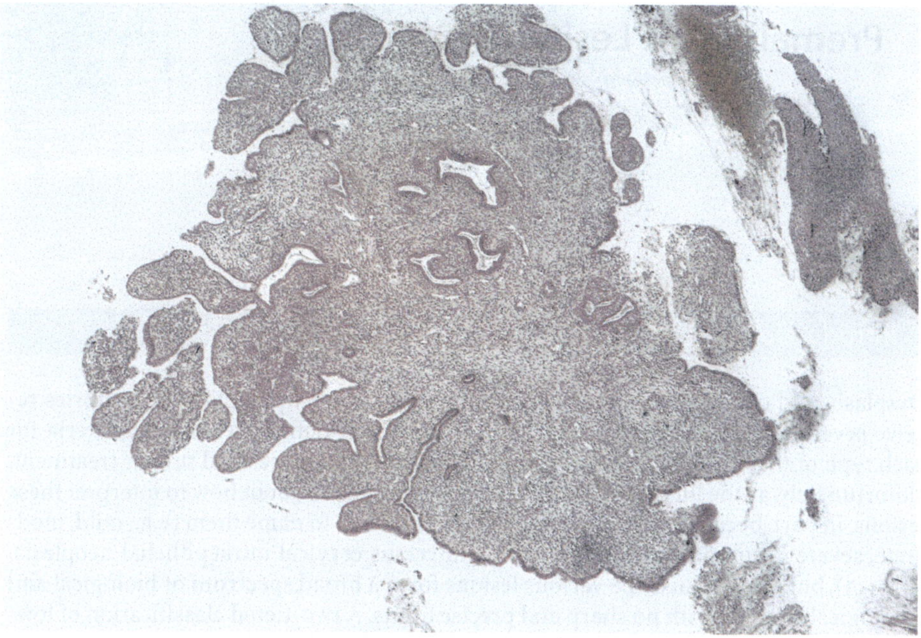

Fig. 98. Papillary adenofibroma of the endocervix. H&E

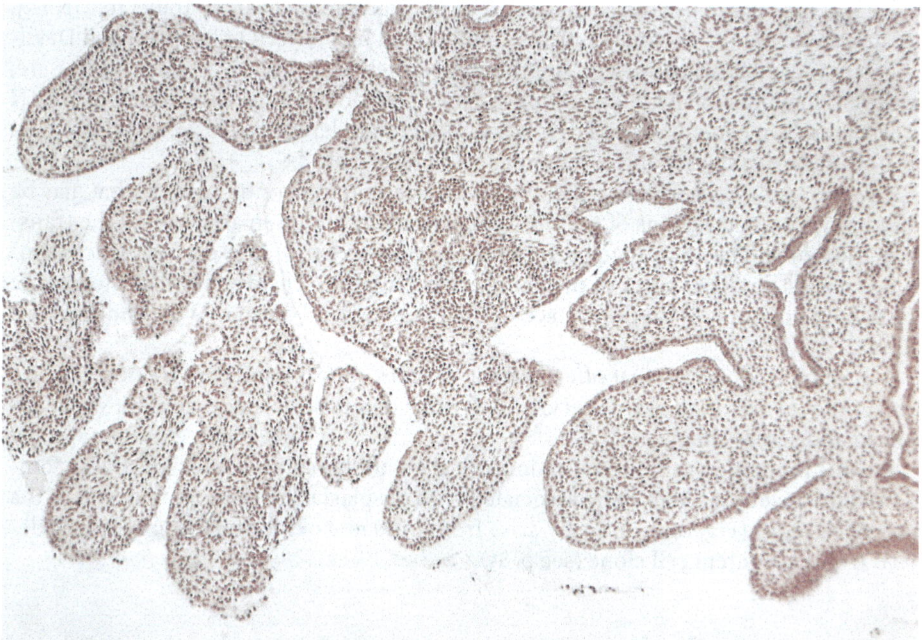

Fig. 99. Papillary adenofibroma of the endocervix. H&E, higher magnification

Premalignant Lesions

Introduction

Dysplasia and carcinoma in situ are common lesions; most pathology laboratories receive several cases weekly. It is important to have well-defined terms and criteria for each type of these lesions, thereby promoting correct diagnoses and proper treatment. Unfortunately, as the literature shows us, there is confusion about how to interpret these lesions, in part, because of disagreement about how best to name them (e.g., mild, moderate, severe dysplasia and carcinoma in situ versus cervical intraepithelial neoplasia, CIN 1–3), but also because the various lesions form a broad spectrum of biological and cytological changes with no sharp and precise limits. A two-tiered classification of low-grade and high-grade squamous lesions (LSIL and HSIL) introduced in the USA for reporting cervical cytology is mainly used in the USA by cytologists and cytopathologists. Its introduction for use in histology parallel to the CIN classification is discussed (Schneider 2003; Crum 2003; for comparison see Table 3).

We have chosen to use the terms dysplasia and carcinoma in situ parallel to CIN 1–3, because these are the original names recommended by the WHO (Tavassoli and Devilee 2003) and most widely used. The differences between the two nomenclatures are, however, small. The WHO classification is a four-step division, the CIN a three-step. CIN 1 corresponds in general to mild dysplasia, CIN 2 to moderate dysplasia, and CIN 3 covers both severe dysplasia and carcinoma in situ (see Table 3).

The spectrum reaches from mild dysplasia to carcinoma in situ, changes that may be found in very small regions of the cervix, but virtually always in and around the transformation zone. They may involve the whole circumference of the cervical orifice to include smaller or larger parts of the endocervical mucosa. The dysplastic or neoplastic epithelium lies not only on the surface, but may also extend down into the endocervical glands.

It must be emphasized that often varying degrees of dysplasia and carcinoma in situ are found together in the same cervix. The prime diagnosis is made from the most advanced and severe change.

Adenocarcinoma in situ of the endocervical glandular epithelium is much less common. Nonetheless, it seems to be associated with dysplasia and carcinoma in situ of the reserve cell type (Fig. 140), and may arise from the same dysplastic primary lesion, derived from one parent cell clone (see p. 85).

Etiology and Pathogenesis

Dysplastic and neoplastic lesions of the uterine cervix are in virtually all cases caused by persistent infections with HR-HPV types (Bosch et al. 2002; Burd 2003). Of the more than 100 types of HPV identified to date, mainly types 16 and 18, but also types 31, 33, 35, 39, 45, 51, 52, 56, 58, 59, 68, 73, and 82 are considered as potentially carcinogenic and are thus referred to as HR-HPV types (Crum et al. 1984; Munoz et al. 2003; deVelliers et al. 2004; see Table 4 and Fig. 100).

High-risk papillomaviruses are generally associated with preneoplastic or neoplastic anogenital lesions. Low-risk HPV types are usually found in benign epithelial lesions as, for example, genital warts (condylomata acuminata), but not in malignant lesions. For the group of probable HR-HPV types, the association is not yet confirmed; they have so far been observed only in incidental preneoplastic lesions.

Table 4. List of the so-far unequivocally classified HPV types (Munoz et al. 2003)

High-risk HPV types	Probable high-risk HPV types	Low-risk HPV types
16, 18, 31, 33, 35, 39, 45, 51, 52, 56, 58, 59, 68, 73, and 82	26, 53, and 66	6, 11, 40, 42, 43, 44, 54, 61, 70, 72, 81, and CP6108

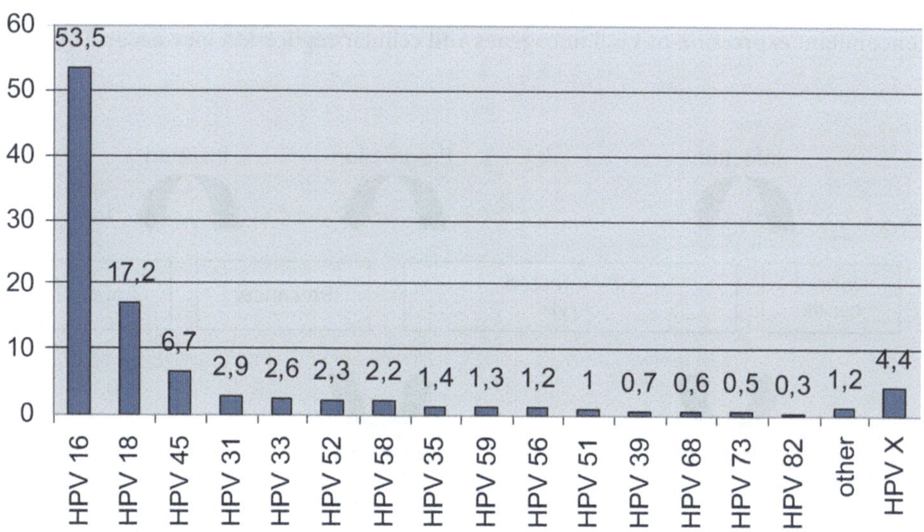

Fig. 100. Relative distribution of individual HR-HPV types in cervical cancers in all world regions combined (in %, modified after Munoz et al. 2004)

Clearly HPV 16 and 18 account for most of the cases; however, there is some geographical variation in the prevalence of the various HPV types, as described in detail by Munoz et al. (2004).

Cervical carcinogenesis is thought to be a multistep event, with HPV as a necessary, but not sufficient carcinogenic agent (Walboomers et al. 1999). From various studies it could be concluded that high parity, smoking (Wyatt et al. 2001), immunodeficiency (Frisch et al. 2000) and, less consistently, long-term use of oral contraceptives are cofactors that may modulate the risk of progression from HPV infection to cervical cancer (Pater et al. 1988; Elson et al. 2000; Moodley et al. 2003; also reviewed in Castellsague and Munoz 2003). Immunological factors may play an important role in the natural surveillance of the early HPV infection, since immunosuppressed patients have significantly higher rates of persisting HR-HPV infections (Palefsky and Holly 2003).

Östör, in his widely cited review paper, reports that CIN 1 progresses to CIN 3 in 10% of cases, and that the likelihood of progression of CIN 3 to invasive cancer is >12%. The percentage of definitive regression, however, seems unpredictable, since CIN3 lesions, once histologically verified, were most likely to be excised in total or erased by surgical or chemical damage (Östör 1993). These observations are in good agreement with the concept that the vast majority of HR-HPV infections remain transient, reflecting a period of active virus replication, and then obviously are defeated by the natural immune response of the infected women (Fig. 101).

Viral gene expression, and particularly that of the viral oncogenes E6 and E7, is in most instances restricted to the intermediate or superficial cell layers. Apparently, control mechanisms suppress their expression in the basal or parabasal cell layers, i.e., in those epithelial cells that retain the capacity to replicate. This mechanism prevents a concomitant expression of viral and cellular genes in genome replication and proliferation (zur Hausen 1994). If these negative regulating mechanisms lose their function, concomitant expression of viral oncogenes and cellular replication may occur. This in-

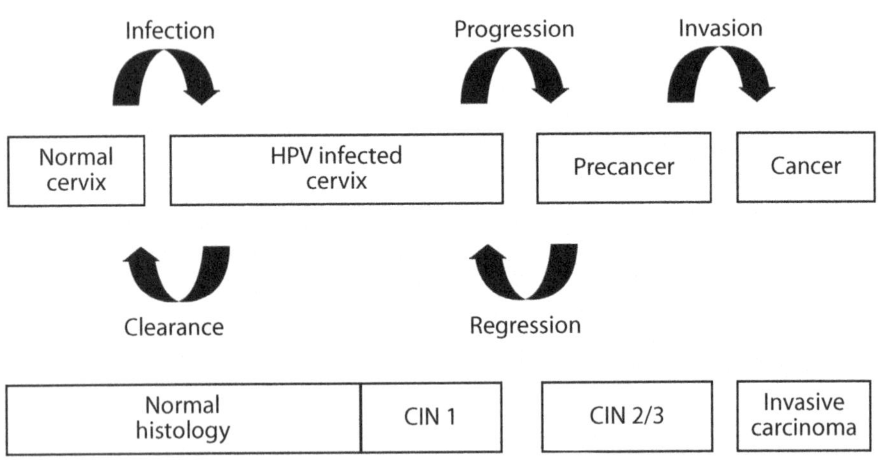

Fig. 101. Natural history of cervical HPV infections (modified after Schiffman and Kjaer, 2003)

duces severe chromosomal instability due to dysregulation of the mitotic spindle apparatus and results in major numerical and structural alterations of the host cell chromosomes (Duensing and Münger 2004).

Histomorphologically, CIN 1 lesions with this deregulated type of viral oncogene expression can initially not be differentiated in H & E stains from the early CIN 1 lesions that still retain the negative regulatory features and are able to suppress viral oncogene expression in the basal and parabasal cell layers. Immunohistochemistry using anti-$p16^{INK4a}$-directed antibodies, however, allows us to monitor the expression of the viral oncogenes in the basal and parabasal cells, since the presence of the E7 oncoprotein in replicating epithelial cells results in strong overexpression of the $p16^{INK4a}$ gene product (see p. 93 and Fig. 107c). This concept of the shift from regulated to deregulated viral gene expression is reflected by the clinical observation that CIN 1 lesions with diffuse $p16^{INK4a}$ gene expression (due to deregulated viral oncogene expression) have a significantly higher risk for progression to higher grades of dysplasia or even invasive carcinomas in comparison to lesions that still retain the regulated pattern of viral gene expression and thus do not display diffuse expression of $p16^{INK4a}$ in the basal and parabasal cell layers (Negri et al. 2004).

Precursors of cervical cancer may develop from the basal layer of regenerating ectocervical squamous epithelium, from proliferating columnar epithelial cells of the endocervical glands, or, most frequently, from hyperplastic reserve cells beneath the endocervical glandular epithelium, located in the transformation zone. Since proliferative activity with high mitotic rates is known to be a prerequisite of cancerogenesis, those cells undergoing proliferation will be most vulnerable to carcinogenic agents. In addition to cellular damage by mechanical or chemical irritation, cellular proliferation here is largely initiated by excessive (mainly exogenous) hormonal stimulation of target cells (see p. 49; Moreno et al. 2002). The bipotential capacity of hyperplastic reserve cells to differentiate into glandular (mucinous) as well as squamous epithelial cells (see Fig. 140a; Tase et al. 1989) is in agreement with the findings that coexisting adenocarcinomas and squamous cell carcinomas are derived from one parent cell clone (see below).

The expression of the viral oncogenes in the replicating basal, parabasal and reserve cell layers results in continuous damage to the host cell genome and ultimately in shifts of the overall DNA content of the host cells. This is reflected by the increasing degree of aneuploidy in these cells. Among those proliferating E6–E7-expressing cell clones, further modified cell clones are selected that stepwise lose their capacity to differentiate in mature squamous epithelia. In consequence the number of cells kept in the active cell cycle increases. This is histopathologically reflected by transition from CIN 1 to CIN 2 and 3 and thickening of the $p16^{INK4a}$-positive cell layer (Figs. 110, 111). At the end of the process, the predominant cell clone has lost its differentiation capacity completely and the lesion impresses as carcinoma in situ with full thickness of replicating diffusely $p16^{INK4a}$-positive cells (Fig. 117). This process of increasing aneuploidization is characterized by increasing chromosomal instability accompanied by continuous recombination of DNA fragments. In frame of these ongoing recombination events, integration of viral genome fragments may occur. The viral genome fragments are predominantly integrated in fragile sites of the host cell genome; however, they do not prefer a specific locus in the human genome (Wentzensen et al. 2004). The majority (up to 80–100%) of carcinomas in situ and invasive cervical carcinomas contain genomically integrated

HPV. Integration of papillomavirus genomes creates unique molecular fingerprints in the genome and unambiguously allows us to identify HPV transformed cells derived from one parent clone (Luft et al. 2001). Using this fingerprinting technique, coexisting adenocarcinomas and squamous cell carcinomas could be identified as being derived from one parent cell clone. This demonstrates that even completely divergent histomorphological structures in different parts of a carcinoma still may be derived from one pre-existing parental cell clone.

Some HPV types, as, for example, the genotype HPV 18 and 45, are found particularly frequently in adenocarcinomas, small cell carcinomas and also in carcinomas of relatively young patients. The genomes of these virus types are found to be integrated in a very high percentage of respective cancers. This may suggest that the damage of the host cell genome conferred by these virus types may be particularly extensive. This is further supported by the clinical observation that the average age of patients with HPV 18 or 45 related carcinomas is about 10 years less than that of patients with cancers associated with less aggressive HR-HPV types, such as 31, 33, 35 or 58, for example. Previous studies have shown that the mean age of patients with invasive carcinoma associated with HPV 16 is 49 years, as contrasted with 37 years for patients with invasive carcinoma associated with HPV 18 (Kurman et al. 1988). Similar observations were made by Walker et al. (1989), who observed rapid recurrences in 45% of patients with carcinomas containing HPV 18 compared with 16% of patients with tumors associated with HPV 16. According to the speed of progression, differences could be observed between several HR-HPV types, e.g., HPV 16 and 18 (Lörincz et al. 1992). The odds ratio indicating the risk of progression to carcinoma for the individual HPV types is different, being highest for HPV 18. Several other reports suggest that the overall survival of patients having cancer associated with HPV 18 or 45 is less in comparison to patients with cancers related to HPV 31 or 33 (Rose et al. 1995; Burger et al. 1996; Lombard et al. 1998; Schwartz et al. 2001). It is therefore of paramount importance to pursue appropriate precautions to prevent an invasive carcinoma from evolving once the diagnosis of a preinvasive lesion is made, by assessing all risk factors and diagnostic tools (see also Trunk et al. 2005).

For routine use, the difference of odds ratios between LR and HR types is clinically more significant, however, than the difference between odds ratios for the individual HR types, warranting testing for risk groups (LR versus HR) rather than for individual HPV types in clinical routine (Munoz et al. 2003).

Histopathology and Immunohistochemistry

Dysplasia and Carcinoma In Situ (CIN 1–3; Figs. 102–140)

The development of dysplasia and carcinoma in situ is a continuum, extending from slight to severe cytological atypia with a gradual loss of epithelial stratification; an increase in nuclear changes, and an increase in the number of atypical mitoses. Because the changes merge into one another, it may be difficult in some instances to differentiate between mild and moderate dysplasia, moderate and severe dysplasia, or severe dysplasia and carcinoma in situ. On the other hand, the distinction between a mild dysplasia and an irregular regenerative or reparative epithelium should not prove difficult. The nuclei of regenerative epithelium may be enlarged, slightly irregular, yet the chromatin pattern normal. The epithelial stratification may be barely altered. On the other hand, the nuclei of dysplastic epithelium are dyskaryotic from the beginning, enlarged, and irregular with chromatin clumping. In addition, abnormal mitotic figures, loss of basal polarity and multinucleated cells may be present. Depending upon the cell of origin and/or the direction of cellular differentiation, structural variations can be observed between squamous and reserve cell intraepithelial neoplasias.

Squamous Cell Differentiation

In *mild* and *moderate dysplasia of squamous cell type* (CIN 1 and 2) (Figs. 102–107), epithelial stratification is only partly lost, with an increasing basal hyperplasia and a general thickening (Figs. 102, 105) or slightly papillomatous change (Figs. 103, 104) of the epithelial layer. Basal polarity and cellular orientation are gradually lost. The nuclei become irregular, hyperchromatic with an abnormal, coarsely granular chromatin pattern. Mitoses increase in number, primarily in the basal and middle epithelial layers. The upper epithelial layers may (Fig. 106) or may not (Fig. 105) show koilocytosis, as a result of viral replication following HPV infection. In mild or moderate dysplasia, the presence of koilocytes may indicate replication of LR-HPV types, e.g., 6 or 11, which will remain episomal; such a dysplasia is virtually always reversible. If, however, the infection is with HR-HPV types, the viral DNA may become integrated into the cellular genome. This, besides mere deregulated expression of the viral E6 and E7 oncogenes in basal or parabasal cells, may further contribute to malignant progression of cervical

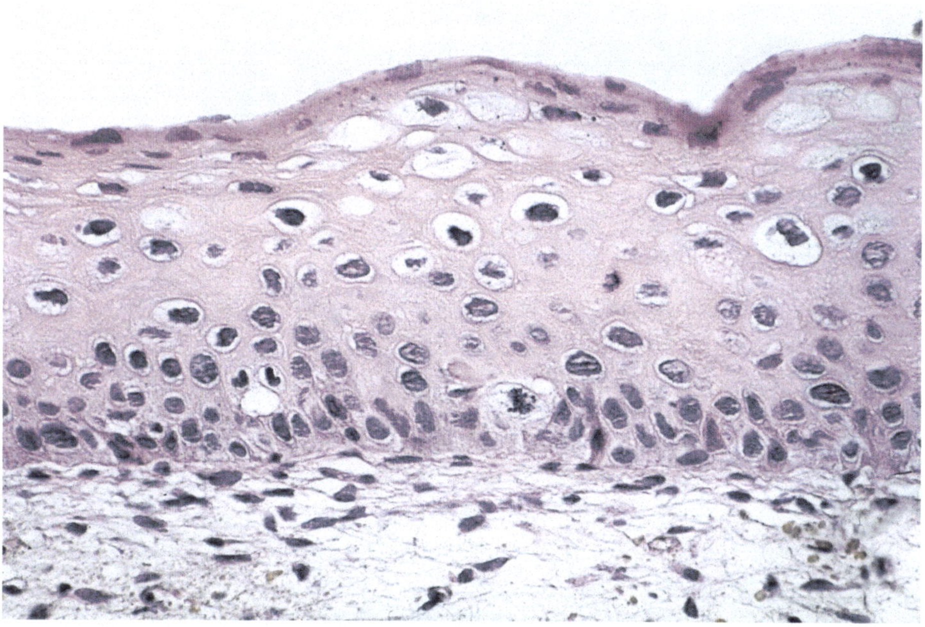

Fig. 102. Mild dysplasia, squamous cell differentiation, koilocytic. H&E

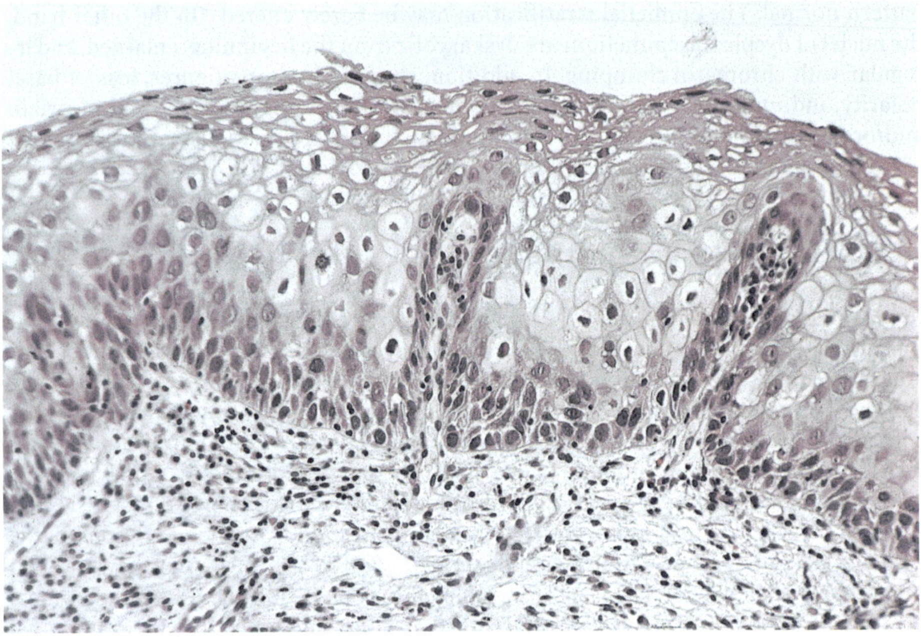

Fig. 103. Mild dysplasia, squamous cell differentiation, slightly papillomatous. H&E

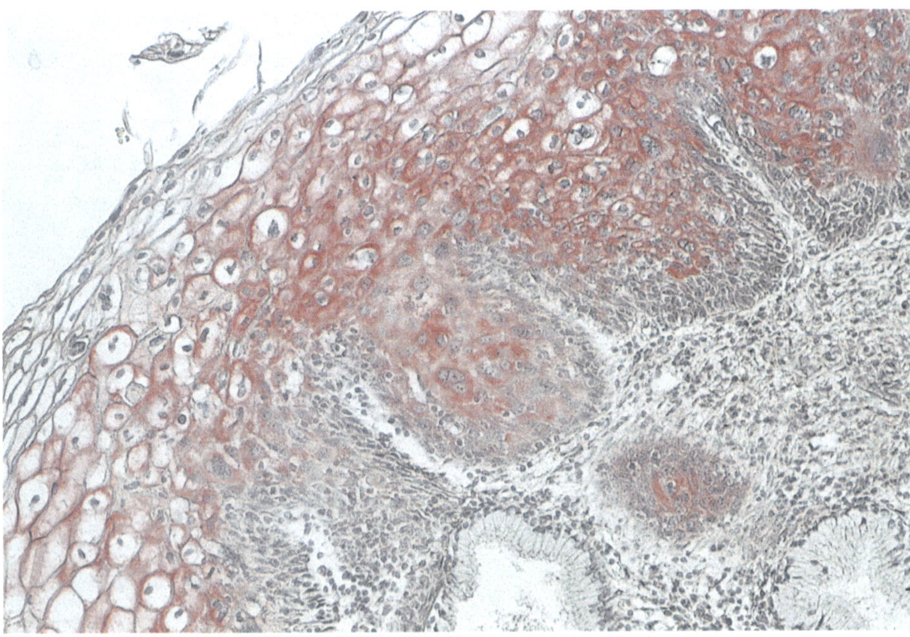

Fig. 104. Mild dysplasia, squamous cell differentiation. Immunohistochemical reaction with anticytokeratin 13

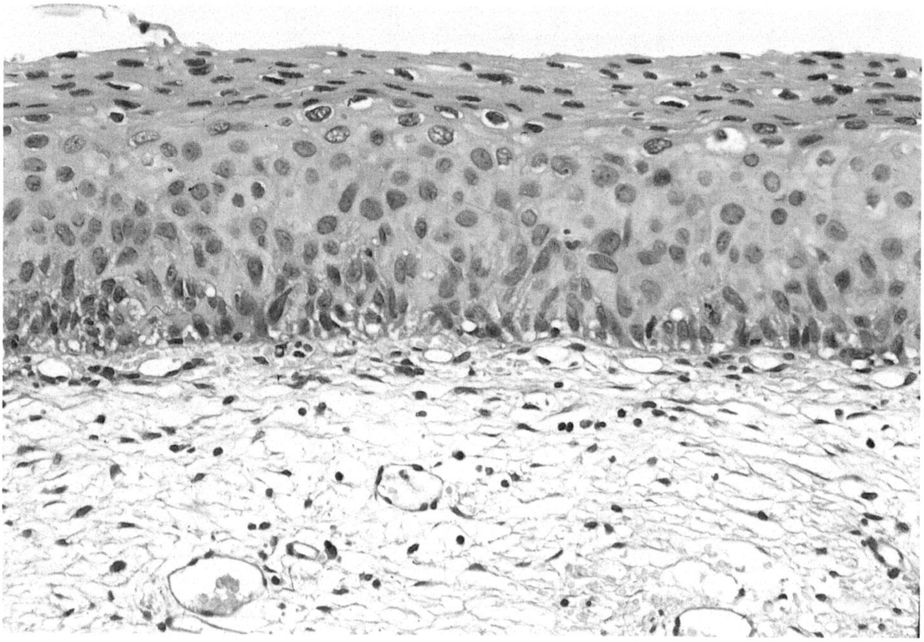

Fig. 105. Moderate dysplasia, squamous cell differentiation, nonkoilocytic. H&E

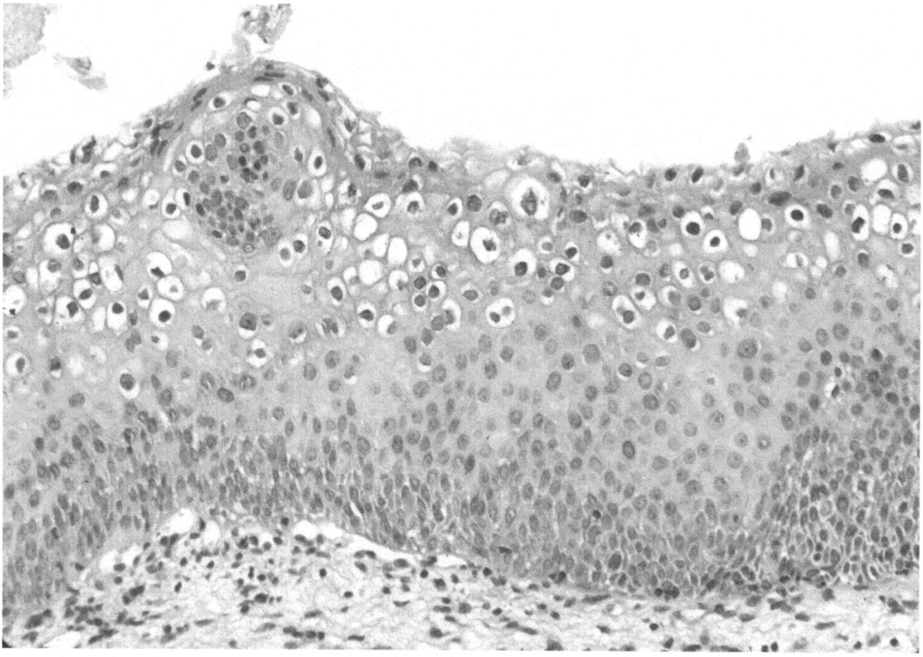

Fig. 106. Moderate dysplasia, squamous cell differentiation, koilocytic. H&E

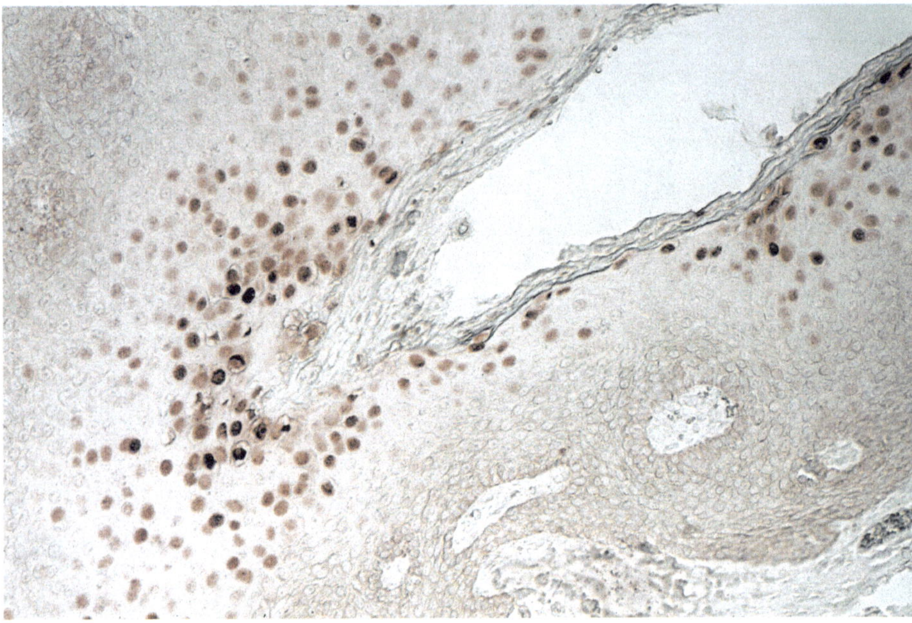

Fig. 107a. Mild to moderate dysplasia, squamous cell differentiation. In situ hybridization with DNA probe HPV 6 and 11

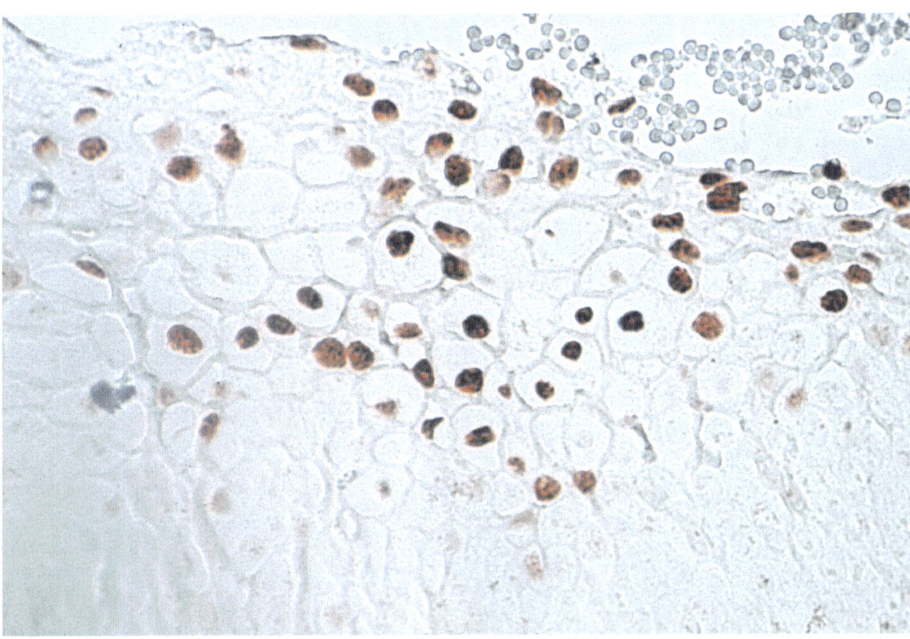

Fig. 107b. Same as Fig. 107a. Positive nuclear signals in koilocytes located in intermediate cellular layers

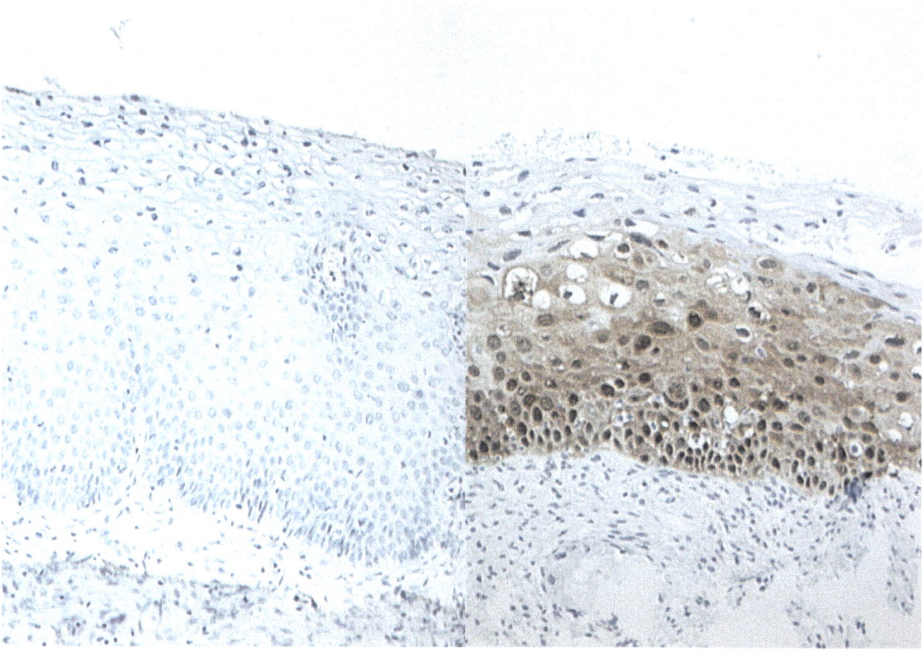

Fig. 107c. Ectocervical epithelium from 2 patients with mild dysplasia (CIN 1) following HPV infection. Immunostaining with $p16^{INK4a}$ shows diffuse reaction (*right*) suspicious of a persisting lesion in contrast to a negative reaction (*left*) suggesting regression

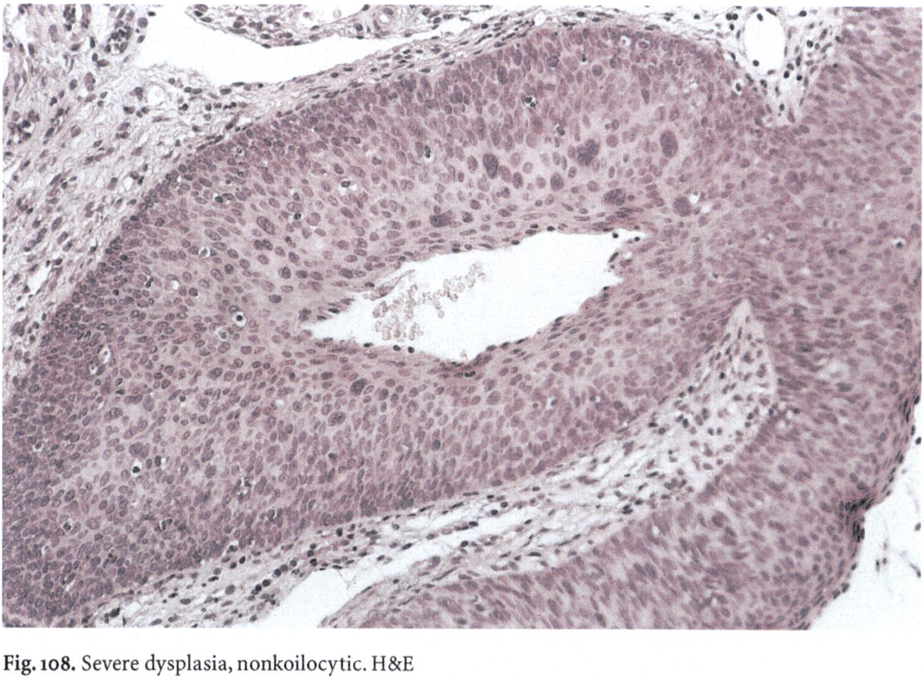

Fig. 108. Severe dysplasia, nonkoilocytic. H&E

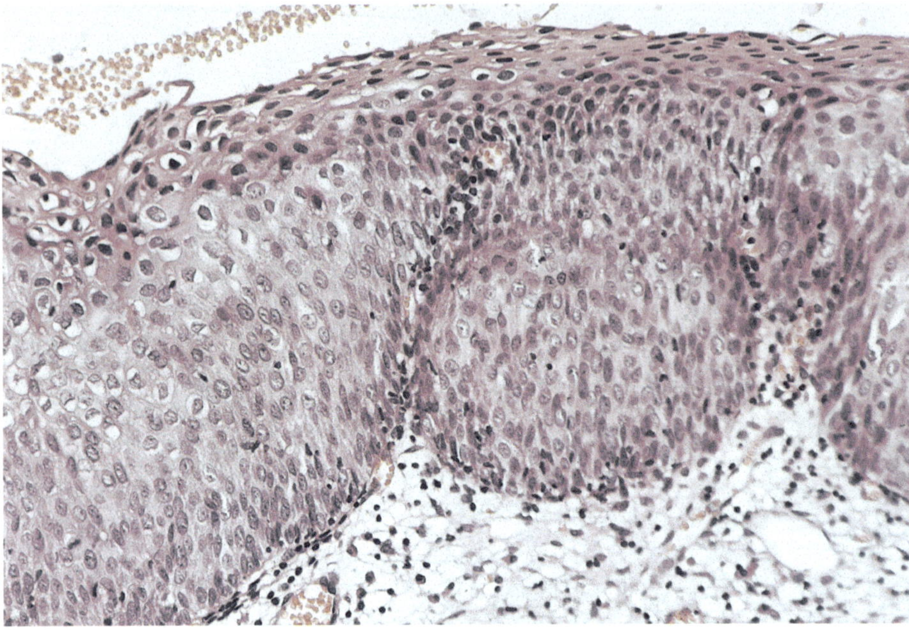

Fig. 109. Severe dysplasia, koilocytic, H&E. Histogenetic type in Figs. 108, 109 cannot be determined without special stains

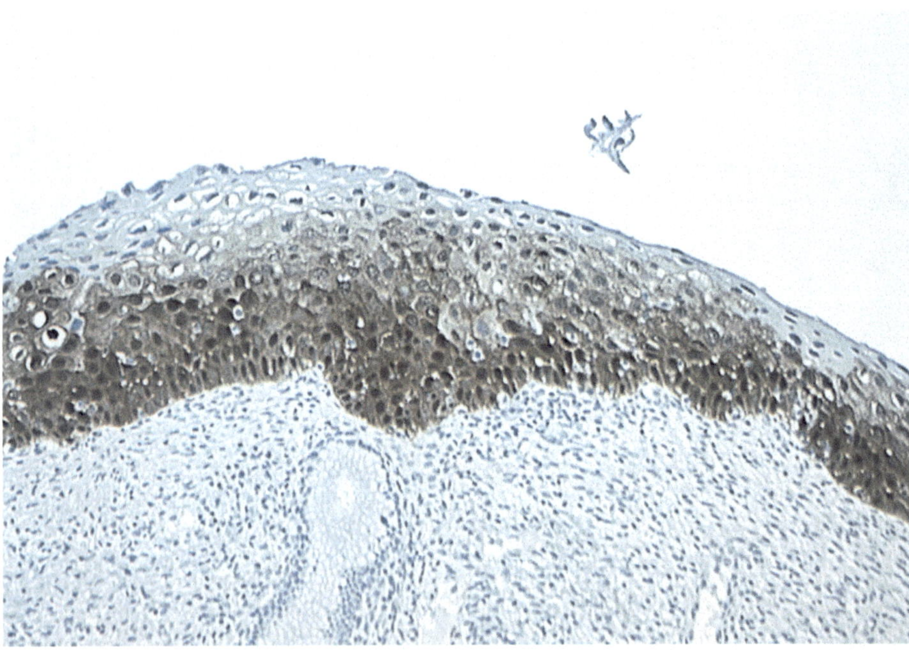

Fig. 110. Moderate dysplasia (CIN 2). Diffuse positivity for $p16^{INK4a}$ in dysplastic cells, koilocytic change in upper epithelial cell layers. $p16^{INK4a}$ immunostain

precancer (Klaes et al. 1999) and initiate malignant change. The dysplastic change starts at the squamocolumnar junction and is usually located there, originating from the basal layer of the regenerated ectocervical epithelium.

Differential Diagnosis. It may be possible to distinguish between reversible and irreversible koilocytic dysplasia at this early stage by identifying the risk type of infective virus (Campion et al. 1986; Fig. 107a and b, 124). If a LR type of HPV is detected, the lesion is to be considered as reversible; if a HR type is identified, it is not possible to make the distinction between reversible and irreversible dysplasia on the assessment of HPV type alone (refer to Fig. 101). The higher the grade of dysplasia, the higher the ratio of HR-HPV infections.

If the decision is not possible, histological (Winkler et al. 1984; Crum et al. 1985) or immunohistochemical (Dallenbach-Hellweg and Lang 1991) distinction should be attempted (see p. 8 f). Dysplasias infected with LR-HPV have dyskaryotic polyploid nuclei but normal mitoses and express cytokeratin 13 only (Fig. 104). Those infected with HR-HPV types have often aneuploid nuclei and atypical mitoses and often, but not always (Fig. 115) show a coexpression of cytokeratins 13, 8, 18, and CEA. Such coexpression of intermediate filaments and CEA may indicate that the dysplasia is most likely of reserve cell type (see below). The distinction is clinically important for deciding how to treat the patient further. According to recent studies (Wang et al. 2004; Negri et al. 2004),

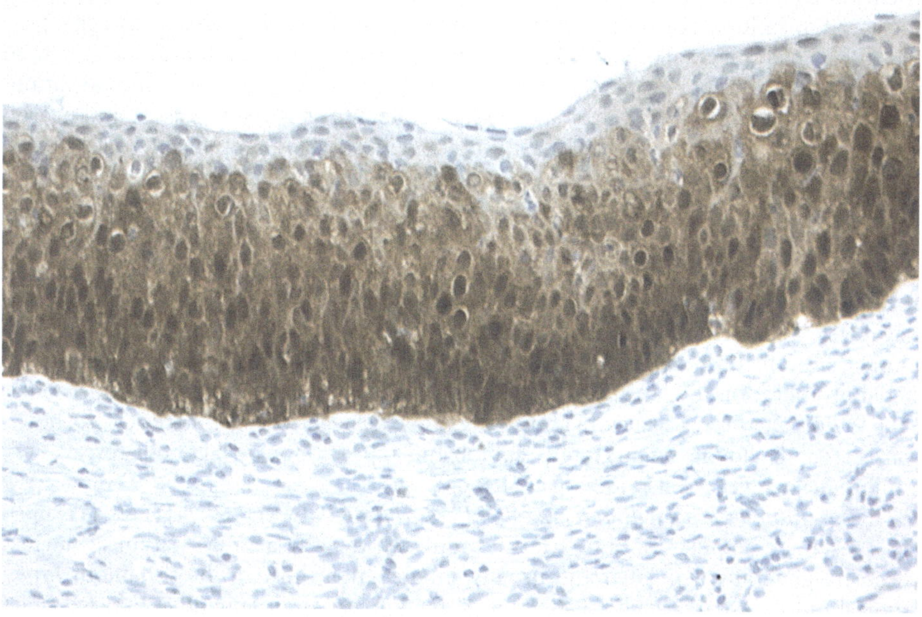

Fig. 111. Severe dysplasia (CIN 3). Diffuse positivity for $p16^{INK4a}$ in dysplastic cells. $p16^{INK4a}$ immunostain

p16^{INK4a}, a cyclin-dependent kinase inhibitor, may be a prognostic marker (see Fig. 107c). Negri showed that CIN 1 lesions with diffuse p16^{INK4a} staining had a significantly higher tendency to progress to a high-grade lesion than p16^{INK4a}-negative cases.

In *severe dysplasia with squamous differentiation* (CIN 3) (Figs. 108–112), loss of epithelial stratification is almost complete. Nuclear changes (enlargement, chromatin clumping, polymorphism, hyperchromasia) and the number of mitoses are considerably increased. Since koilocytes can only develop in maturing cells, they will be less numerous than in mild or moderate dysplasia. The dysplastic epithelium is usually quite high, may be covered by a thick layer of parakeratosis (Fig. 112), and may form broad papillae that extend downwards into the underlying stroma (Fig. 109) or into the mouths of endocervical glands (Fig. 108).

Carcinoma in situ with squamous differentiation (CIN 3) [8070/2] (Figs. 113–117) shows a complete loss of stratification. The entire epithelium consists of poorly differentiated neoplastic cells, which contain disorganized, large, atypical, hyperchromatic nuclei surrounded by little cytoplasm. Atypical mitoses are frequent in all layers; koilocytes are not present. This neoplastic epithelium originates at the squamocolumnar junction and from there may grow out to replace large areas of the ecto- and endocervical surface epithelium. It is usually covered by a layer of atypical parakeratosis. Its spread into glands is much less pronounced than that of carcinoma in situ with reserve cell differentiation.

Reserve Cell Differentiation

Mild, moderate or severe dysplasia with reserve cell differentiation (CIN 1–3) [8077/2] (Figs. 118–133) develops from the reserve cell layer of the endocervical epithelium and is usually preceded by a reserve cell hyperplasia. The gradual increase in cytological and nuclear atypicality corresponds closely to the various degrees of squamous-type dysplasia. Because the reserve cells are bipotential, irregular maturation towards mucin formation, often monocellular (Fig. 122), clear cell change (Figs. 118, 123), or maturation towards keratinization (Fig. 119) may be seen. Koilocytosis is often present and nearly always caused by infection with HR-HPV types (Fig. 124). Topographically, reserve cell dysplasia is not always concentrated at, but rather above the squamocolumnar junction, and may also arise anywhere within the endocervical mucosa (surface epithelium and glands; Figs. 118, 119).

In rare instances reserve cell dysplasia may form papillary structures resembling a pedunculated papilloma of the ectocervix (Figs. 130, 131). Since an invasive carcinoma may develop at their base, the papillomatous growths should be excised in total and examined carefully (Randall et al. 1986). Because of the histological resemblance of its epithelial proliferation to transitional metaplasia, this lesion has been called transitional cell papilloma (Albores-Saavedra and Young 1995). Its negative reaction for CK 20, however, casts some doubts on this interpretation and appears more in favor of a reserve cell (Müllerian) origin (see also Koenig et al. 1997).

The *carcinoma in situ with reserve cell differentiation* (CIN 3) [8077/2] (Figs. 134–140) also presents a complete loss of stratification with densely arranged atypical nuclei. These are generally elongated and usually smaller than those of the squamous type. Atypical mitotic figures such as three-group metaphases are frequently observed (Fig. 136, 137). Koilocytes are not seen, because no mature cells are present in the upper layers. The very sparse cytoplasm of the tumor cells may show incomplete differentiation in

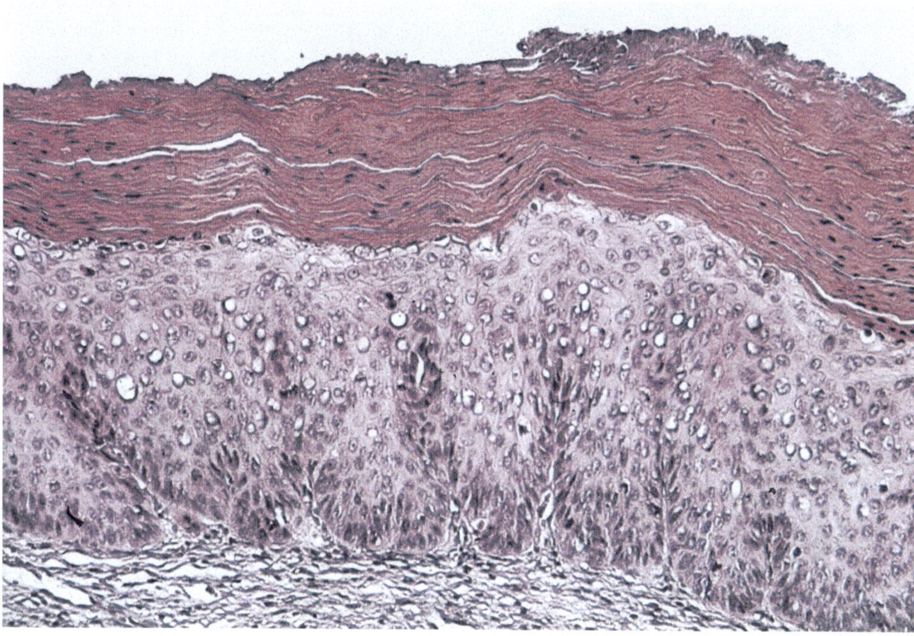

Fig. 112. Severe dysplasia, squamous cell differentiation, covered by a broad layer of parakeratosis. H&E

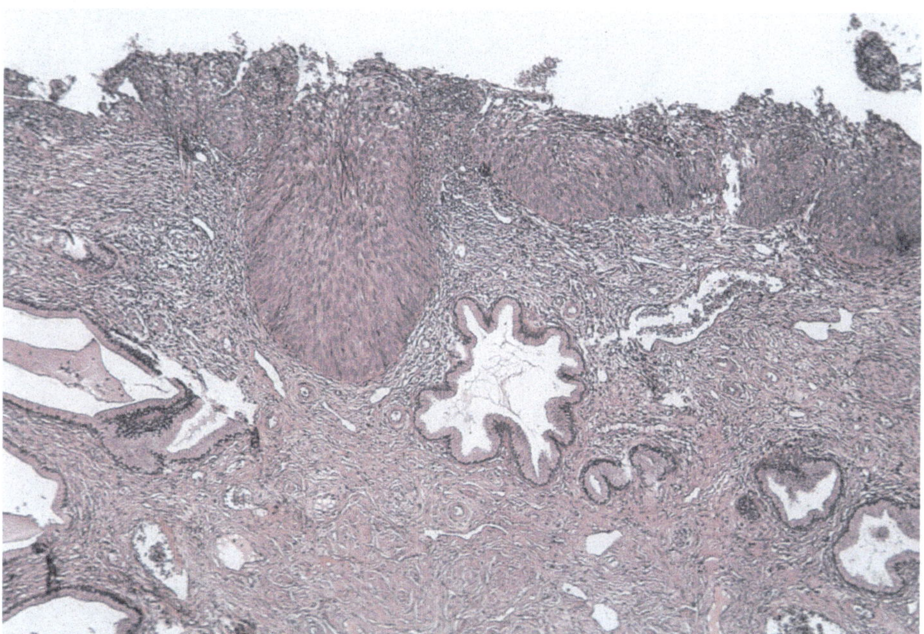

Fig. 113. Carcinoma in situ. H&E

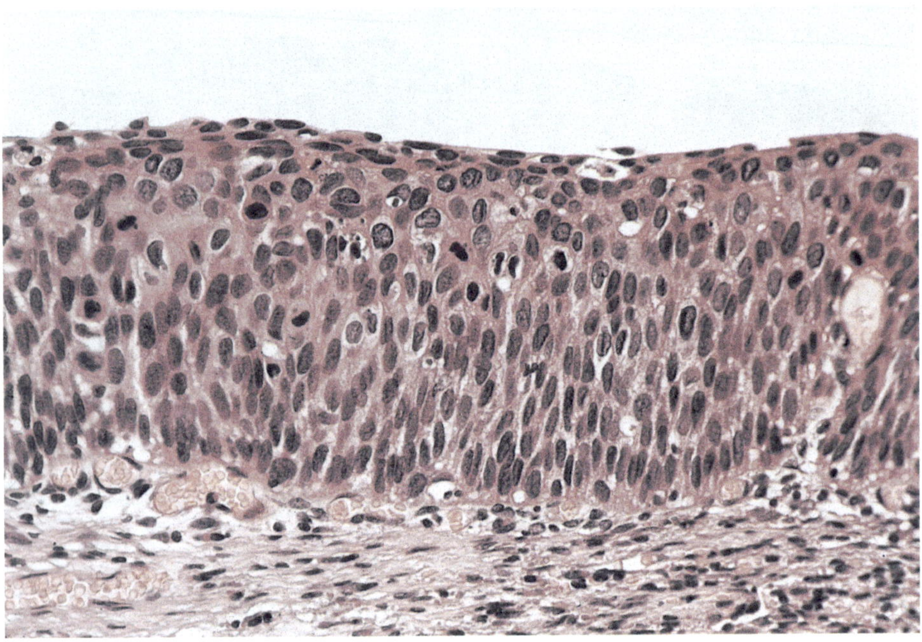

Fig. 114. Carcinoma in situ. H&E, higher magnification

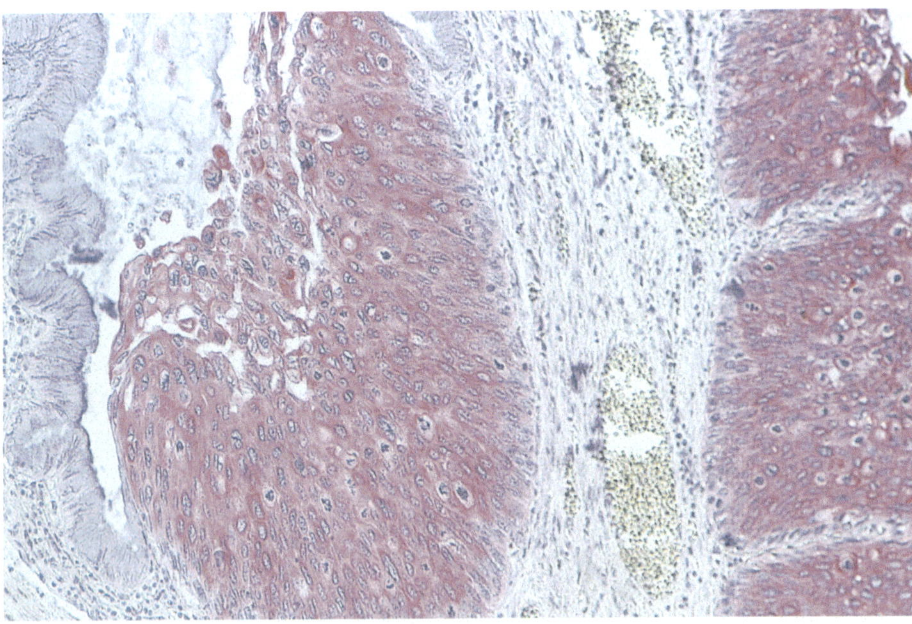

Fig. 115. Carcinoma in situ. Immunohistochemical reaction with cytokeratin 13 only

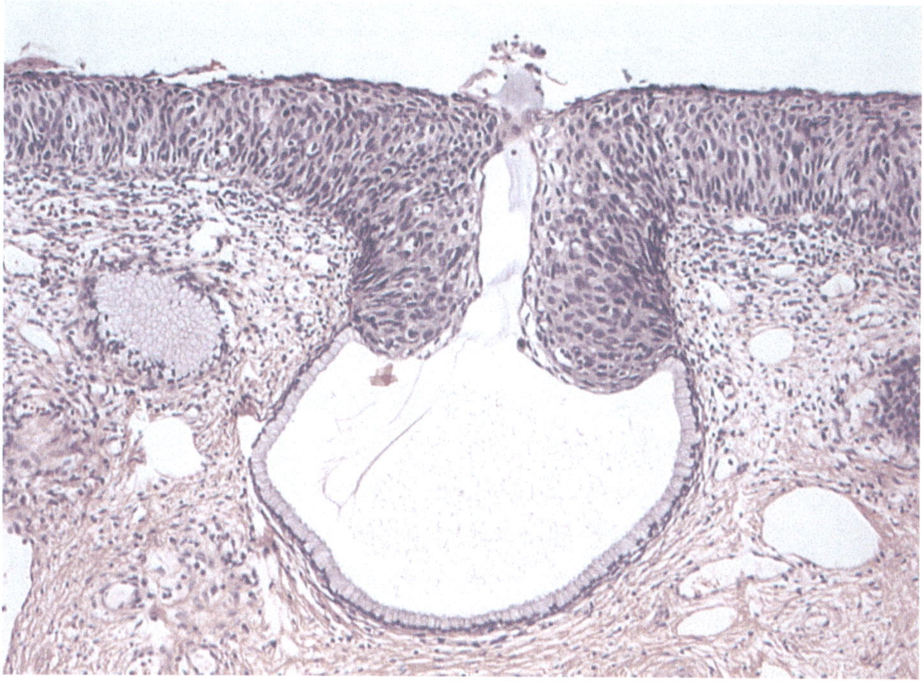

Fig. 116. Carcinoma in situ (CIN 3). H&E

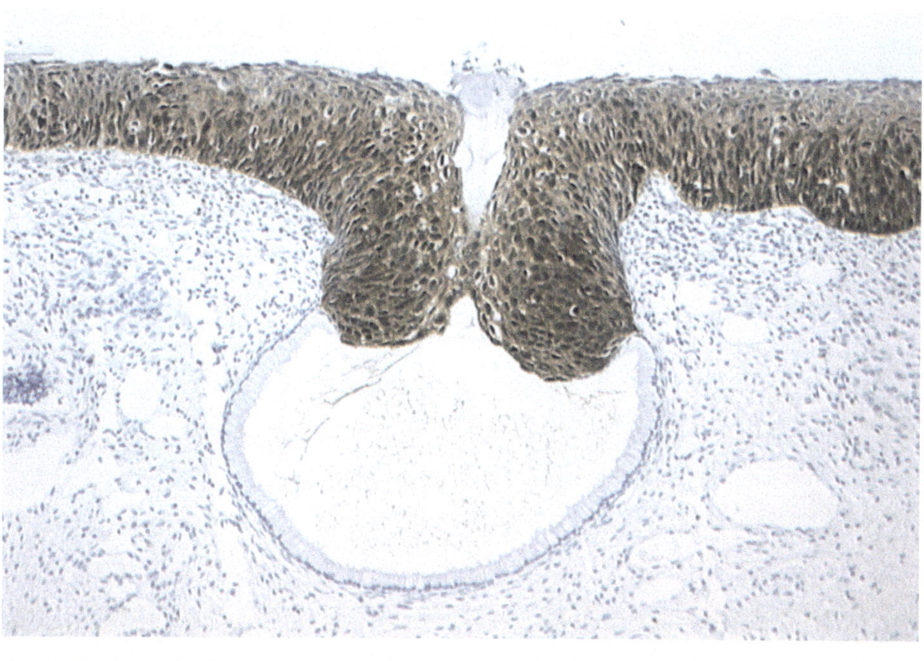

Fig. 117. Carcinoma in situ (CIN 3), same case as in Fig. 115. Diffuse positivity for p16^{INK4a} in dysplastic cells. p16^{INK4a} immunostain

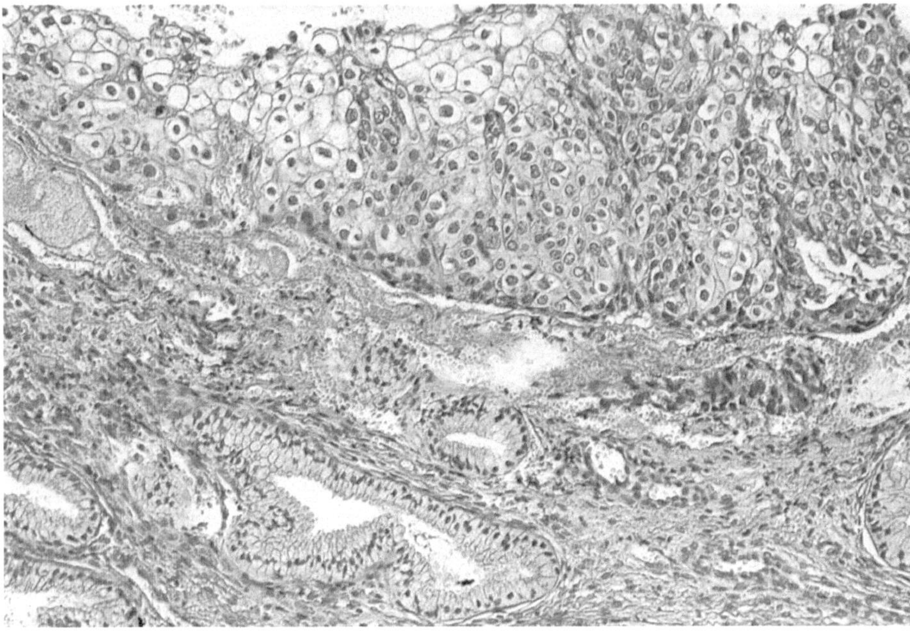

Fig. 118. Mild dysplasia, reserve cell differentiation with koilocytes. H&E

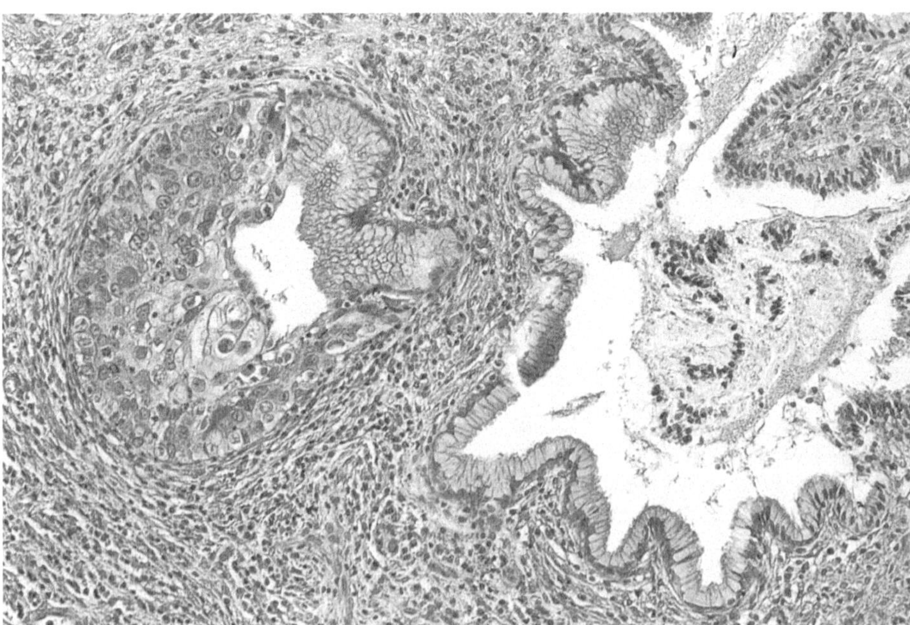

Fig. 119. Mild dysplasia, reserve cell differentiation with koilocytes in endocervical gland. H&E

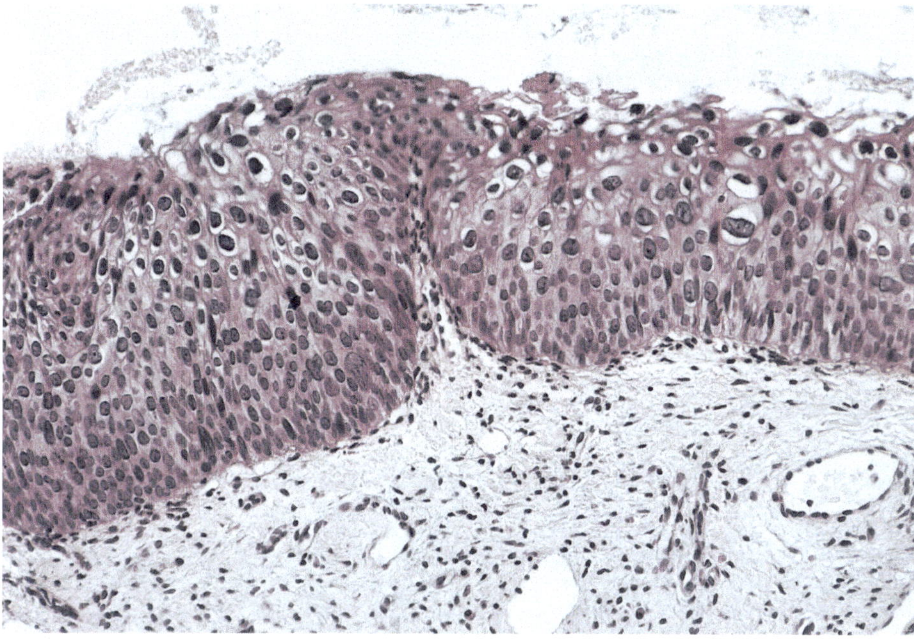

Fig. 120. Severe dysplasia with koilocytes. H&E

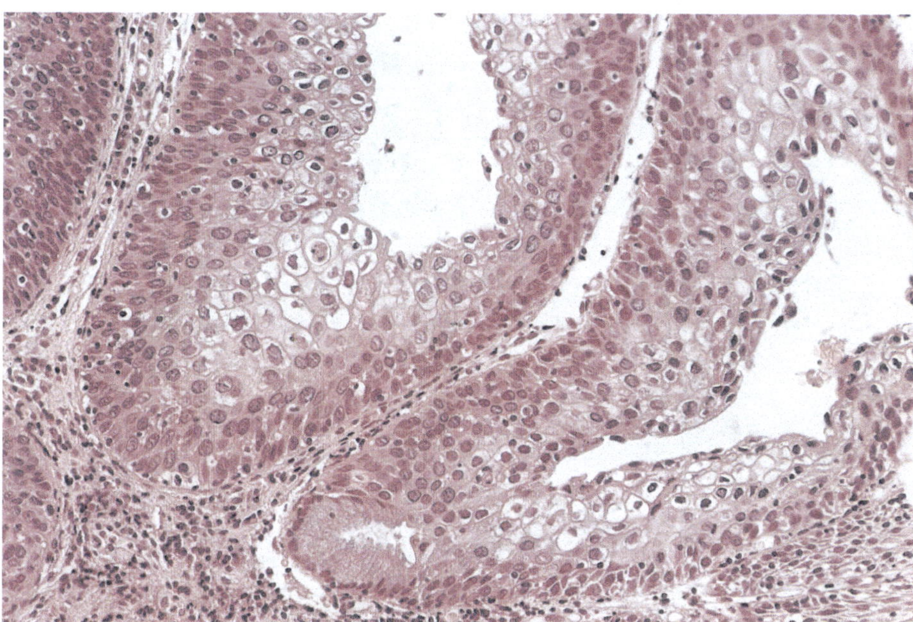

Fig. 121. Moderate koilocytic dysplasia, reserve cell differentiation, in endocervical glands. H&E

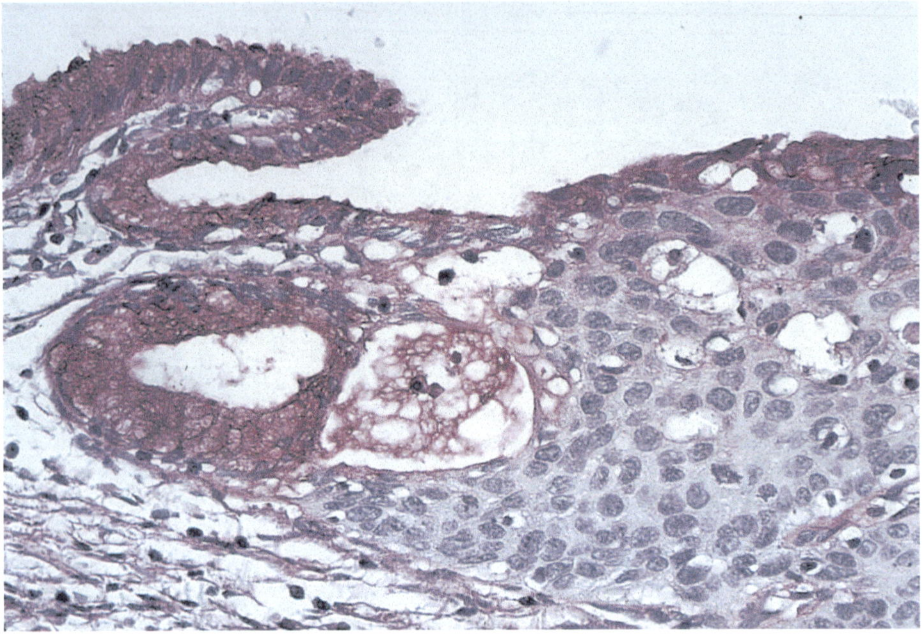

Fig. 122. Moderate dysplasia, reserve cell differentiation with monocellular mucin formation. PAS reaction

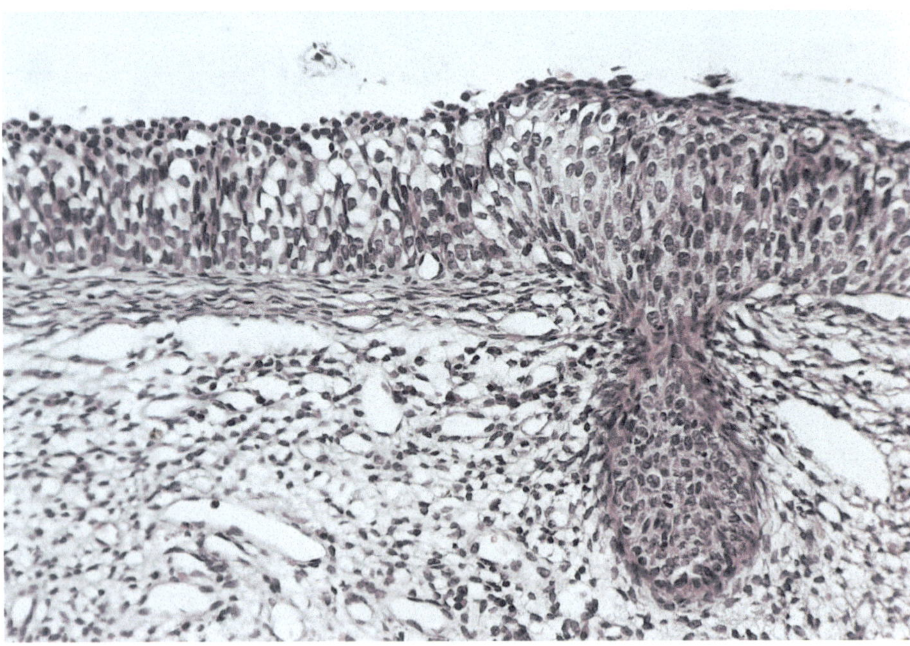

Fig. 123. Severe dysplasia, reserve cell differentiation, with clear cell change and with protrusion towards stroma. H&E

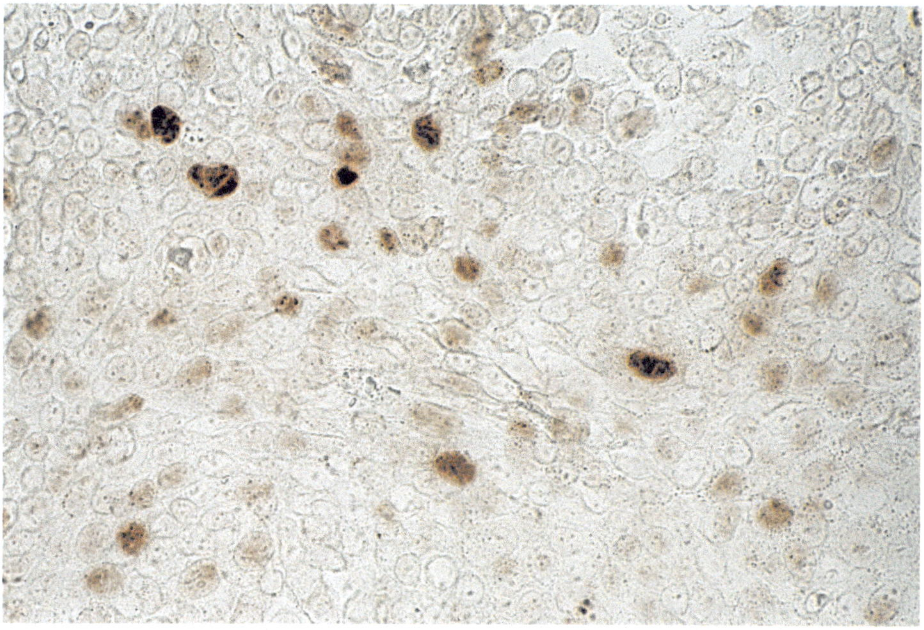

Fig. 124. Koilocytic dysplasia, reserve cell differentiation. In situ hybridization with DNA probe for HPV 16 and 18

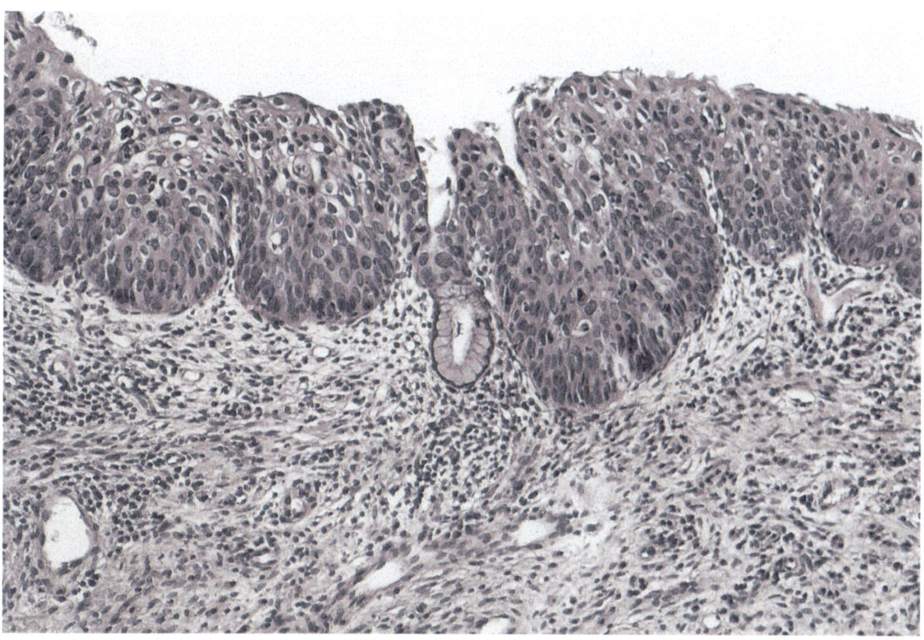

Fig. 125. Severe dysplasia, reserve cell differentiation, almost complete loss of stratification. H&E

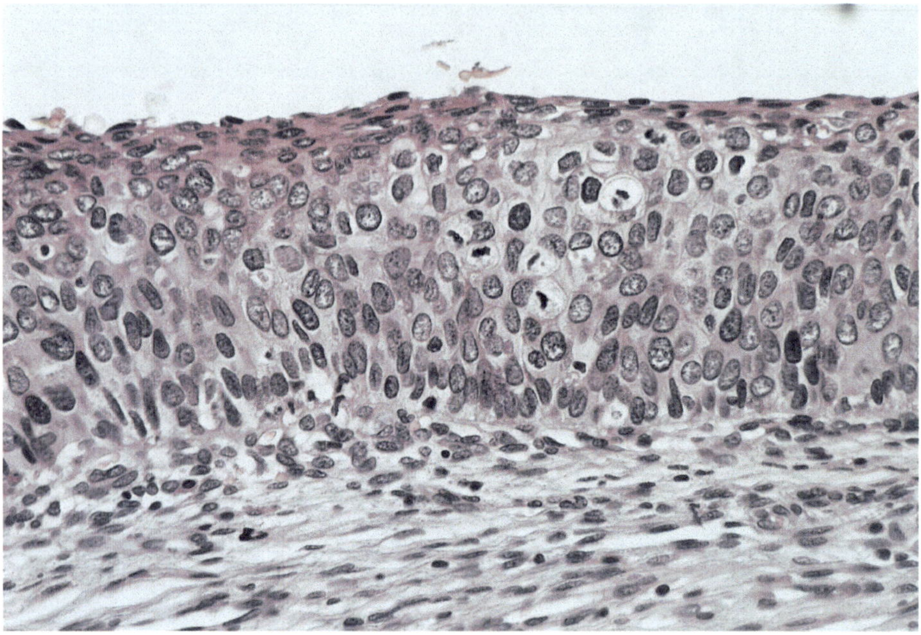

Fig. 126. Severe dysplasia, reserve cell differentiation with frequent mitoses. H&E

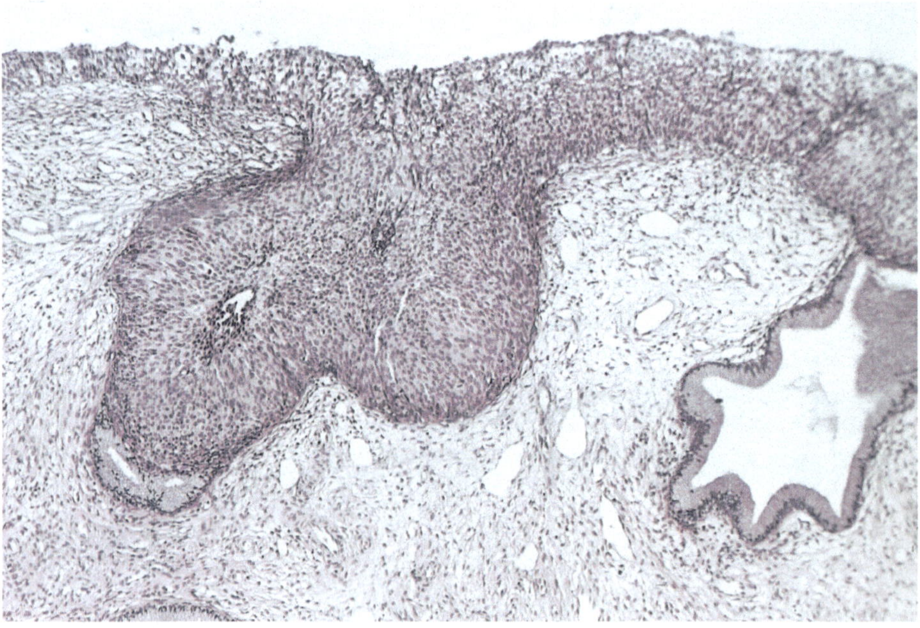

Fig. 127. Severe dysplasia, reserve cell differentiation, with transition to carcinoma in situ. H&E

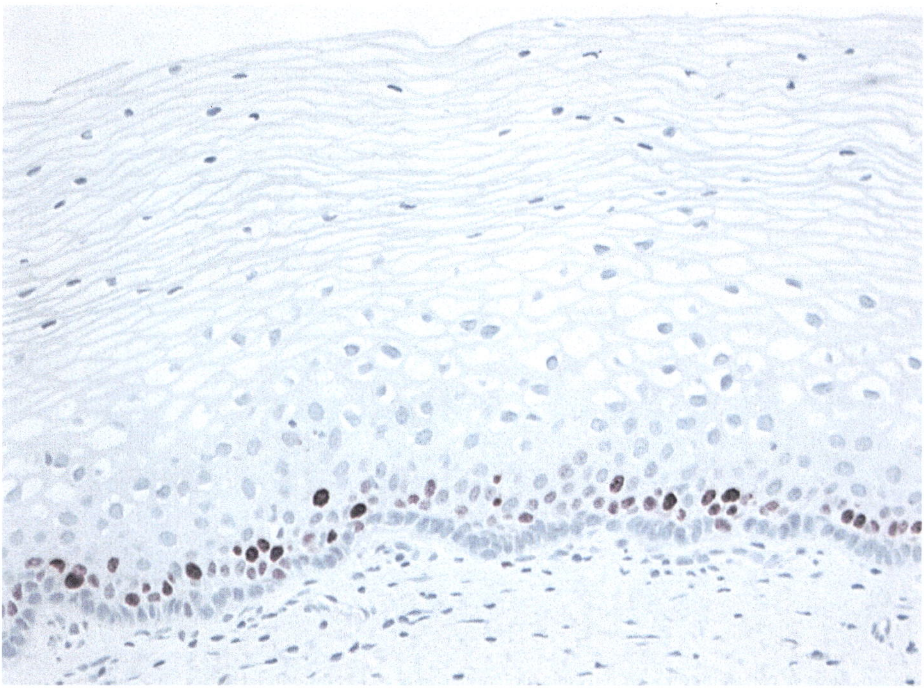

Fig. 128. Normal squamous epithelium, ectocervix. Nuclear positivity for proliferation marker MIB-1 mostly in parabasal cell layer. MIB-1 immunostain

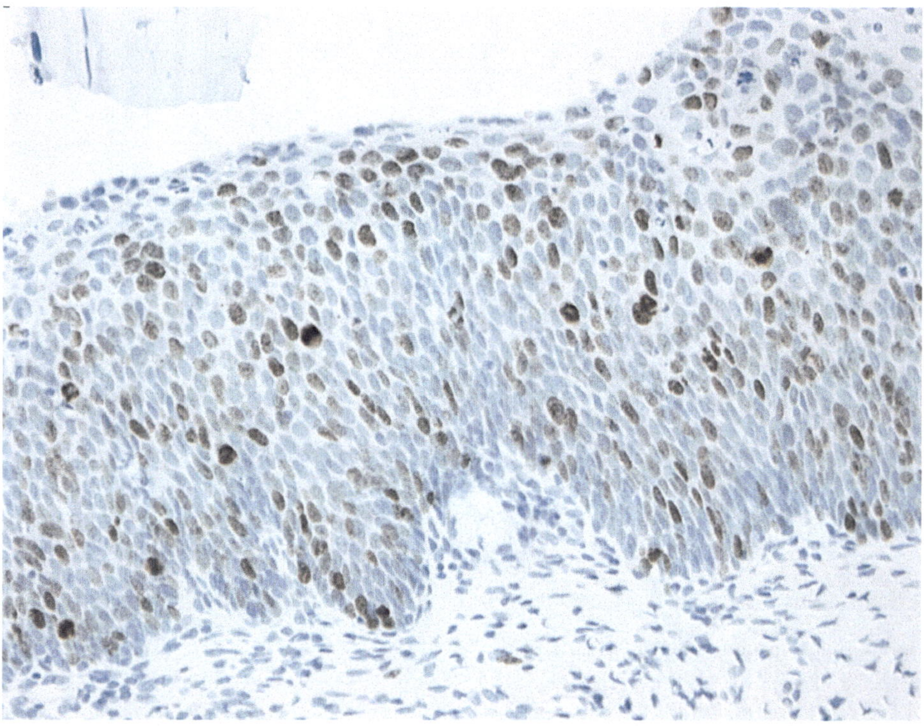

Fig. 129. Severe dysplasia (CIN 3). Nuclear positivity for proliferation marker MIB-1 throughout the epithelium. MIB-1 immunostain

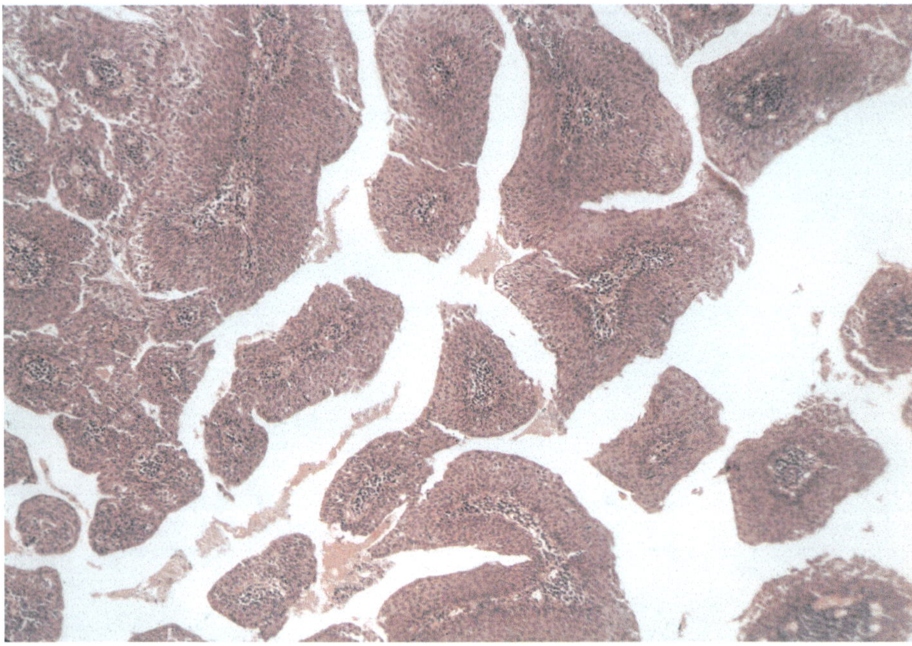

Fig. 130. Reserve cell papilloma with dysplasia (transitional cell papilloma). H&E

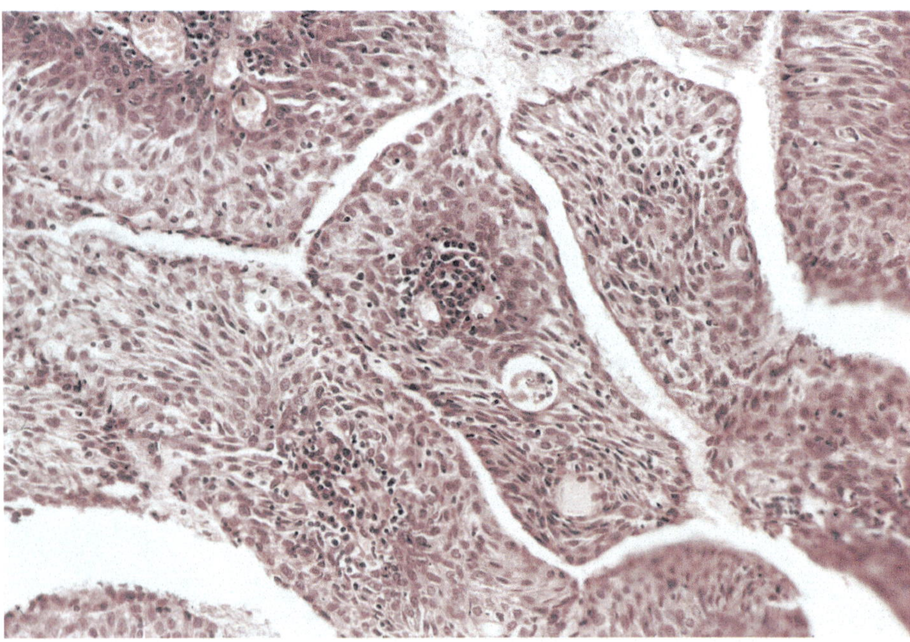

Fig. 131. Higher magnification of Fig. 127. H&E

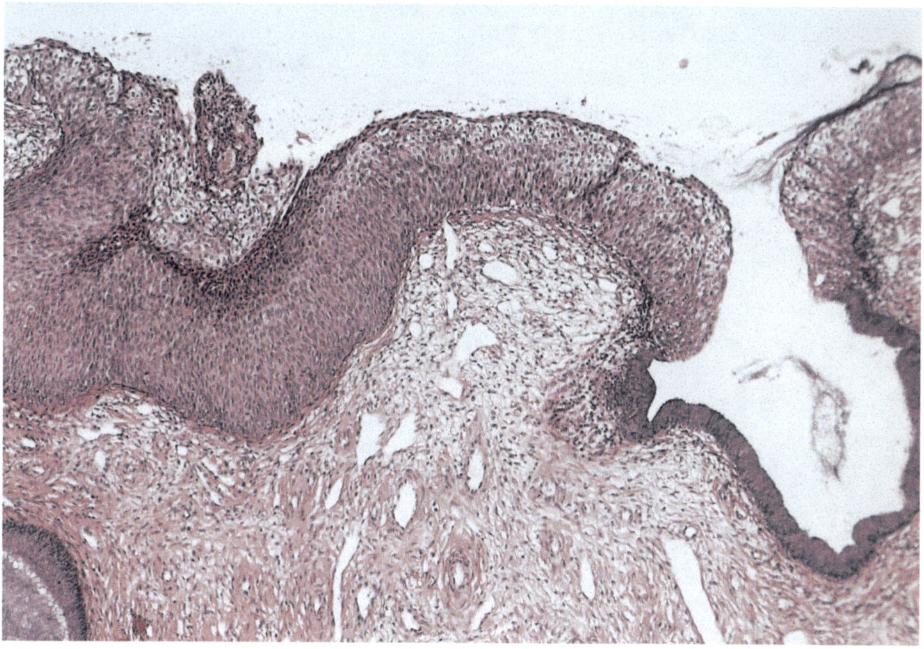

Fig. 132. Severe dysplasia, reserve cell differentiation, with transition to carcinoma in situ. H&E

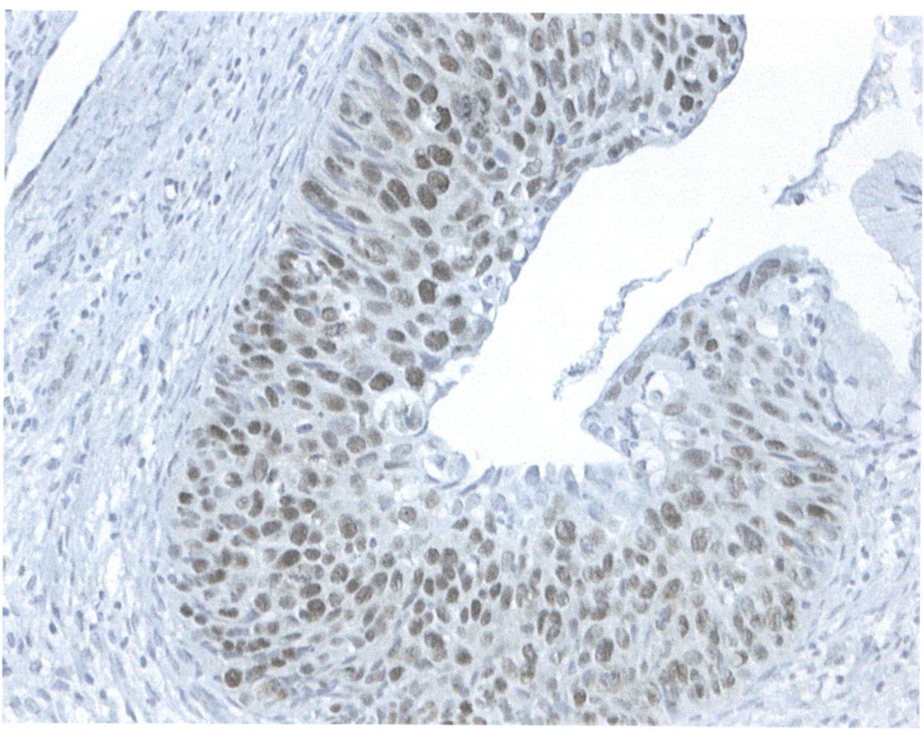

Fig. 133. Severe dysplasia (CIN 3). Nuclear positivity for proliferation marker mcm5. Immunostain with mcm5

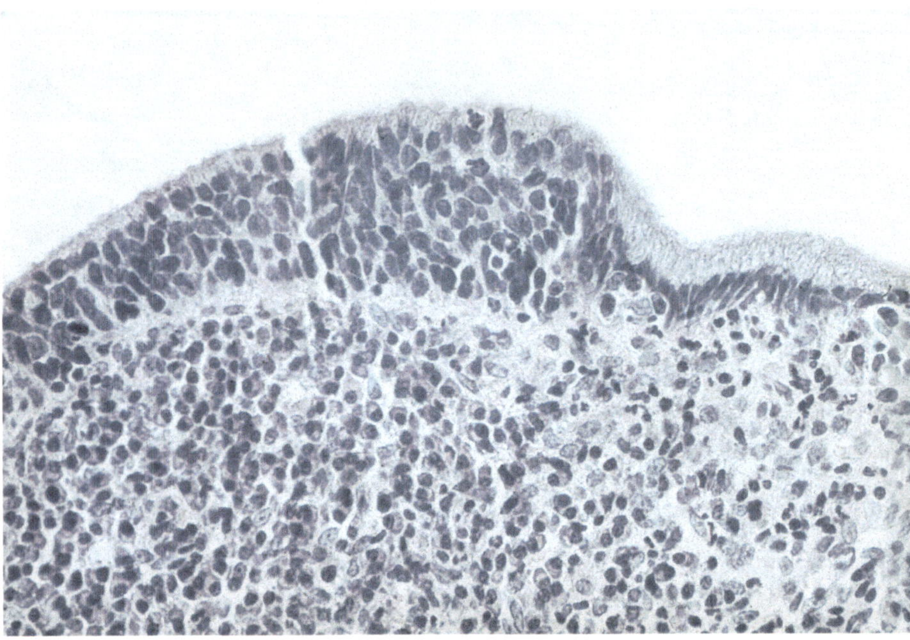

Fig. 134. Carcinoma in situ, early change from atypical reserve cell hyperplasia. H&E

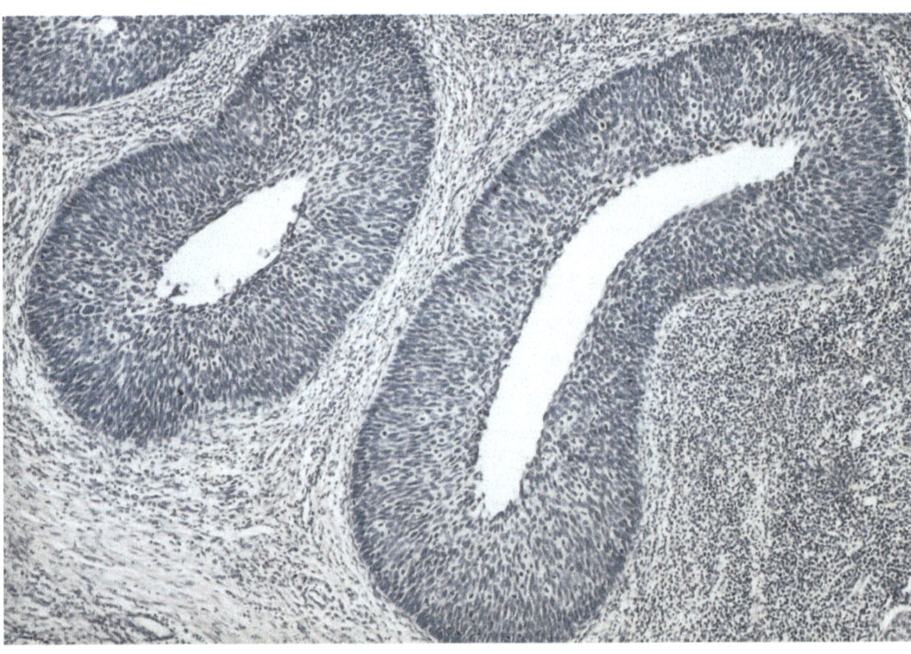

Fig. 135. Carcinoma in situ, reserve cell differentiation, intraglandular spread. H&E

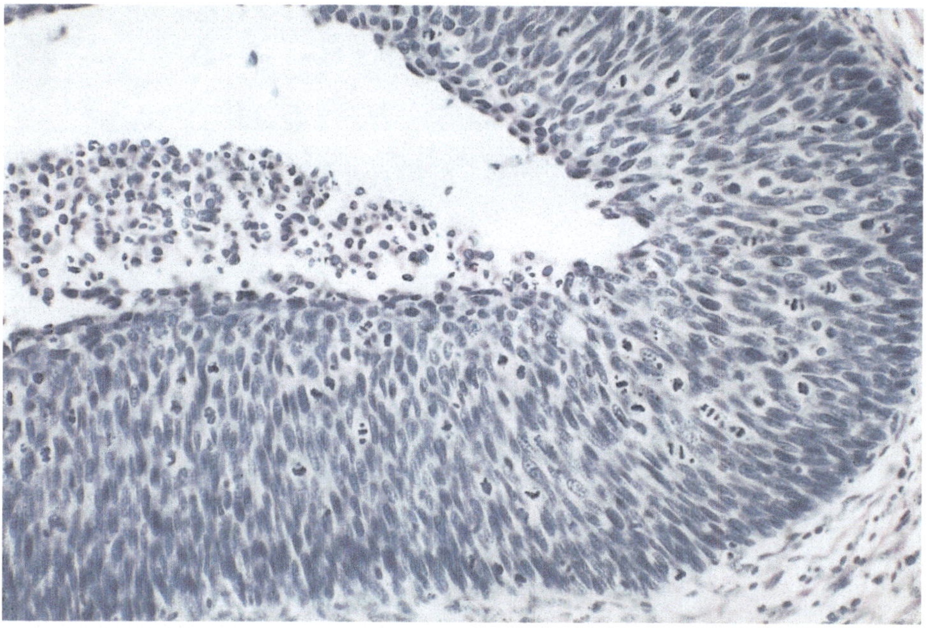

Fig. 136. Carcinoma in situ, reserve cell differentiation, three group metaphases. H&E

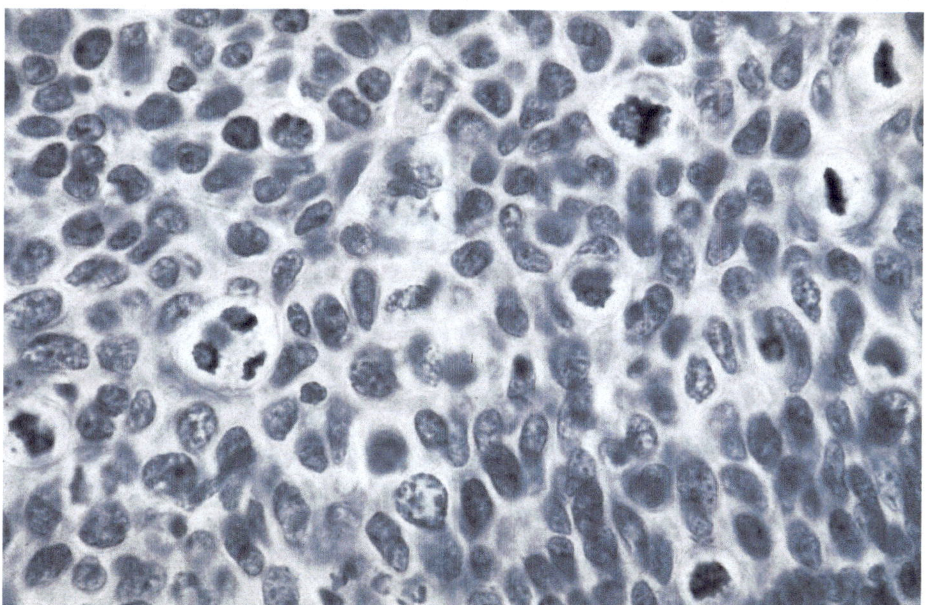

Fig. 137. Carcinoma in situ, reserve cell differentiation. H&E, higher magnification

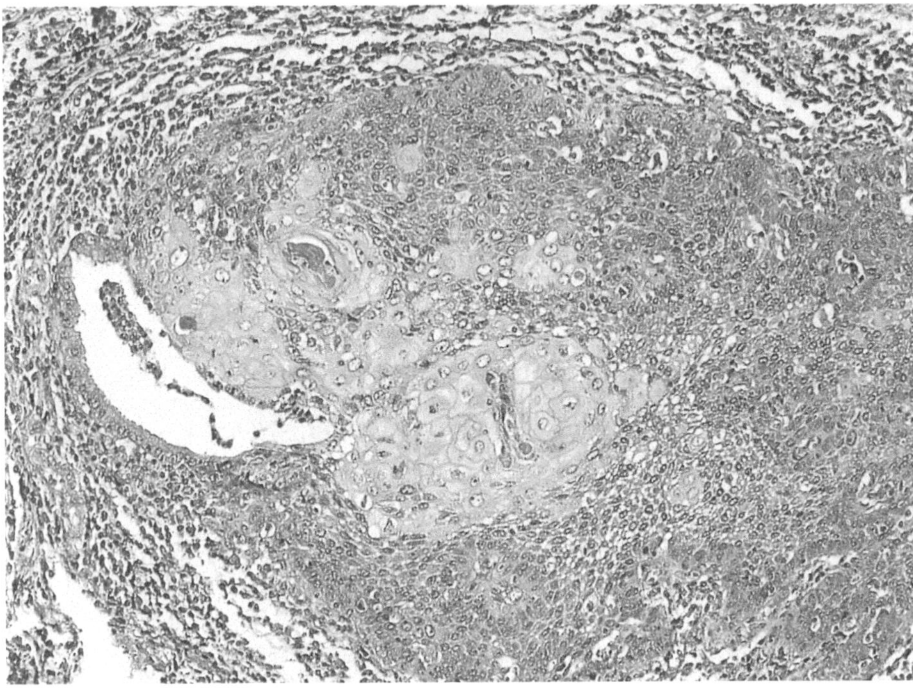

Fig. 138. Carcinoma in situ, reserve cell differentiation, with metaplastic squamous differentiation and formation of microglands (*lower middle*). H&E

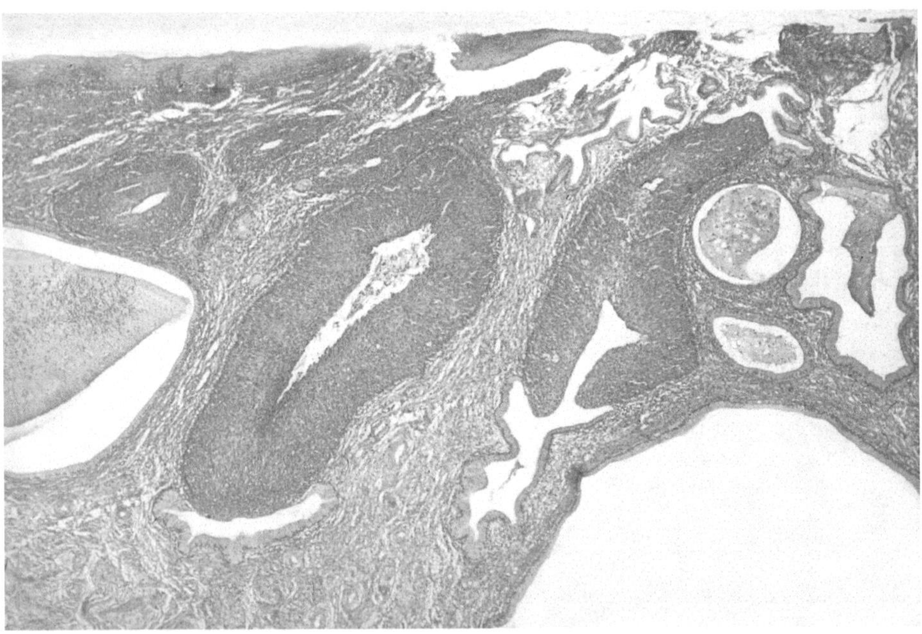

Fig. 139. Carcinoma in situ, reserve cell differentiation, intraglandular spread with deep extension. H&E

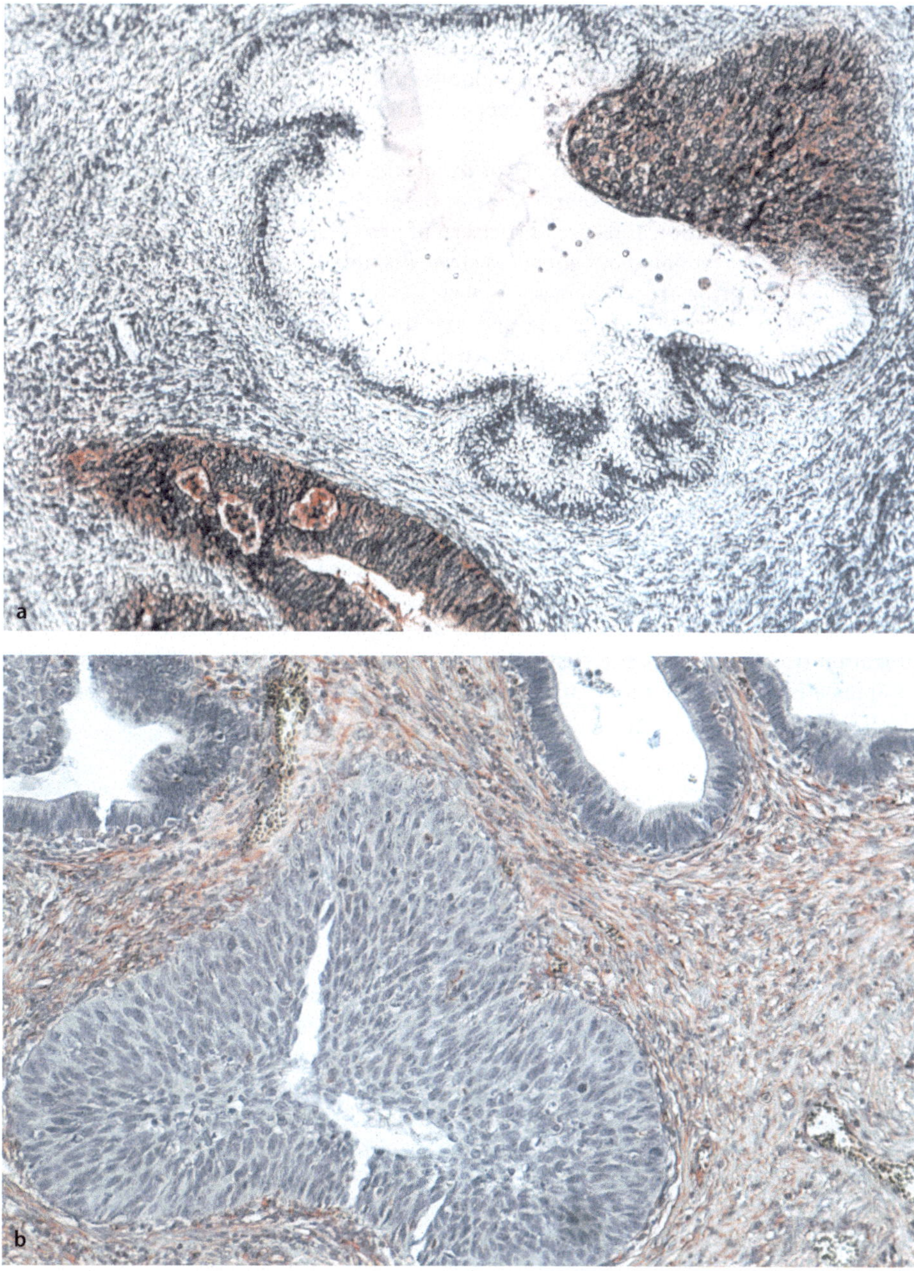

Fig. 140. a Carcinoma in situ, reserve cell differentiation. Positive immunohistochemical reaction for CEA (*upper right corner*) and with coexisting adenocarcinoma in situ (*lower left corner*), demonstrating that both precancerous lesions derive from one parent cell clone (s. p. 85f). **b** Carcinoma in situ, reserve cell differentiation, with coexisting adenocarcinoma in situ. Van Gieson

some areas, forming either keratin or mucin or presenting cytoplasmic clearing (Fig. 138). In contrast to that with squamous differentiation, carcinoma in situ with reserve cell differentiation often grows into glands, and in the noninvasive stage may even spread out over large areas of the endocervical mucosa (Fig. 139).

■ **Differential Diagnosis.** The two types of dysplasia and carcinoma in situ with squamous or with reserve cell differentiation can be distinguished in most cases by their topographical localization and spread (pattern of growth), and by the variation in their nuclear structure, as pointed out above. In some instances, both types develop simultaneously in neighboring areas. There are, however, intermediate lesions in which it is difficult to make a distinction (Figs. 108, 109, 113, 114). In those instances immunohistochemistry will be of considerable help, since both types have different compositions of intermediate filaments in their cytoplasm: the dysplasias and carcinoma in situ with squamous differentiation react positively with cytokeratin 13 (Fig. 115), but negatively with cytokeratin 8 and 18 and with CEA. The in situ lesions with reserve cell differentiation, on the contrary, show a coexpression of cytokeratin 13, 8 and 18 and are also positive with CEA (Fig. 140a). The distinction between the two is clinically important, since the reserve cell type, which is most frequently observed in young women, progresses more rapidly and frequently recurs in the infected mucosa of the endocervix, despite its complete removal by conization. Such recurrences are explained by the fact that normal epithelium around the carcinoma in situ may already be infected by HPV at the time of conization (Colgan et al. 1989). Distinction of carcinoma in situ from transitional cell metaplasia is obvious by the regular nuclear structure of the metaplastic lesion (see p. 34).

Adenocarcinoma In Situ [8140/2] (Figs. 141–149)

In *adenocarcinoma in situ* the normal columnar epithelium of the endocervical glands may be replaced by two types of abnormal epithelial cells. In the first type, one sees a pseudostratified or even multilayered atypical glandular epithelium with enlarged, elongated, hyperchromatic nuclei surrounded by a sparse undifferentiated cytoplasm. Mitoses are frequent. Mucin formation is absent or minimal (uniform type of Gloor and Ruzicka 1982; Figs. 141, 142). The glandular lumina are preserved, but may show intraglandular budding or bridging (Fig. 144). This atypical change is usually focal and may be limited to only one part of the gland (Fig. 141). In the second type, seen less frequently, the glands may be lined by strikingly disorganized, irregular cells with enlarged depolarized, pleomorphic nuclei with disordered chromatin. The cytoplasm is clear, foamy, and PAS negative (pleomorphic type of Gloor and Ruzicka; Figs. 145, 146). Occasional goblet cells may be found. These two types of ACIS may replace smaller or larger portions of normal glandular epithelium of the endocervical mucosa. Occasionally, the surface epithelium of the endocervix may also be involved (Fig. 147).

Adenocarcinoma in situ of the endocervix was once a rare lesion (Friedell and McKay 1953; Abell and Gosling 1962; Krimmenau 1966; Barter and Waters 1970; Sachs et al. 1975; Werner and Waidecker 1975), but has since increased in frequency (Jaworski et al. 1988; Hemminki et al. 2002; Wang et al. 2004), like invasive adenocarcinoma (see p. 136), and, like this, contains HPV 18 in a high percentage (Farnsworth et al. 1989; Tase

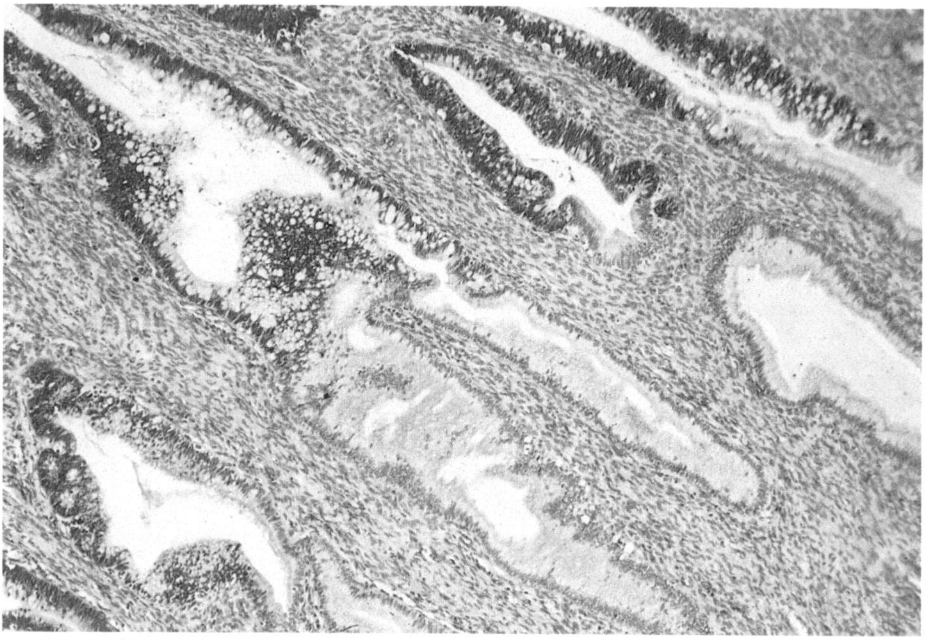

Fig. 141. Adenocarcinoma in situ, uniform type. H&E

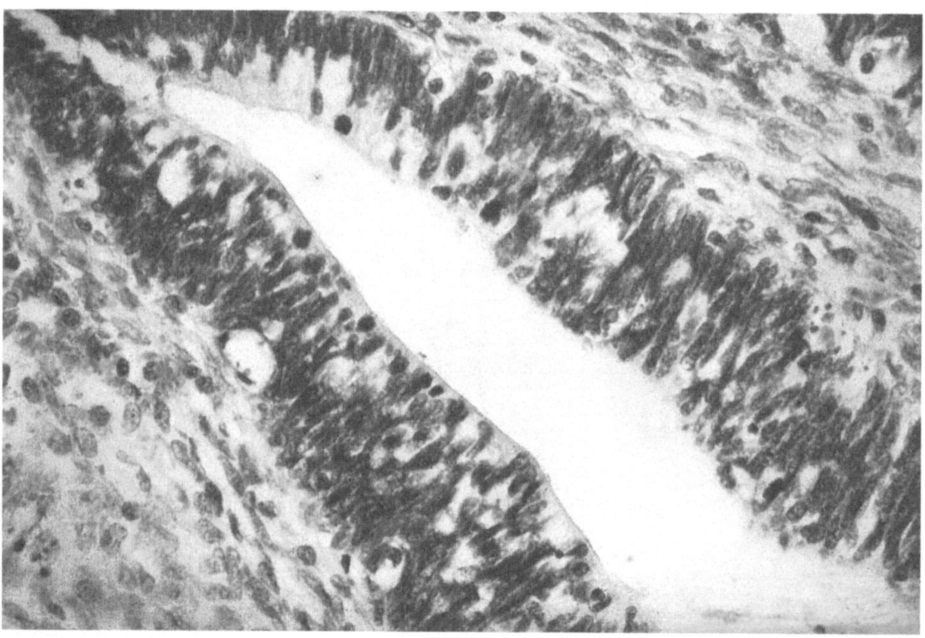

Fig. 142. Adenocarcinoma in situ, uniform type. H&E, higher magnification

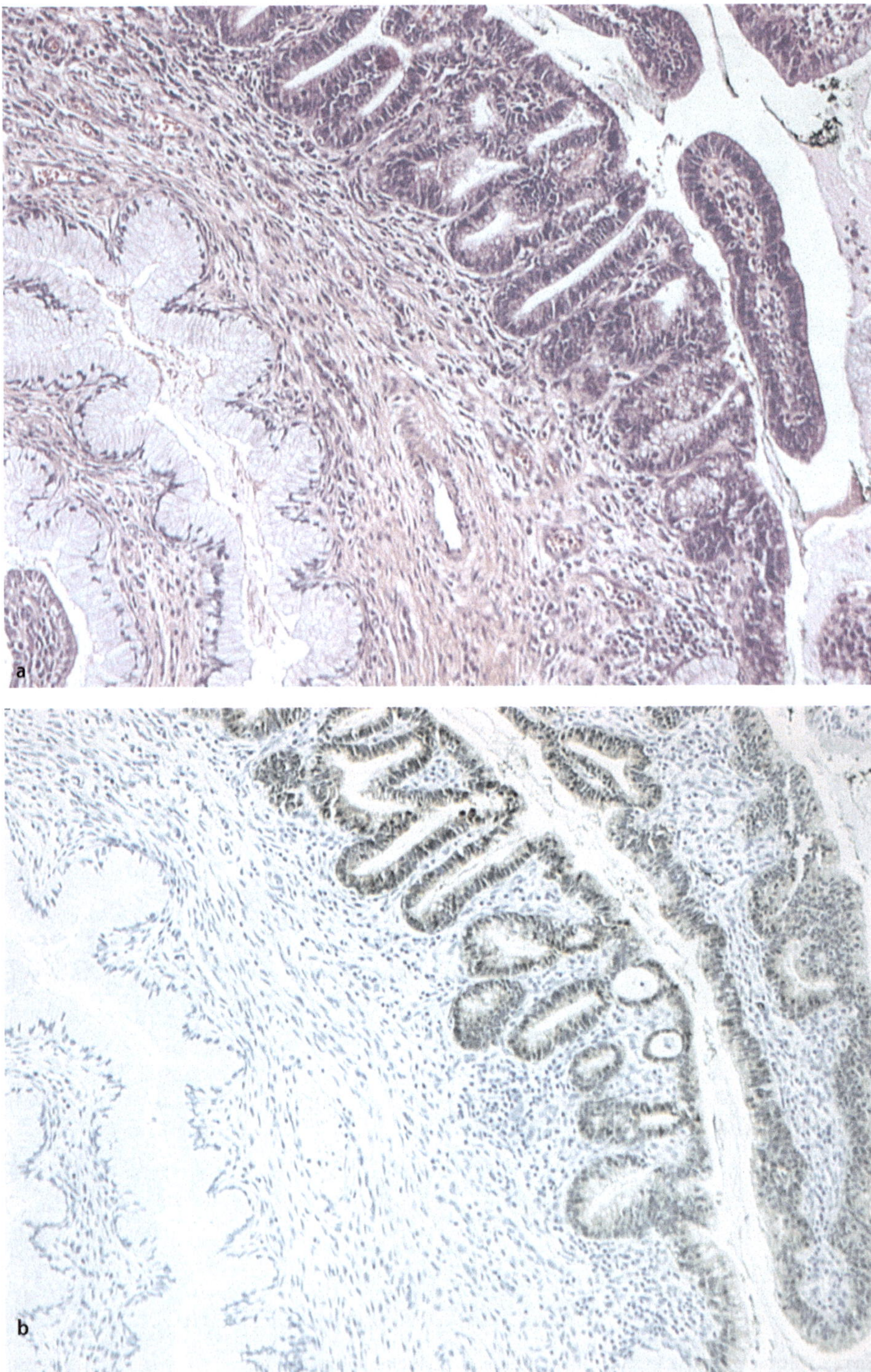

Fig. 143a,b. Adenocarcinoma in situ. **a** H&E; **b** $p16^{INK4a}$. Diffuse, continuous positivity for $p16^{INK4a}$ in atypical epithelium, negative reaction in normal endocervical epithelium

et al. 1989). Since only a few glands may be affected and be focally distributed, they may be overlooked unless serial sections of a cone biopsy are examined. If the lesion is overlooked or incompletely excised, it will progress to invasive adenocarcinoma (Boon et al. 1981; Wells and Brown 1986; Östör et al. 2000). Since both glandular and squamous cells of the endocervix may originate from the subcolumnar reserve cell (Alva and Lauchlan 1975; Christopherson et al. 1979; Boon et al. 1981; Tase et al. 1989), their precancerous and neoplastic changes are often closely related. Consequently, they often show an identical or a very similar expression of intermediate filaments (Fig. 140). When dealing with a dysplasia or carcinoma in situ of the endocervix, it is essential to search carefully for a coexistent ACIS.

Differential Diagnosis. Adenocarcinoma in situ can be distinguished from adenomatous and microglandular hyperplasia of the endocervix immunohistochemically: in most cases ACIS reacts positively with $p16^{INK4a}$ (Fig. 143b) and CEA (Fig. 148), whereas adenomatous and microglandular hyperplasias react negatively (compare also Hurlimann and Gloor 1984; Gloor and Hurlimann 1986; Cameron et al. 2002; Negri et al. 2003). Distinction from invasive adenocarcinoma is not possible from a small biopsy, but rather requires examination of larger areas of the endocervical mucosa. In contrast to invasive carcinoma, ACIS is limited to the glands; a stromal response is lacking, and normal glands are constantly admixed with neoplastic glands (Östör et al. 1984).

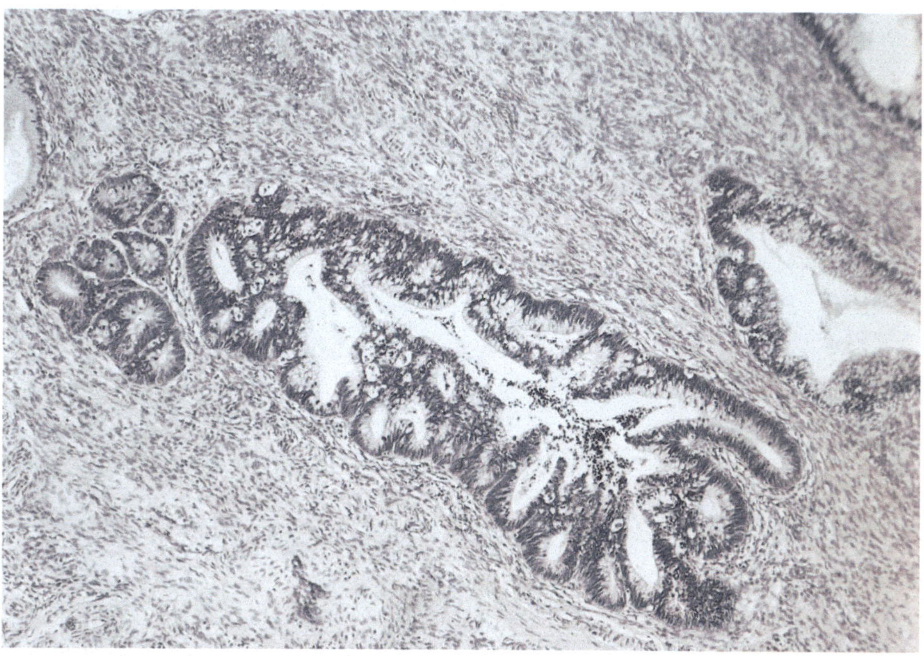

Fig. 144. Adenocarcinoma in situ, with intraglandular budding. H&E

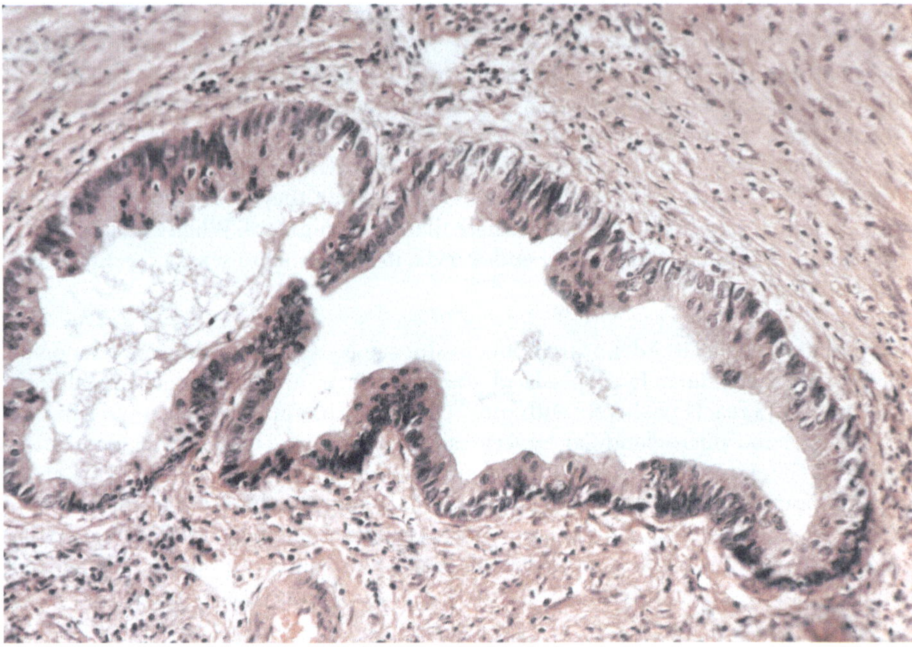

Fig. 145. Adenocarcinoma in situ, pleomorphic type. H&E

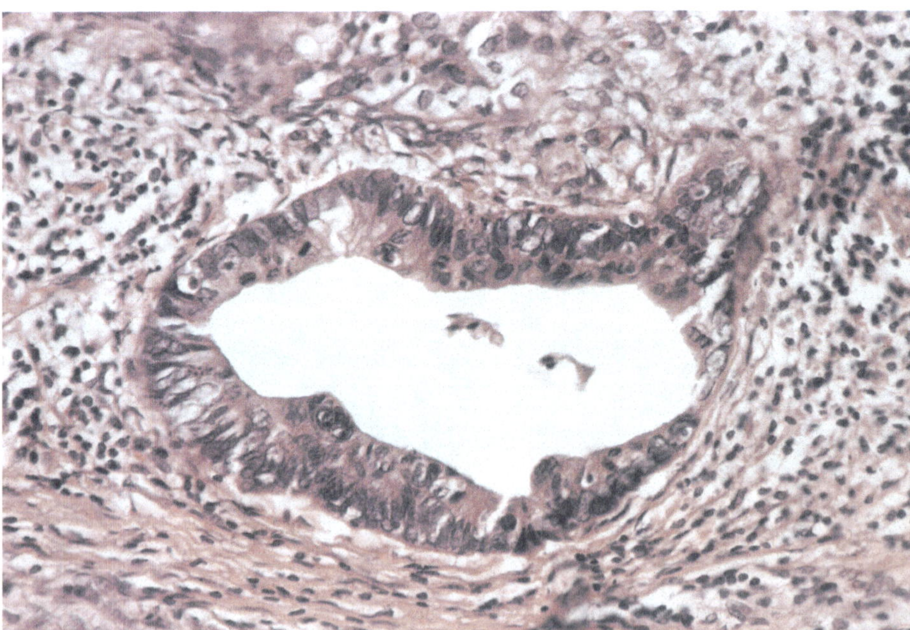

Fig. 146. Adenocarcinoma in situ, pleomorphic type. H&E

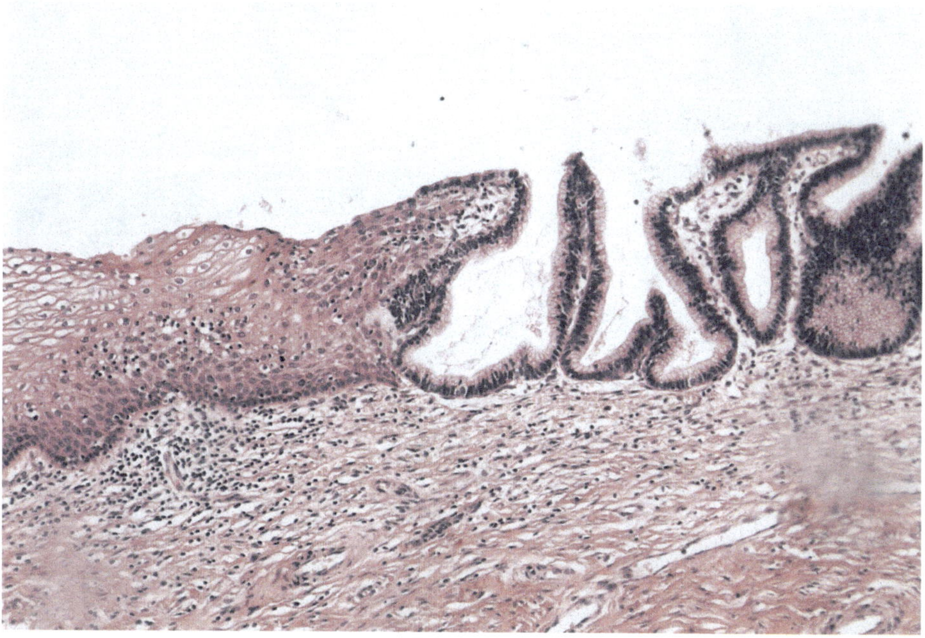

Fig. 147. Adenocarcinoma in situ, involving the surface epithelium. H&E

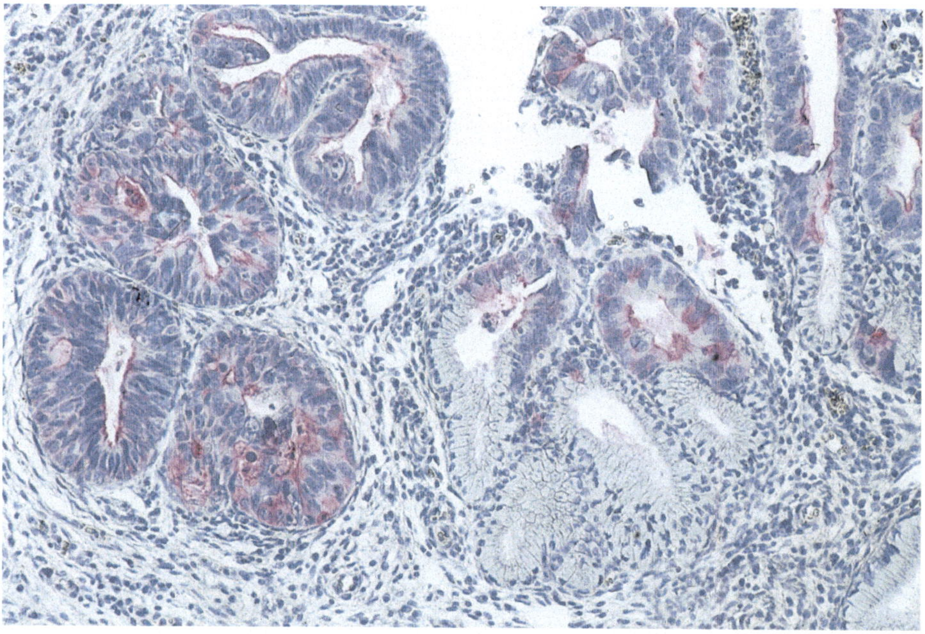

Fig. 148. Adenocarcinoma in situ, positive reaction for CEA (normal glands react negatively)

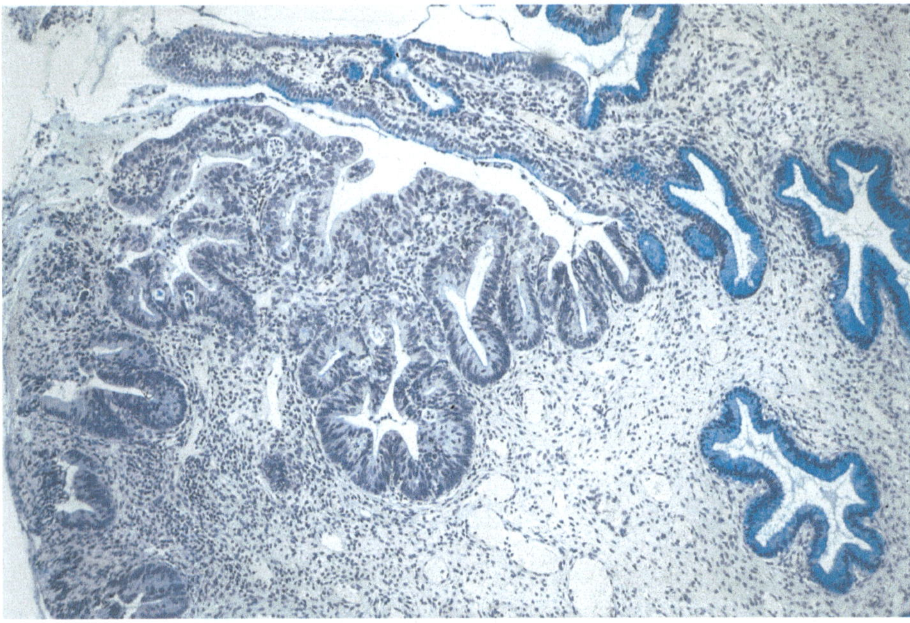

Fig. 149. Adenocarcinoma in situ, negative reaction with alcian blue (normal glands react positively)

Malignant Tumors

Epithelial Tumors

Squamous and Reserve Cell Types (Figs. 150–177)

Microinvasive Carcinoma [8076/3] (Figs. 150–157)

A *microinvasive carcinoma* (MIC; FIGO stage IA, TNM 1a1 and 1a2) was originally defined as an early invasive carcinoma that could not be detected grossly, only histologically (Mestwerdt 1947). Attempts to define its maximal size in millimeters in order to distinguish it from frank invasive carcinoma resulted in controversial opinions (Ferenczy and Winkler 1987). Since microinvasion often develops from precancerous epithelium located on the surface, as well as from that located in the glands, measurements cannot be made from the mucosal surface, but instead must be made from the intact basal membrane of the dysplastic epithelium bordering the carcinoma. According to the 1985 modification of FIGO staging, a MIC was defined as a carcinomatous invasion not exceeding 5 mm in depth and 7 mm in horizontal spread. Despite these strictures, the clinical outcome of patients with MIC was found to vary considerably, depending upon the variations in depth of stromal invasion, and upon the presence or absence of vascular invasion. To date – according to the TNM classification (UICC 2002) – it is widely accepted that a microinvasive squamous carcinoma stage 1a1 is a lesion that invades no greater than 3 mm (as measured from the basement membrane of its point of origin) and does not show vascular invasion (Tsukamoto et al. 1989). In stage 1a2 the invasion is limited to 5 mm in depth. The horizontal spread in both stages must be limited to 7 mm. According to several large clinical studies (cited by Ferenczy and Winkler 1987), when these criteria for MIC are applied, the rate of recurrence or of pelvic node metastases is less than 1% in stage 1a1, but 2% in stage 1a2 with a recurrence rate of 4% (Östör 1995).

The type of stromal invasion of the carcinoma depends upon the type of cell from which it arises: MIC developing from dysplasias and carcinoma in situ with squamous cell differentiation generally shows an early branching invasion, whereby tumor cells separate, ramify, and form slender cords that penetrate between the stroma cells (Figs. 150–152).

In contrast, MIC developing from a carcinoma in situ with reserve cell differentiation grows as a plump bulky coherent infiltration, which bulges out from the confines of the endocervical glands, breaking through the basal membrane and pushing the surrounding stroma aside (Figs. 153–157). Both types of invasion show similar characteristic cel-

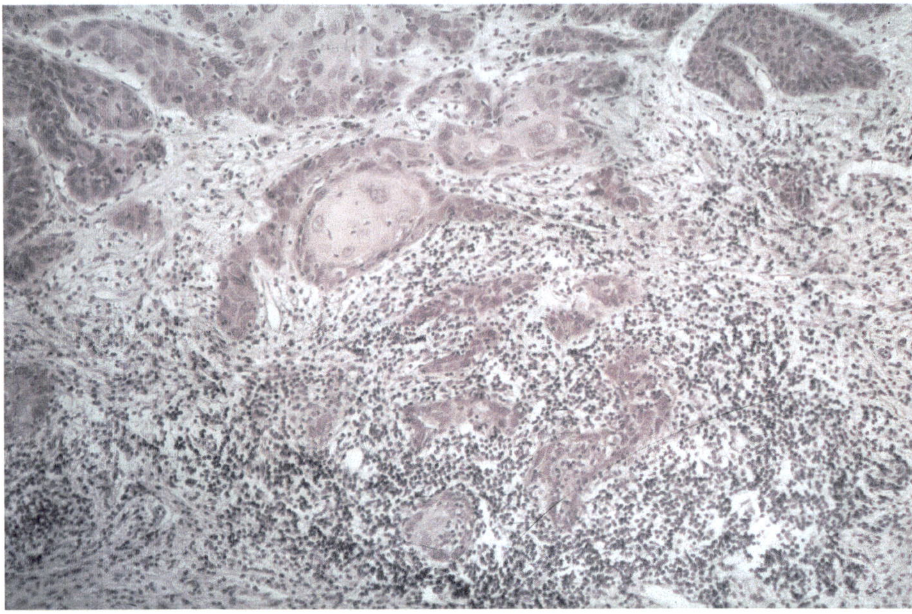

Fig. 150. Microinvasive carcinoma, netlike infiltration. H&E

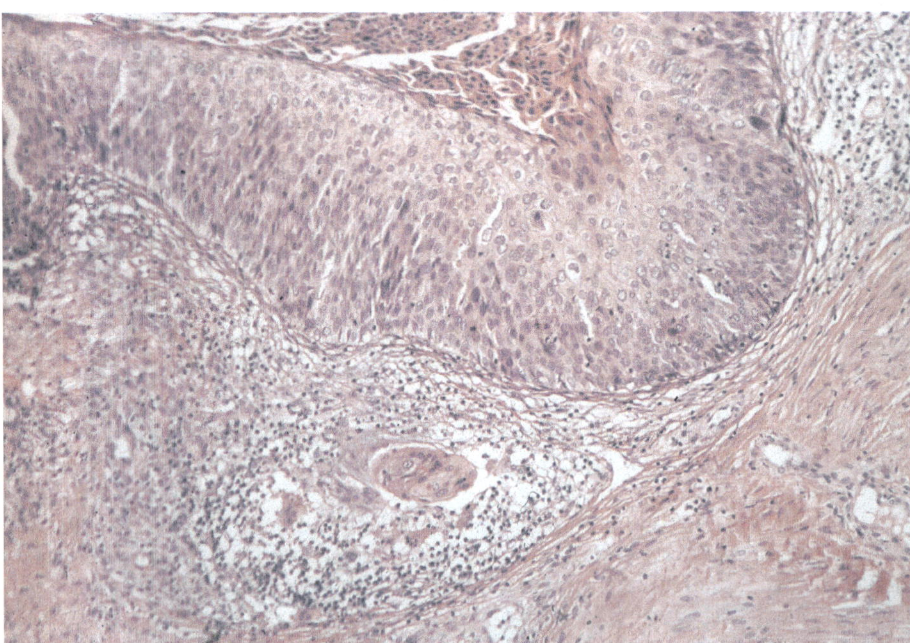

Fig. 151. Microinvasive carcinoma, netlike spread of individual cells. H&E

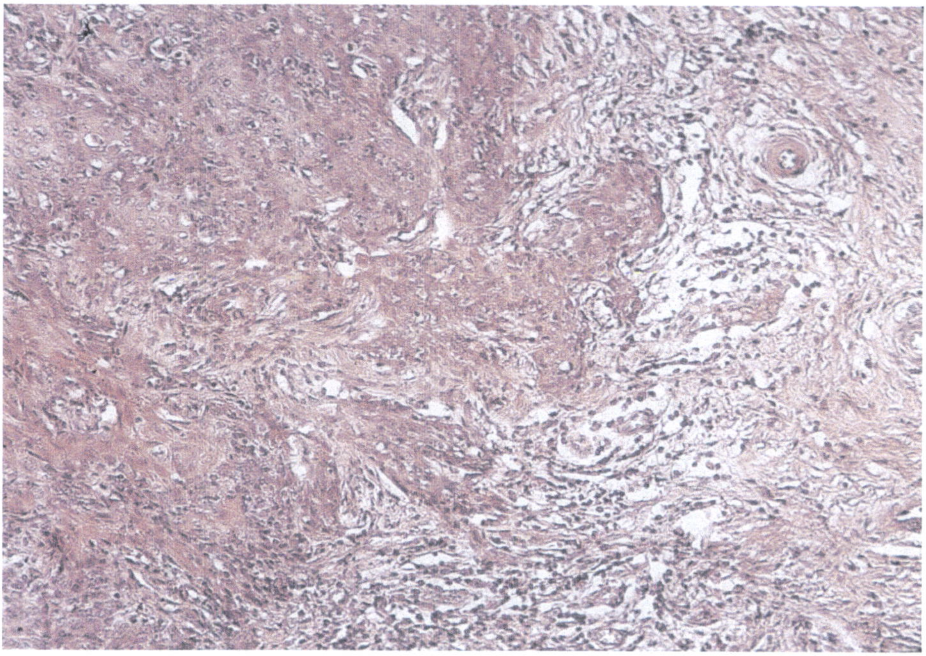

Fig. 152. Microinvasive carcinoma, netlike spread. H&E

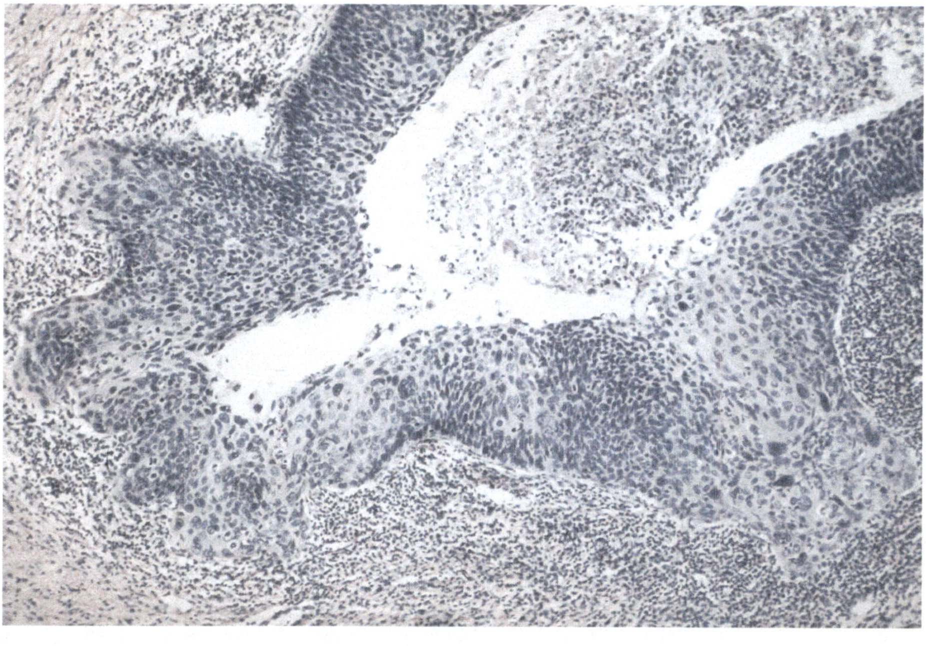

Fig. 153. Microinvasive carcinoma, plump infiltration. H&E

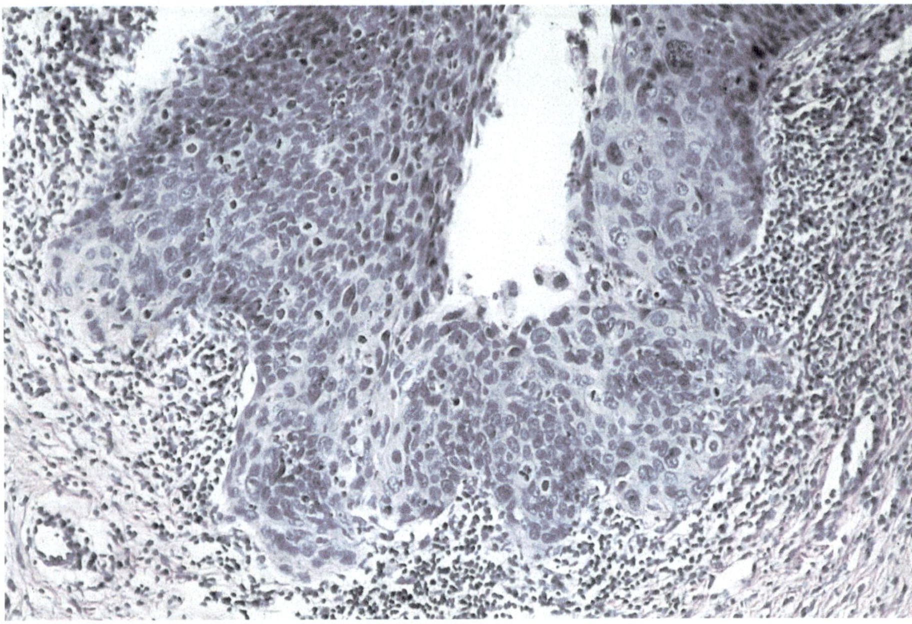

Fig. 154. Microinvasive carcinoma, plump infiltration. H&E

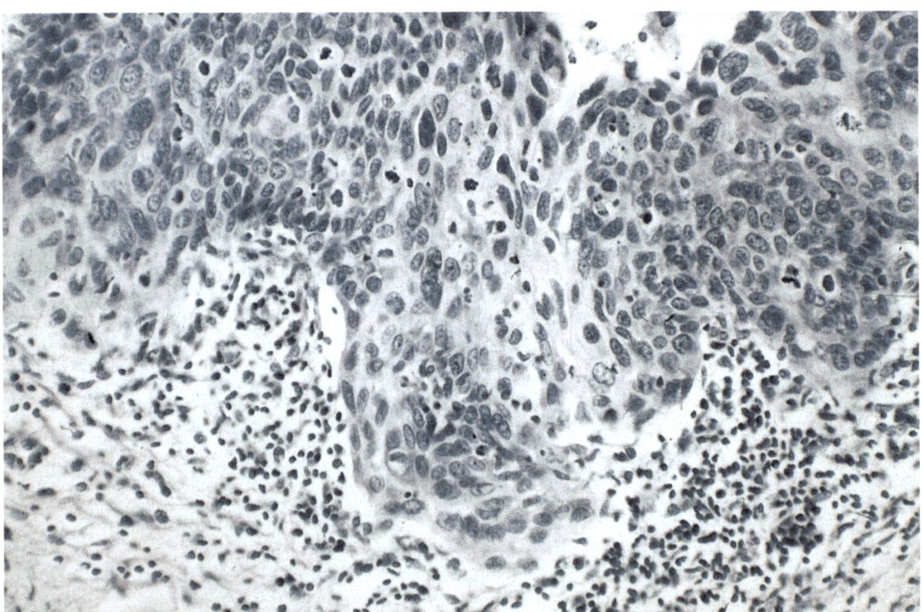

Fig. 155. Microinvasive carcinoma, plump infiltration. H&E, higher magnification

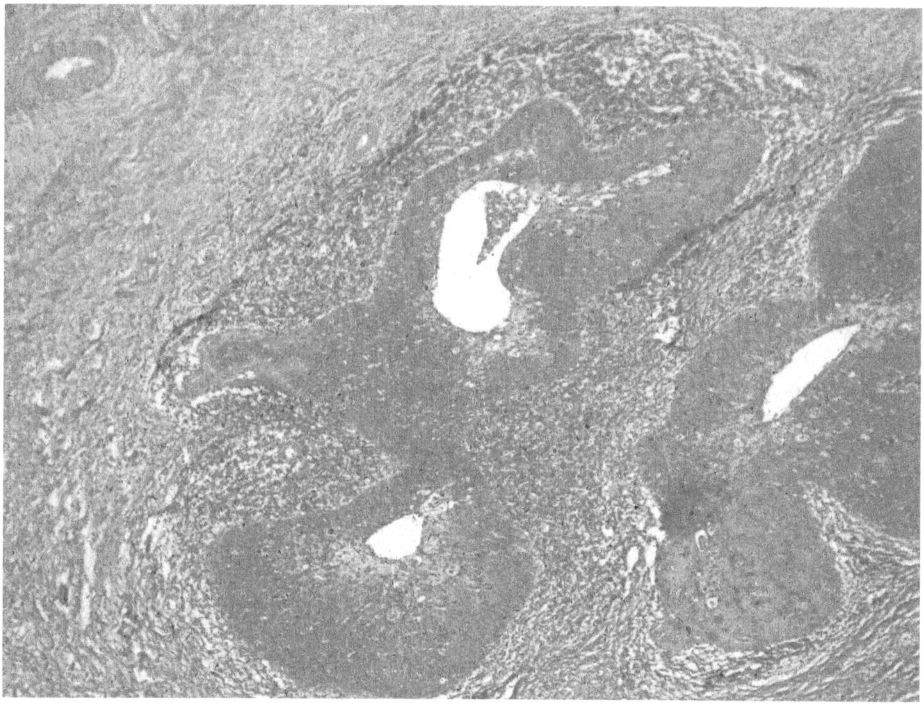

Fig. 156. Microinvasive carcinoma, extensive plump infiltration. H&E

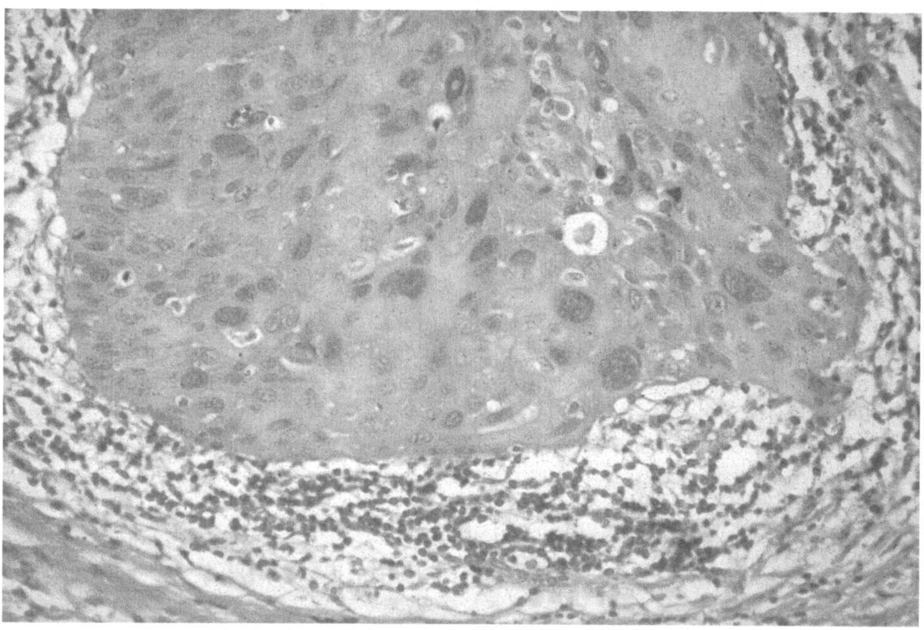

Fig. 157. Microinvasive carcinoma, plump infiltration. H&E, higher magnification

lular changes at the site of early invasion. The nuclei become larger with prominent nucleoli, and the abundant eosinophilic cytoplasm may even start to keratinize. As a result, the invading carcinoma cells appear to be more differentiated than those of their non-invasive counterparts. In addition, the sites of microinvasion are often surrounded by dense lymphoplasmocytic infiltrates. Detection of lymphatic or vascular invasion is important for recognizing a more advanced stage of carcinoma (1b) and for differentiating it from a microinvasion. As one might expect from these differences in type of invasion, the reserve cell type carcinoma may extend over large areas of the cervix within an expanded field of endocervical glands, yet still be microinvasive (Fig. 156), whereas a carcinomatous invasion of the squamous cell type penetrating more than 3 mm in depth and invading vascular channels has to be classified as invasive carcinoma stage 1b1. In our experience, this staging seems justified, since the netlike invasion of the squamous cell type often involves the lymphatic vessels early, whereas the bulky infiltration of reserve cell type spreads widely, but usually invades lymphatic vessels late. As our studies show, at least 80% or even more of all invasive carcinomas are of the reserve cell type. This corresponds to the observation that up to 90% of all squamous cell carcinomas of the cervix start in the glandular area of the endocervix (Clement and Scully 1982).

■ **Differential Diagnosis.** For deciding appropriate surgical therapy, it is of clinical importance to distinguish between stage 1a1 and 1a2 by measuring the depth of invasion and the horizontal spread (see p. 117), and by searching for vascular invasion. If the depth of invasion reaches more than 5 mm, and/or vascular invasion is seen, the neoplastic lesion has already reached stage 1b1, and a hysterectomy is clinically indicated. A hysterectomy appears advisable, too, in stage 1a2 because of the higher recurrence rate. On the other hand, a large cone with tumor-free borders will almost always be sufficient for a MIC with stage 1a1.

The two types of microinvasion can be distinguished histologically or immunohistochemically. As in the dysplasias preceding the carcinoma, the squamous cell type is positive with anticytokeratin 13 only; in contrast, the reserve cell type shows a coexpression of cytokeratin 13, 8, 18, and CEA.

Differentiation from benign or preinvasive lesions is possible by noting whether or not the basal membrane is intact, as well as by noting an absence of stromal reaction or cellular maturation at the base of the atypical epithelium.

Invasive Carcinoma [8070/3] (Figs. 158–177)

Invasive carcinomas also show a broad spectrum, from microinvasion (up to 3 mm in depth) to clinically occult invasive carcinoma (measuring from 3 mm to more than 1 cm in depth; Boyes et al. 1970), and to grossly visible invasive carcinoma with endophytic or exophytic growth and spread throughout the cervical wall. As in the preinvasive stages, HPV DNA has also been detected in virtually all cervical squamous cell carcinomas and has been considered a necessary cause of invasive cervical cancer worldwide (Gissmann 1984; Lörincz et al. 1987; Walboomers et al. 1999).

On histological examination, two major types can be distinguished: small or large cell nonkeratinizing carcinoma, and large cell keratinizing carcinoma.

Small Cell Type of Nonkeratinizing Carcinoma [8083/3]

The *small cell type of nonkeratinizing carcinoma* (representing approximately 5%), as the least differentiated type, consists of diffusely infiltrating small or larger strands and nests of tumor cells with hyperchromatic oval nuclei in a sparse cytoplasm, resembling basal-type or undifferentiated reserve cell-type cells (Figs. 158–161). An intense stromal inflammatory reaction is characteristic (Fig. 159), and there is usually extensive lymphatic invasion (Figs. 160, 161).

Large Cell Type of Nonkeratinizing Carcinoma [8072/3]

The *large cell type of nonkeratinizing carcinoma* (representing about 70%) is composed of broader cords of moderately differentiated tumor cells with large, often irregular nuclei. The cytoplasm varies in amount and differentiation (Figs. 162–167). Some of these carcinomas grow in rather uniform strands, whose spindle-shaped cells are vertically oriented towards the basal membrane resembling the preceding carcinoma in situ with reserve cell differentiation (Fig. 163).

Large Cell Keratinizing Carcinoma [8071/3]

The *large cell keratinizing carcinoma* (representing about 25%) consists of small or large nests of mature epithelial tumor cells that adhere to one another by intercellular bridges. The nuclei are large, round or irregular, often hyperchromatic. The cytoplasm is abundant, eosinophilic or pale. Besides the keratin pearls in the center of epithelial nests (Fig. 170), a scattered monocellular keratinization is frequently seen (Figs. 168, 169).

As to be expected, these types do not always occur alone. Combinations or mixtures may be seen, indicating again that we are dealing with a spectrum of biological changes. An intermediate form between small cell and large cell carcinoma is shown in Figs. 174 and 175; a special form consisting of nonkeratinizing and keratinizing carcinoma may result in a pleomorphic type of carcinoma (Fig. 176).

With invasive carcinoma, it is difficult to trace the cell of origin and to distinguish on routine histological examination between squamous cell and reserve cell differentiation. The bipotential reserve cells, like in benign metaplasia, may differentiate to keratinizing squamous as well as to glandular epithelial cells with mucin production. With immunohistochemistry, such a distinction is possible in the majority of carcinomas (Moll et al. 1983). As in the preinvasive stages, the invasive carcinoma with reserve cell differentiation shows a coexpression of cytokeratin 13, 8, 18, and CEA (Figs. 165, 166, 171), whereas the invasive carcinoma with squamous cell differentiation reacts positively only for the squamous epithelial cytokeratins and negatively for cytokeratin 8 and 18 and for CEA in immunohistochemistry (Dallenbach-Hellweg and Lang 1991). In applying these stains, of which the CEA reaction is the most important, it becomes apparent that most invasive cervical carcinomas arise from reserve cells, which are the most susceptible cells for HR-HPV infections, mainly types 16 and 18.

Despite their structural alteration, they retain the cytokeratin pattern shown by their cells of origin. The reserve cell carcinomas acquire a coexpression for CEA just as the adenocarcinomas, which also arise from reserve cells. The expression of CEA indicates malignant change. To determine the rate of growth (cell proliferation index) in each type of carcinoma, Ki-67 (MIB-1) is the most reliable marker for measuring not only cells in mitosis, but in all stages of cell division not detectable in routine stains (Fig. 177). $p16^{INK4a}$ is diffusely positive in most invasive carcinomas of both squamous and reserve cell differentiation; a focal staining pattern indicates a benign behavior of the lesion (Klaes et al. 2001).

Mode and speed of invasion and spread varies from early root- or netlike stromal infiltration with rapid lymphatic invasion and spread beyond the uterus, to bulky infiltration, which usually remains confined to the uterine cervix until it has largely replaced the cervical wall. None of the conventional histological parameters, such as degree of keratinization, nuclear pleomorphism, number of mitoses, cell size, or stromal reaction, however, can reliably predict patient survival (Beecham et al. 1978; Crissman et al. 1987; Stock et al. 1994).

■ **Differential Diagnosis.** The small cell type of nonkeratinizing carcinomas must be distinguished from the small cell neuroendocrine type of carcinoma [8041/3] (see p. 165). This is possible with neuroendocrine markers such as CD 56, chromogranin A and synaptophysin or with a Grimelius stain, which is positive in neuroendocrine tumors but negative in the small cell type carcinoma of reserve cell origin. Primitive neurogenic tumors closely resembling small cell carcinomas are negative with all markers for cytokeratin and for CEA, but show a distinctly positive reaction for neuron-specific enolase (NSE; see p. 166).

Lymphoepithelioma-like Carcinoma [8082/3]

A large cell variant of nonkeratinizing carcinoma with extensive lymphocytic infiltration has been classified *lymphoepithelioma-like carcinoma* with a more favorable prognosis. Epstein–Barr virus has been detected in some of these carcinomas (Tseng et al. 1997). Occasionally, a chronic granulomatous inflammation may be confused with a small cell carcinoma. A careful cytological evaluation should help to reveal the nature of such granulomas, which will give negative reactions for cytokeratins.

Verrucous Carcinoma [8051/3]

Verrucous carcinoma is a rare variant of cervical CEA-negative squamous cell carcinoma composed of very well-differentiated keratinizing squamous cells growing in frondlike papillae. Stromal invasion is always bulky; lymphatic involvement or distant spread is rare. This tumor is more common in the vulva and vagina.

Distinction from large papillomas, on one hand, and from the large cell keratinizing type of invasive carcinoma, on the other hand, may be difficult unless the entire tumor is studied (Rorat et al. 1978). Pronounced nuclear atypia and the presence of small groups of anaplastic cells in the underlying stroma exclude verrucous carcinoma. Verrucous carcinoma has a tendency to recur locally, and the therapy of choice is wide local excision.

Warty (Condylomatous) Carcinoma [8051/3]

The *warty (condylomatous) type* is a squamous cell carcinoma with obvious cellular signs of HPV infection, e.g., koilocytosis, and with a warty surface.

Papillary Squamous Cell Carcinoma [8052/3]

Papillary squamous cell carcinoma is another rare variant of cervical squamous cell carcinoma, presenting the gross and histological appearance of a benign papilloma undergoing dysplastic cellular change (compare Figs. 128 and 129). Beneath the papillary dysplasia, strands of invasive carcinoma can be detected (Randall et al. 1986; Brinck et al. 2000). Diagnosis of invasion, therefore, depends upon examining the entire papillary lesion.

This papillary carcinoma of squamous cell type should not be confused with the serous papillary carcinoma (serous adenocarcinoma) of glandular type (see p. 153).

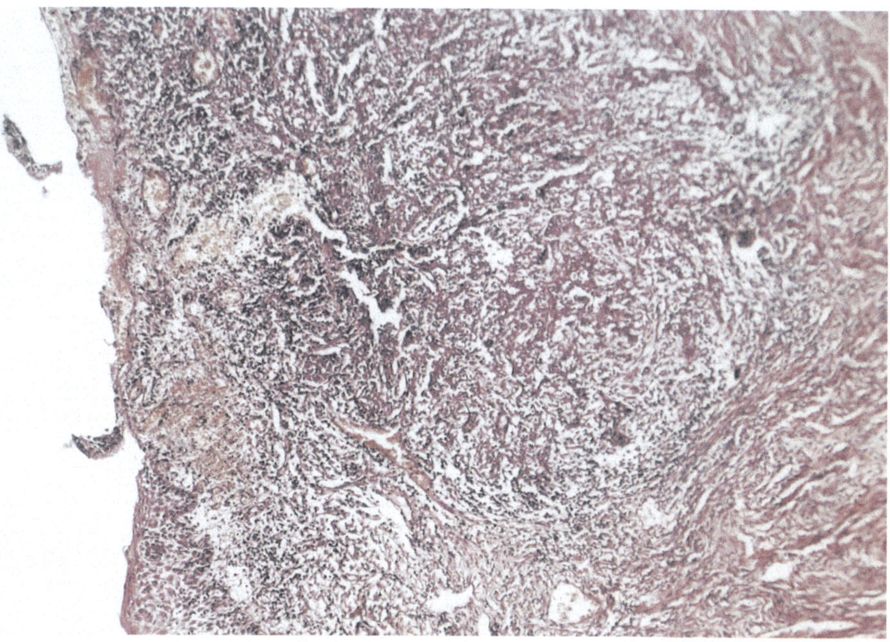

Fig. 158. Small cell carcinoma. H&E

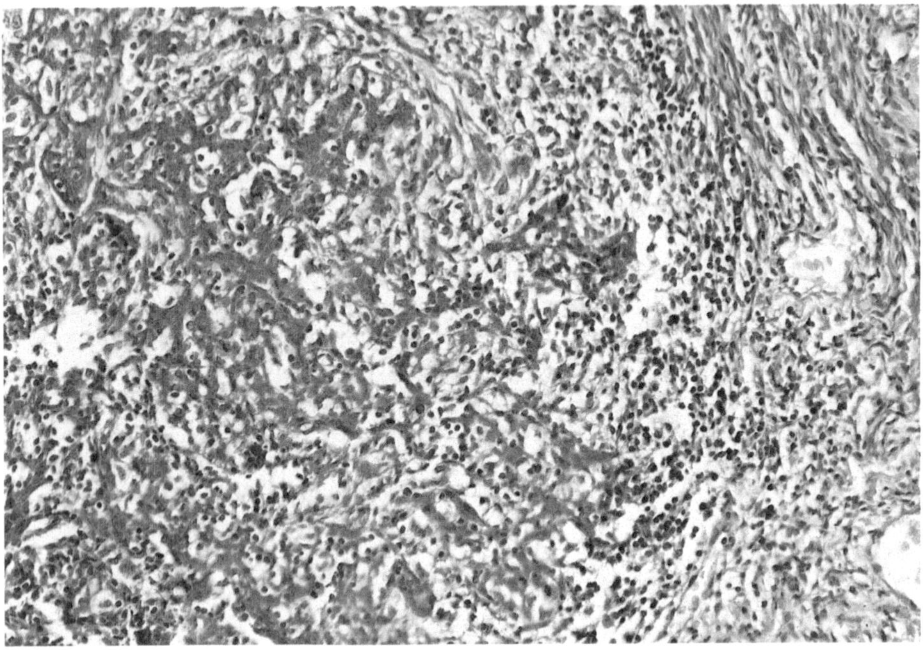

Fig. 159. Small cell carcinoma. H&E, higher magnification

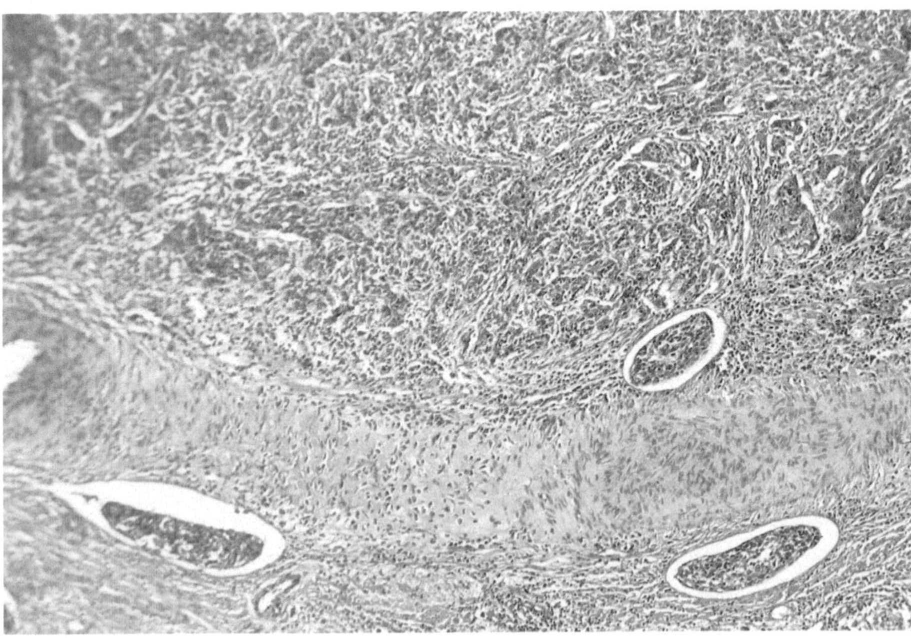

Fig. 160. Small cell carcinoma, extensive lymphatic invasion. H&E

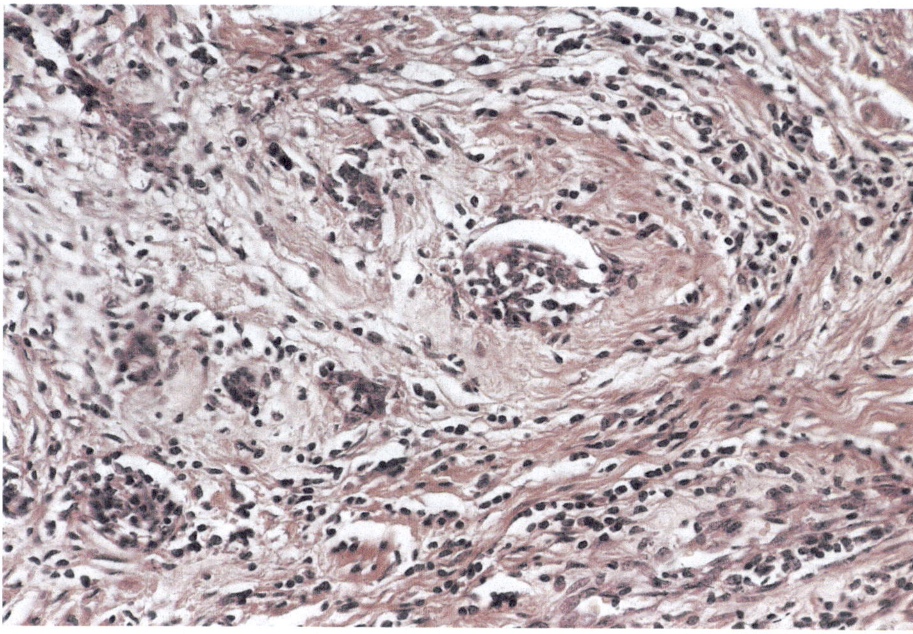

Fig. 161. Small cell carcinoma, extensive lymphatic invasion. H&E

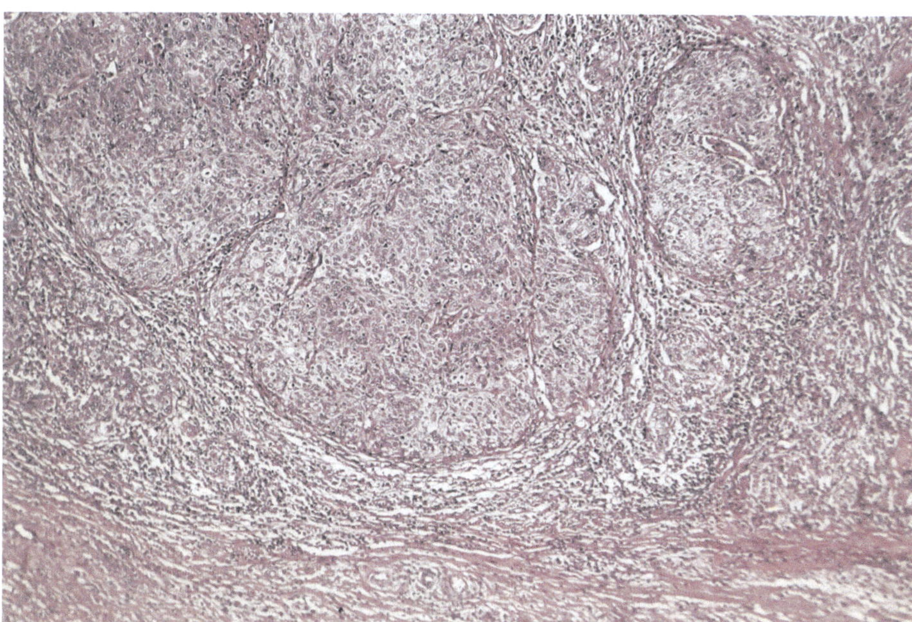

Fig. 162. Large cell nonkeratinizing carcinoma. H&E

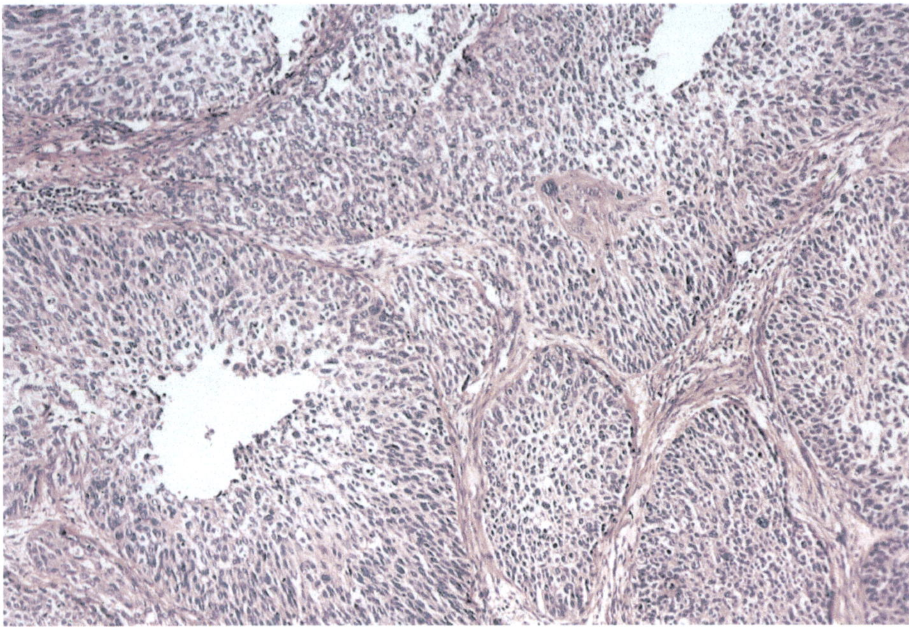

Fig. 163. Large cell nonkeratinizing carcinoma, poorly differentiated, with spindle-shaped cellular appearance. H&E

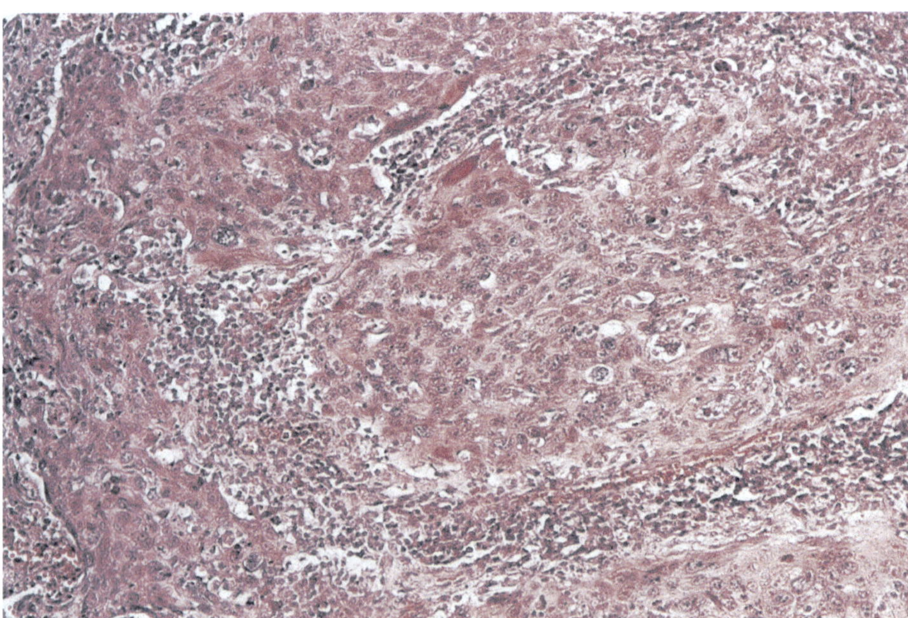

Fig. 164. Large cell nonkeratinizing carcinoma with slight nuclear polymorphism. H&E

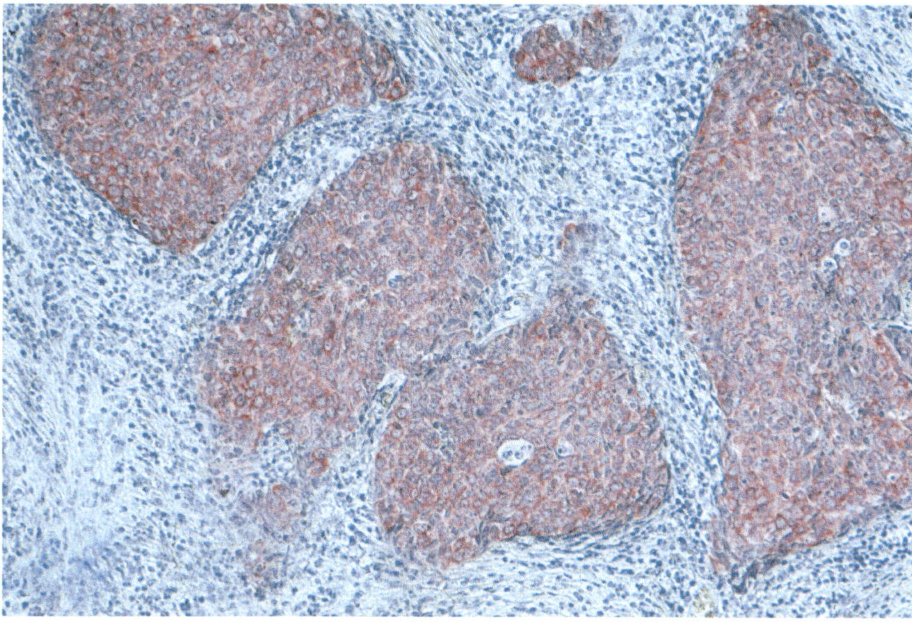

Fig. 165. Same as in Fig. 164. Immunohistochemical reaction with anticytokeratin 8

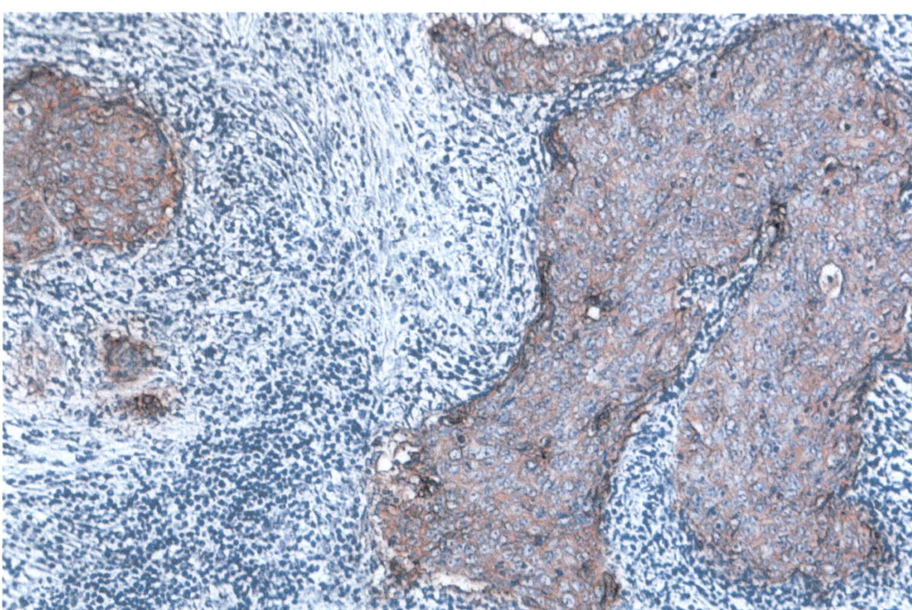

Fig. 166. Large cell carcinoma of reserve cell type. Immunohistochemical reaction with CEA

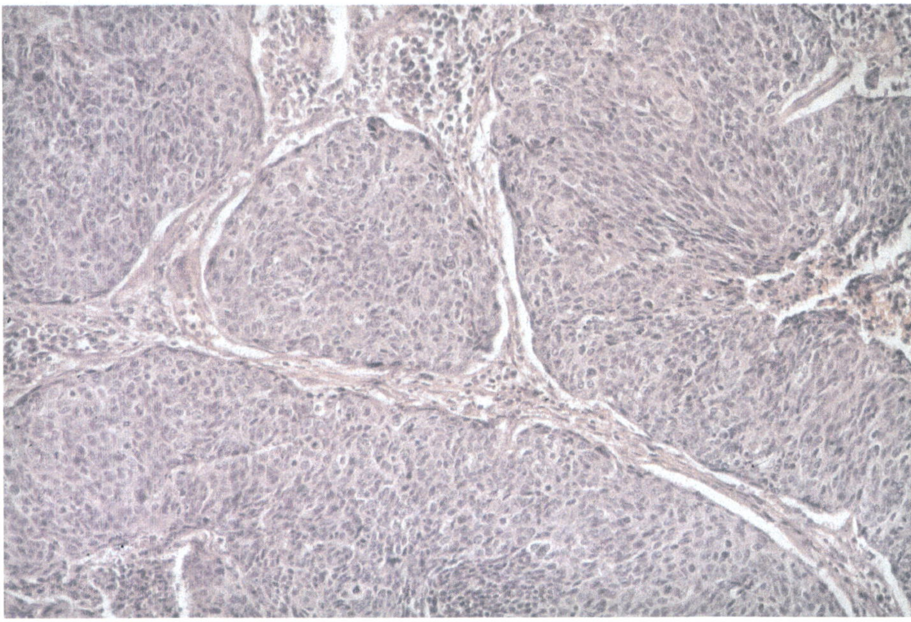

Fig. 167a. Large cell nonkeratinizing carcinoma, moderately differentiated. H&E

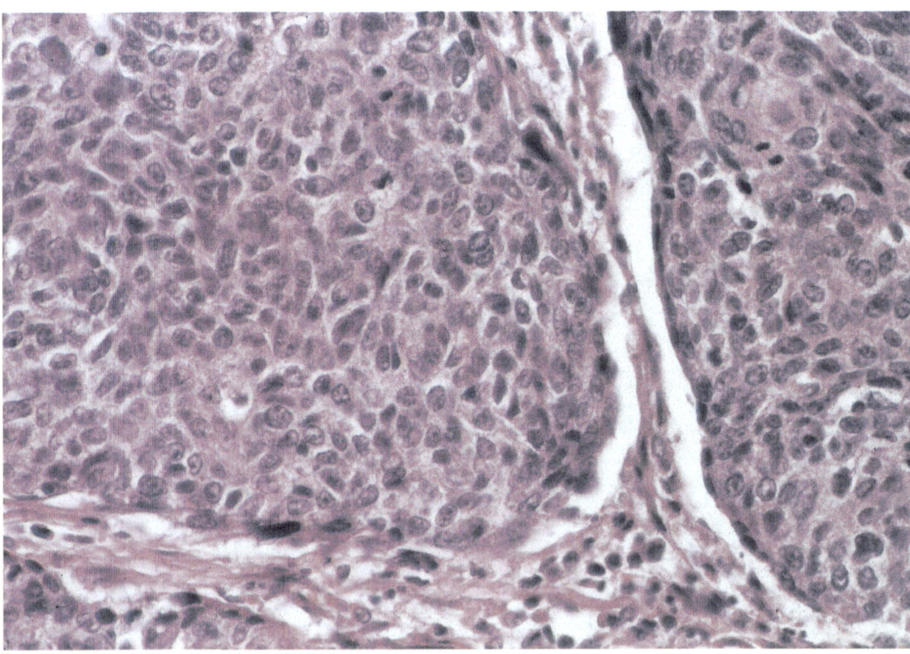

Fig. 167b. Same as Fig. 167a. H&E, higher magnification

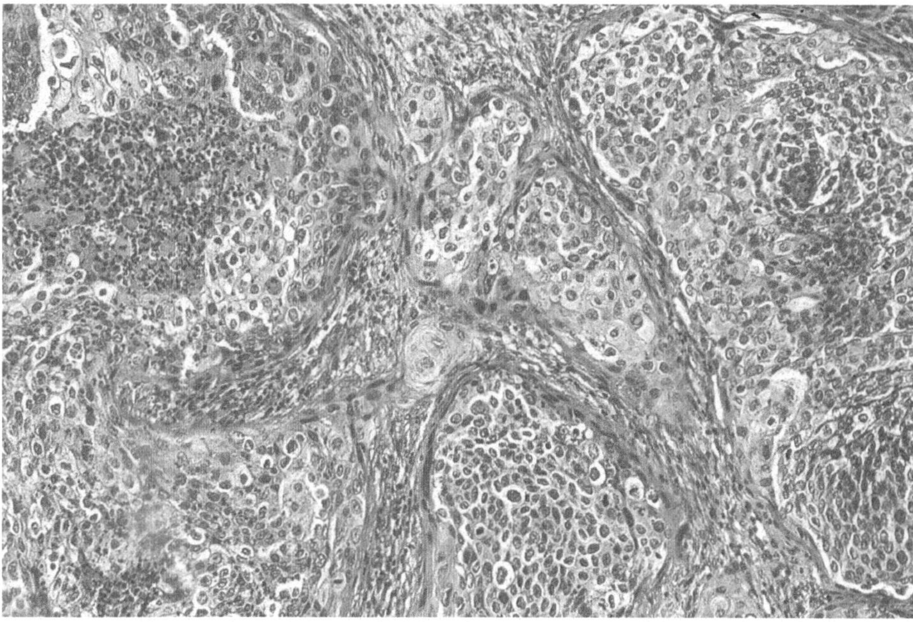

Fig. 168. Large cell keratinizing carcinoma. H&E

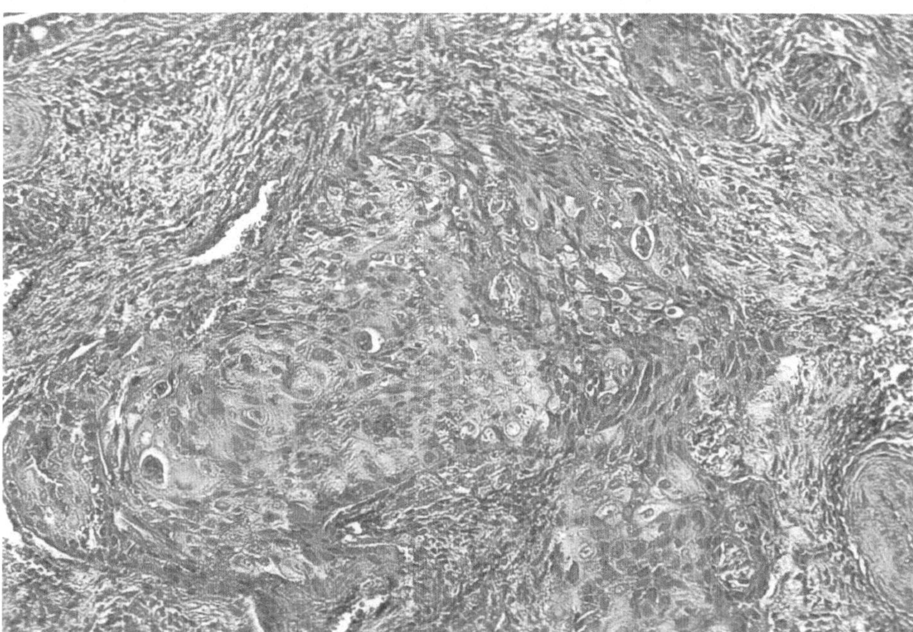

Fig. 169. Large cell keratinizing carcinoma. H&E

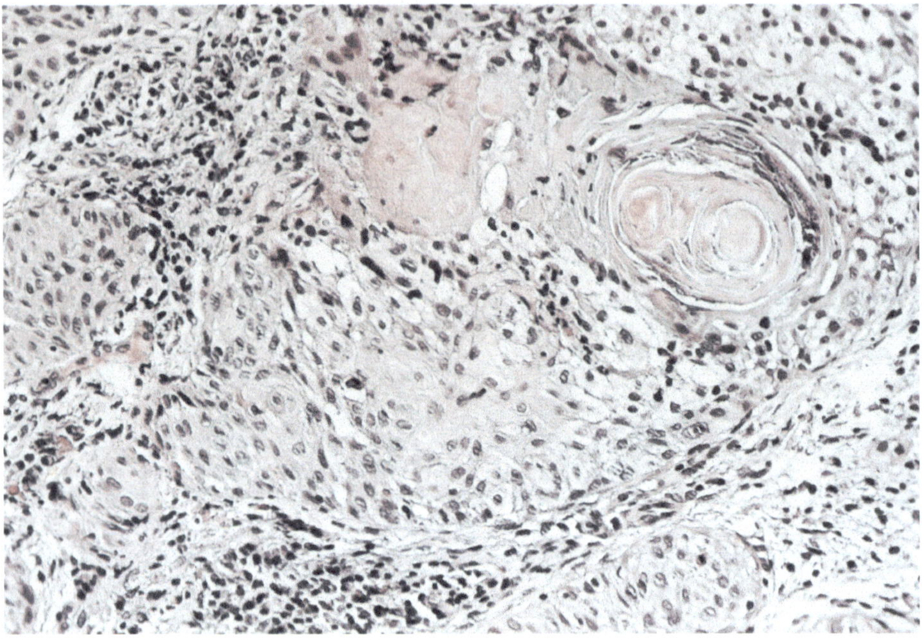

Fig. 170. Large cell keratinizing carcinoma. H&E

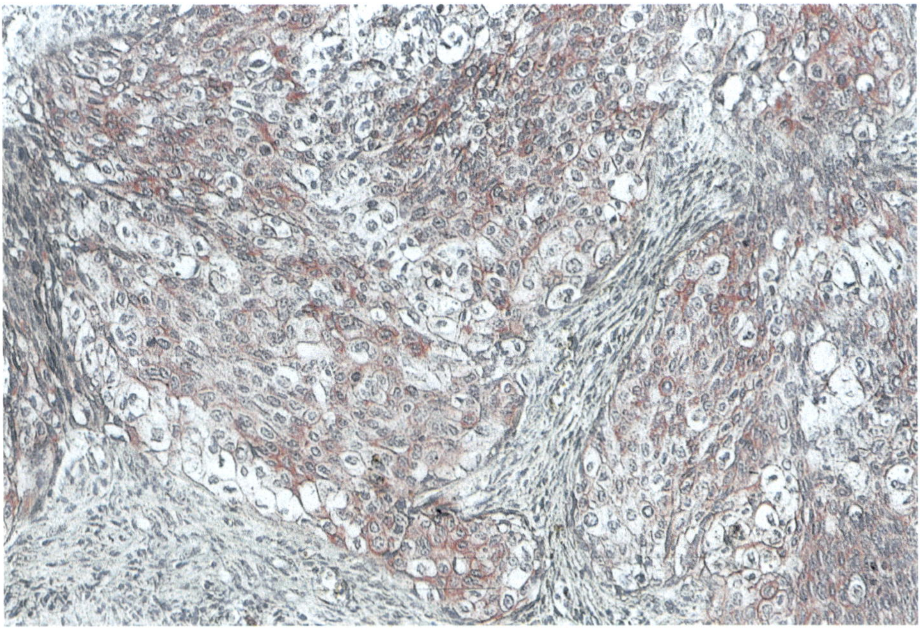

Fig. 171. Large cell keratinizing carcinoma of reserve cell type. Immunohistochemical reaction for CEA

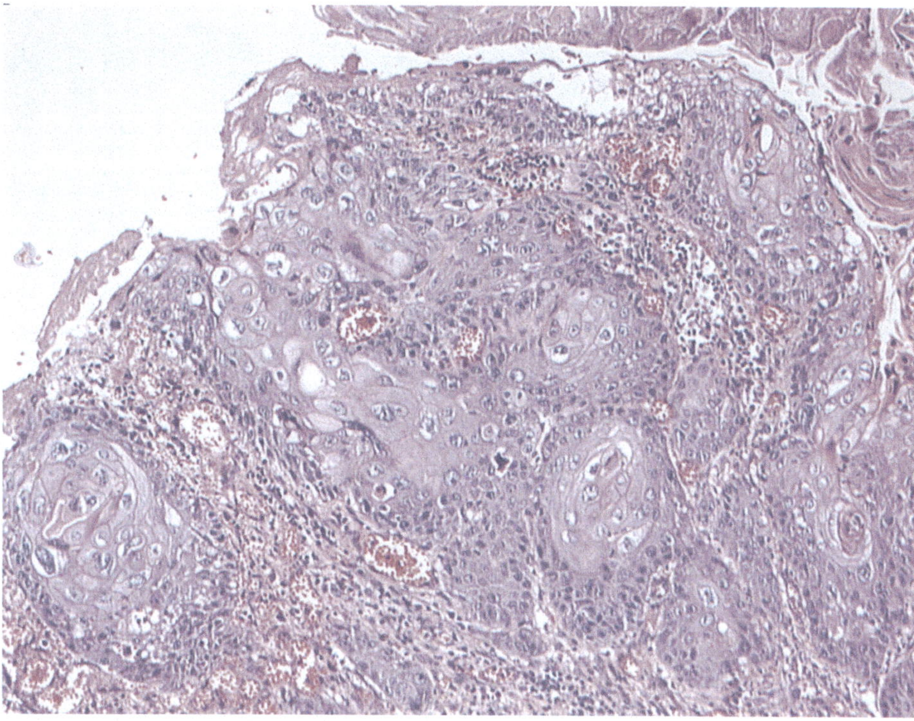

Fig. 172. Large cell keratinizing carcinoma. H&E

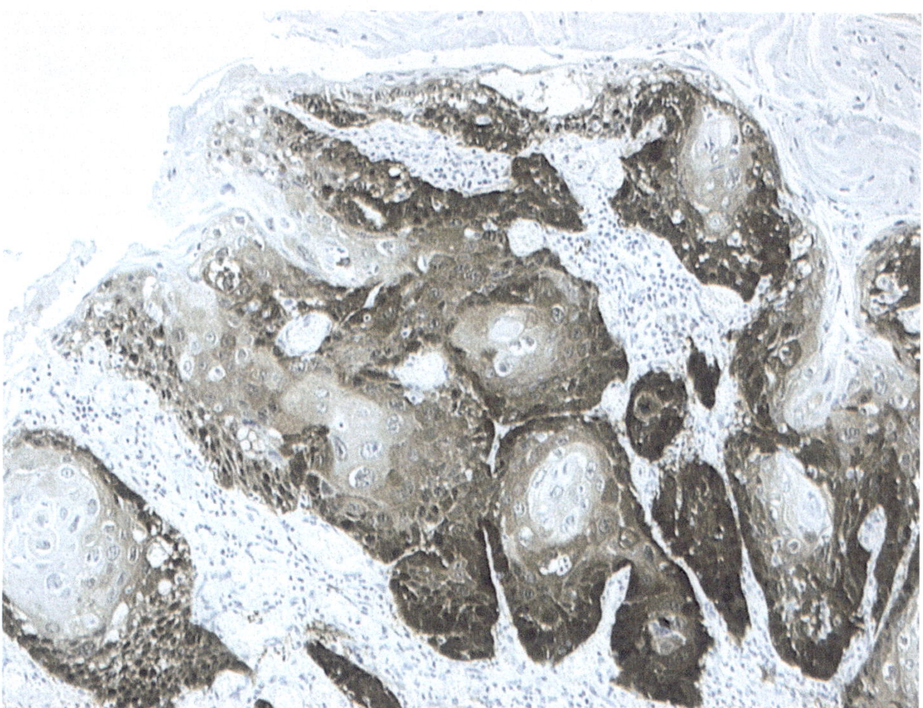

Fig. 173. Large cell keratinizing carcinoma, same case as in Fig. 171. Diffuse positivity for p16^{INK4a}, negative reaction in squamous pearls. p16^{INK4a} immunostain

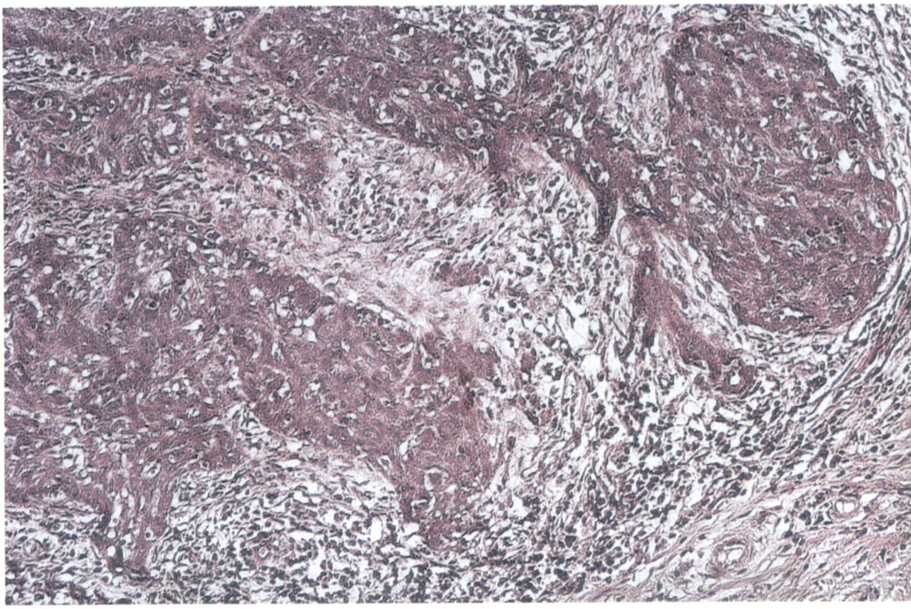

Fig. 174. Intermediate form between small and large cell carcinoma. H&E

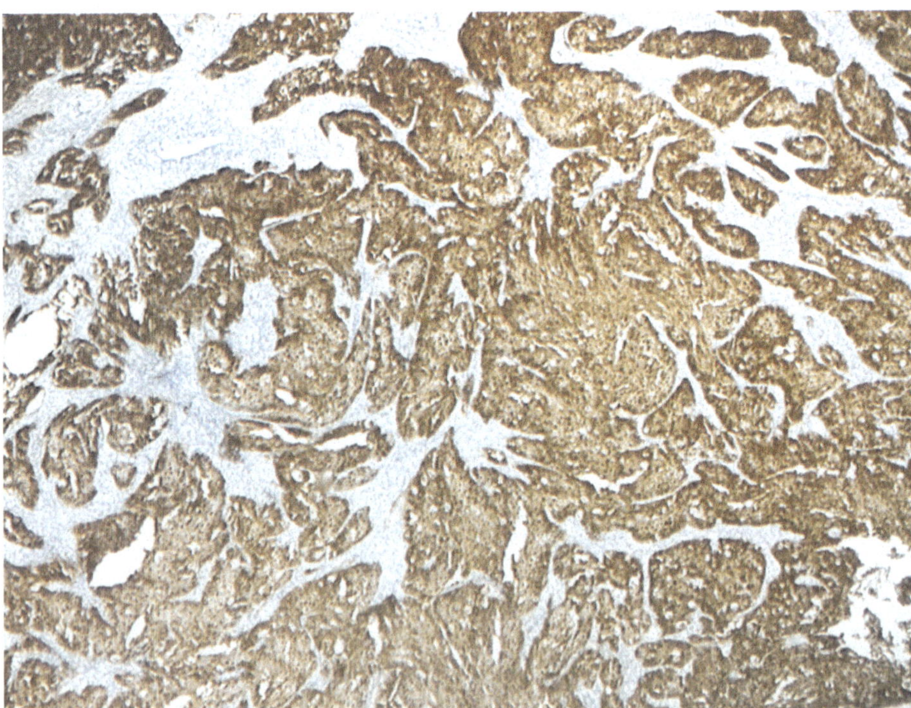

Fig 175. Invasive carcinoma, strong diffuse positivity for $p16^{INK4a}$. $p16^{INK4a}$ immunostain

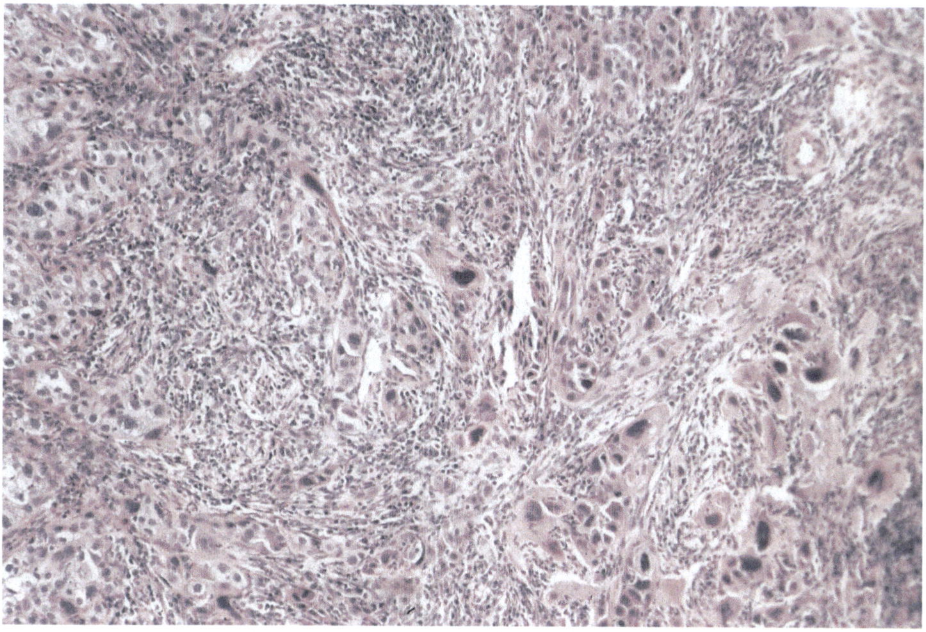

Fig. 176. Large cell pleomorphic carcinoma. H&E

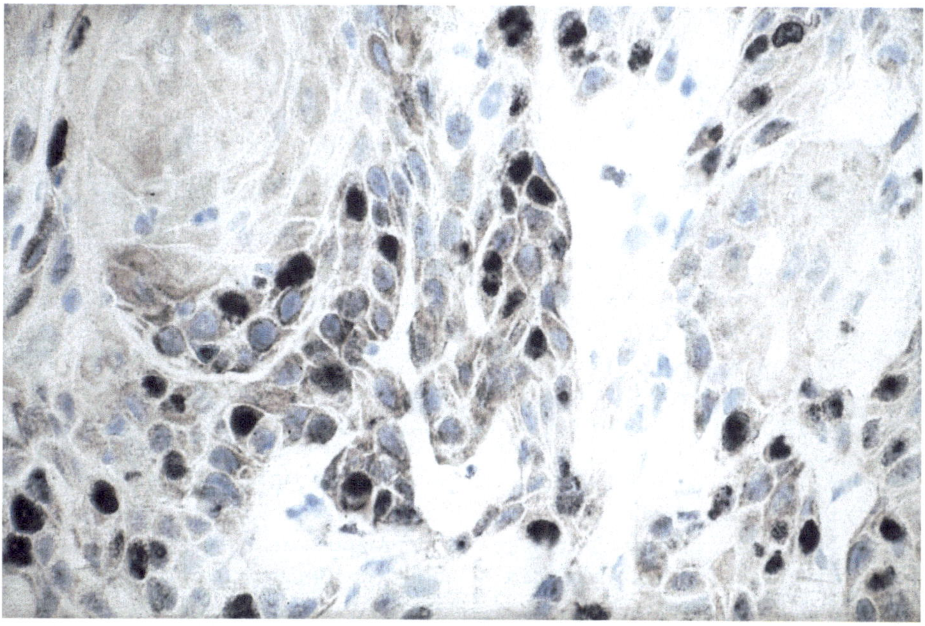

Fig. 177. Large cell keratinizing carcinoma. Immunohistochemical reaction with Ki-67

Squamo-Transitional Cell Carcinoma [8120/3]

This term has been introduced because of the histologic similarity of the cervical neoplasm to transitional cell carcinoma of the urinary tract. Like in transitional cell metaplasia, some doubts on this interpretation have been raised in several aspects (Koenig et al. 1997; Lininger et al. 1997, 1998). Unlike transitional cell carcinoma of the urinary tract, the endocervical "transitional cell carcinoma" shows a Müllerian immunoprofile, e.g., by its negative immunoreaction with CK 20 and uroplakin. In addition, it is almost always admixed with squamous, glandular or clear cell patterns, suggesting a bipotential behavior, as frequently seen in carcinomas of reserve cell type. Also, a large percentage of endocervical "transitional cell carcinomas" is positive for HPV 16.

Detailed molecular analysis of papillomavirus DNA integration sites revealed convincing evidence that the squamous and glandular part of these tumors were derived from one identical precursor cell clone (Luft et al. 2001). The papillary architecture of this rare type of endocervical carcinoma appears to be the most distinctive, objective feature rather than its superficial resemblance to urothelial transitional cell carcinomas. This type of endocervical carcinoma should rather be classified as a papillary variant of reserve cell (squamous or adenosquamous) carcinoma. Consequently, the dysplastic reserve cell papilloma (p. 94, Figs. 130, 131) should be considered as its preinvasive stage.

Glandular Type (Figs. 178–208)

All types of adenocarcinomas [8140/3] of the endocervix have become more common over the past three decades (Schwartz and Weiss 1986; Vizcaino et al. 1998), especially in young women (Bulk et al. 2005). Their proportion among all cervical cancers has increased from 4.6% to over 30% in some studies. As already mentioned, the great majority of endocervical adenocarcinomas contain HPV 18 or 45. This virus infects both the reserve cells and the glandular epithelial cells mainly when these are hyperplastic, that is, excessively stimulated, as, for instance, under the growth-promoting action of synthetic gestagens taken as the major component of oral contraceptives (Gallup and Abell 1977; Dallenbach-Hellweg 1984). This concept is in agreement with epidemiological studies (Brinton et al. 1986; Peters et al. 1986). Both infected and hyperstimulated cell types – reserve cells and glandular cells, may under such conditions develop into in situ and invasive adenocarcinoma, often with coexistent carcinoma in situ of reserve cell type (Maier and Norris 1980).

The prognosis of all types of endocervical adenocarcinomas is generally less favorable than that of squamous carcinomas (Eide 1987; Quinn 1997). It depends more on the degree of nuclear ploidy, the stage of the disease, and the lymph node status than on the histological appearance (Fu et al. 1982; Hopkins et al. 1988; Alfsen et al. 2001).

In *early invasive adenocarcinoma* [8140/3], microinvasion must be limited to 5 mm in depth with extension beyond the normal glandular field. Stromal response may be present, but is not mandatory for diagnosis. The prognosis and, in consequence, treatment of this type of microinvasive carcinoma is very similar to that of its squamous counterpart (Östör 2000).

Mucinous Adenocarcinoma [8480/3]

The *mucinous (endocervical) type of adenocarcinoma* (Figs. 178–194) is most frequently encountered. All degrees of differentiation can be found. The amount of mucin roughly follows the degree of differentiation. Most of the mucinous adenocarcinomas are well or moderately differentiated. Their interbranching glands may show microglandular changes (Young and Scully 1992, Fig. 186) and contain variable amounts of intracytoplasmic mucin (Tambouret et al. 2000, Fig. 189). In the poorly differentiated type (Figs. 187, 188), solid strands of tumor cells predominate with pseudorosette formation or palisading of nuclei. There is very little intracytoplasmic mucin, but monocellular or microcystic accumulation of mucin may be found scattered within cellular strands. All types of mucinous carcinomas, regardless of their degree of differentiation, almost always stain positively for CEA (Figs. 190, 191).

Minimal Deviation Adenocarcinoma [8480/3] (adenoma malignum, Figs. 178, 179) is extremely well differentiated, but nonetheless has a poor prognosis, often despite radical therapy (Kaku and Enjoji 1983; Kaminski and Norris 1983; Michael et al. 1984). This particular type of endocervical adenocarcinoma may be associated with a Peutz–Jegher syndrome and with a second primary ovarian mucinous adenocarcinoma (Young and Scully 1988; Gilks et al. 1989). Cytological abnormalities are absent or subtle, consisting of slight nuclear enlargement, chromatin clumping, loss of nuclear polarity, and increased mitotic activity. The carcinomatous glands are lined by a single layer of columnar mucinous epithelium generally similar to that seen in normal glands. There may be a weak desmoplastic or edematous reaction around some glands. Necrosis is absent. Architectural abnormalities are the main distinguishing features: the endocervical

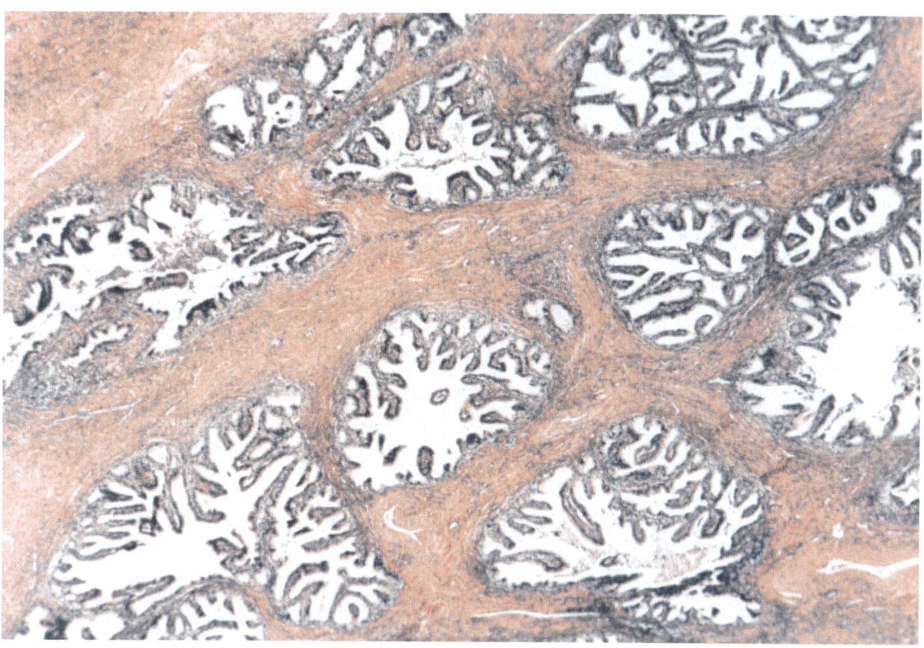

Fig. 178. Minimal deviation adenocarcinoma. H&E

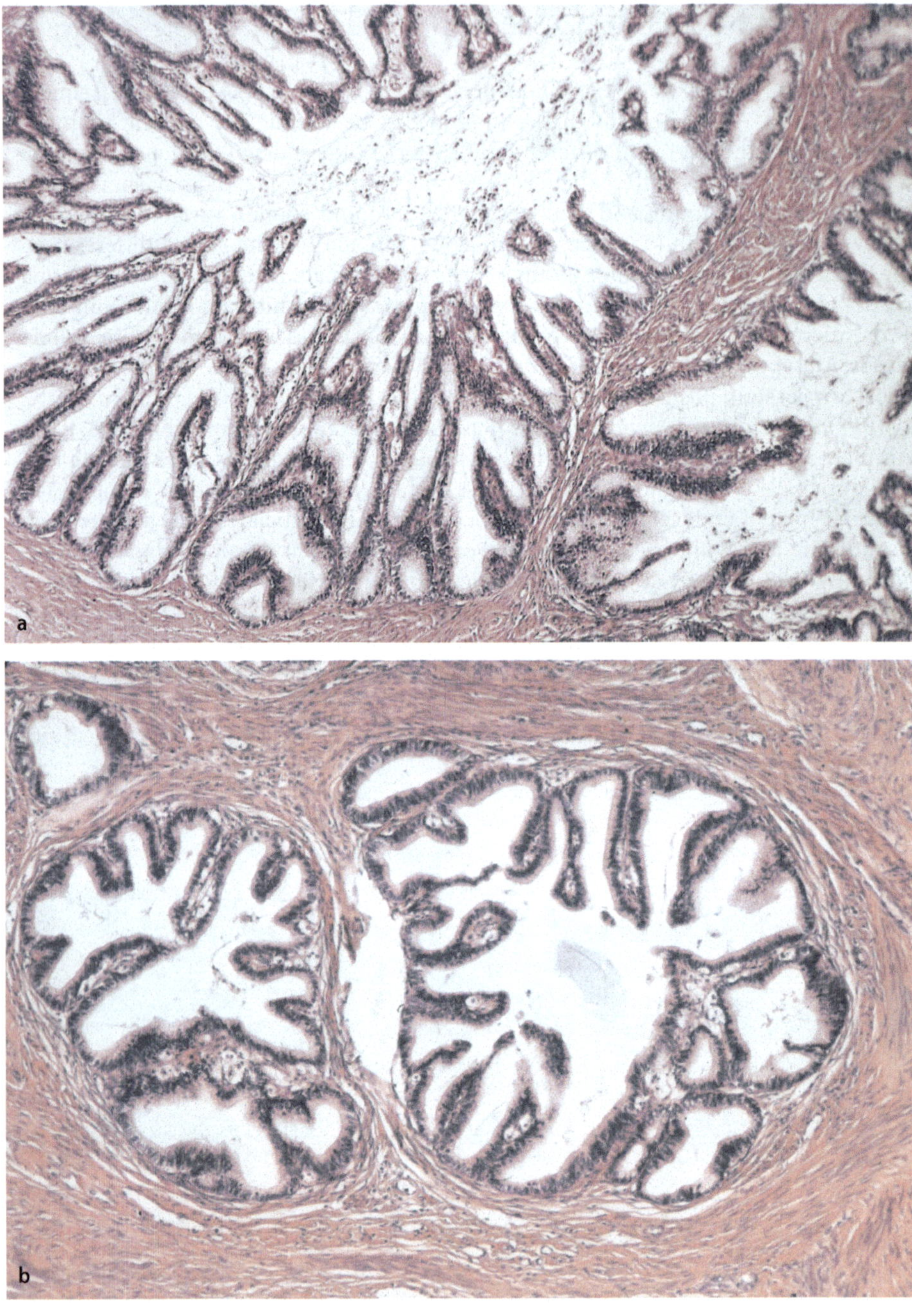

Fig. 179. Minimal deviation adenocarcinoma. H&E, higher magnification

glands, excessively convoluted with papillary projections into their lumina, are randomly distributed in the cervical wall, which they invade beyond the area in which glands are normally found. In most cases, vascular and perineural invasion is already evident.

Differential Diagnosis. It may be very difficult to distinguish carcinomatous glands from normal or hyperplastic endocervical glands, e.g. focal or diffuse laminar glandular hyperplasia (Jones et al. 1991), endocervicosis or adenomyoma of endocervical type and even impossible if only a small biopsy is available. In such cases, immunohistochemical stains with CEA may be very helpful: all or part of the carcinomatous glands are positive for CEA in most instances, whereas normal and hyperplastic endocervical glands stain negatively (Steeper and Wick 1986; Nanbu et al. 1988; Gilks et al. 1996; Nucci et al. 1999; Young and Clement 2000). Immunohistochemistry with $p16^{INK4a}$ is also helpful in distinguishing adenocarcinoma from benign mimics; it shows a diffuse positivity in malignancy, whereas the benign lesions are negative or show focally weak staining for $p16^{INK4a}$ (Cameron et al. 2002, Negri et al. 2003, Ishikawa et al. 2003). In larger specimens, deep infiltration of carcinomatous glands around the thick-wall vessels is always highly suggestive if not diagnostic of invasive carcinoma (see Fig. 181b; cf. to Wheeler and Kurman 2005).

Intestinal Mucinous Adenocarcinoma [8144/3]. The intestinal type of mucinous adenocarcinoma (Fig. 193) contains goblet cells resembling those of adenocarcinoma of the colon, and occasionally argentaffin and Paneth's cells. Such an intestinal-type change may be found diffusely or only focally within a mucinous carcinoma, which has developed from an intestinal metaplasia of the endocervical mucosa. A signet-ring cell type [8490/3] is very rare (Haswani et al. 1998).

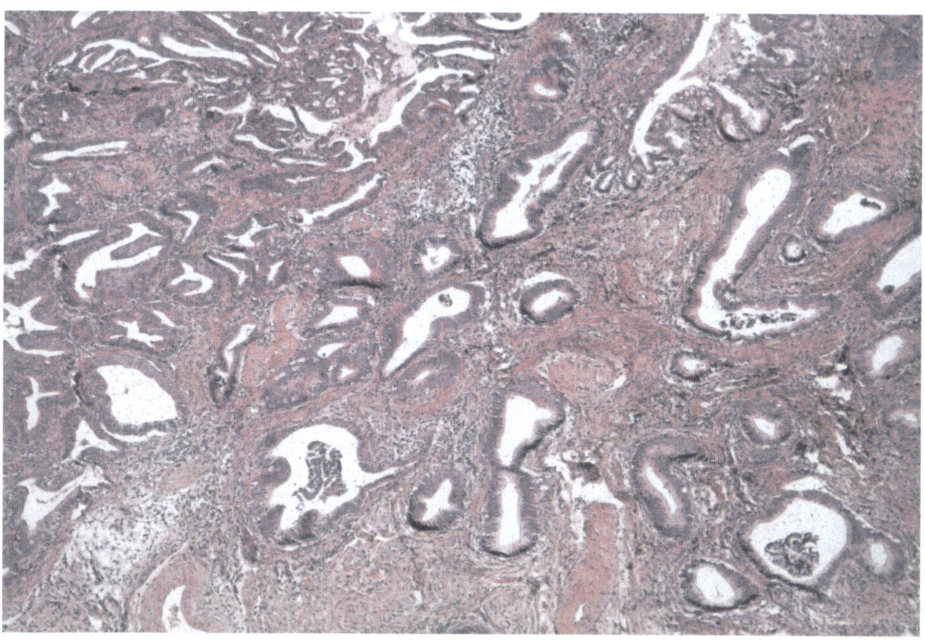

Fig. 180. Mucinous adenocarcinoma, grade 1. H&E

Various other types of Müllerian metaplasia may give rise to special forms of endocervical adenocarcinomas (Lauchlan 1984). A combination of mucinous adenocarcinoma and epidermoid carcinoma may be seen and should be distinguished from adenosquamous carcinoma.

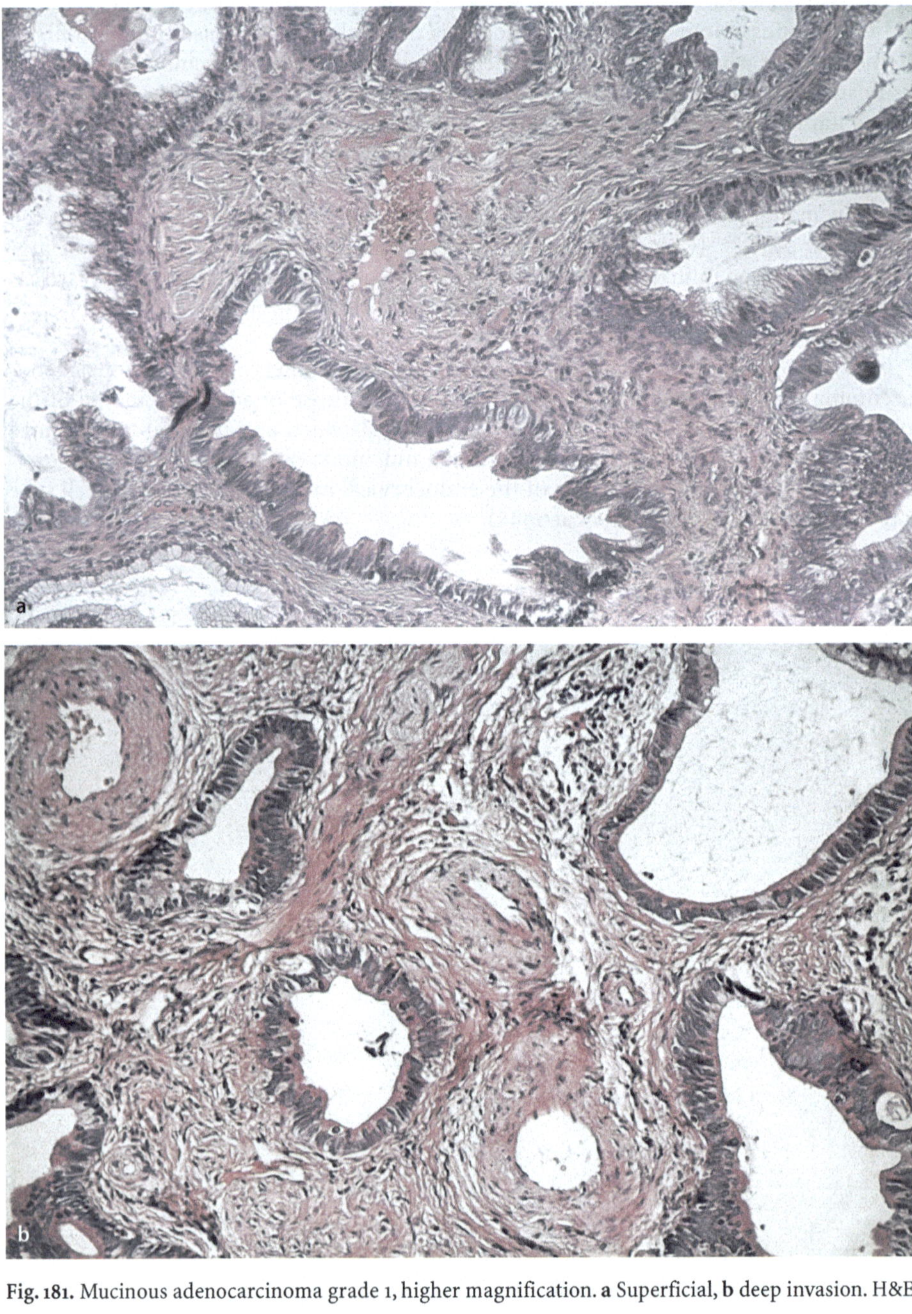

Fig. 181. Mucinous adenocarcinoma grade 1, higher magnification. **a** Superficial, **b** deep invasion. H&E

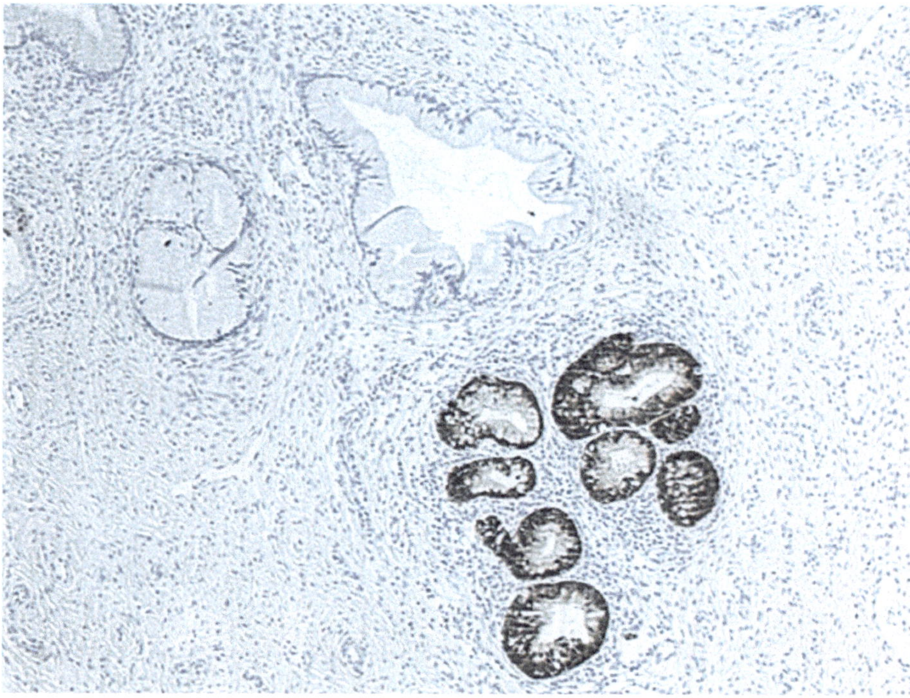

Fig. 182. Adenocarcinoma in situ. Diffuse, continuous positivity for p16^{INK4a} in atypical glands, negative reaction in normal endocervical glands. p16^{INK4a} immunostain

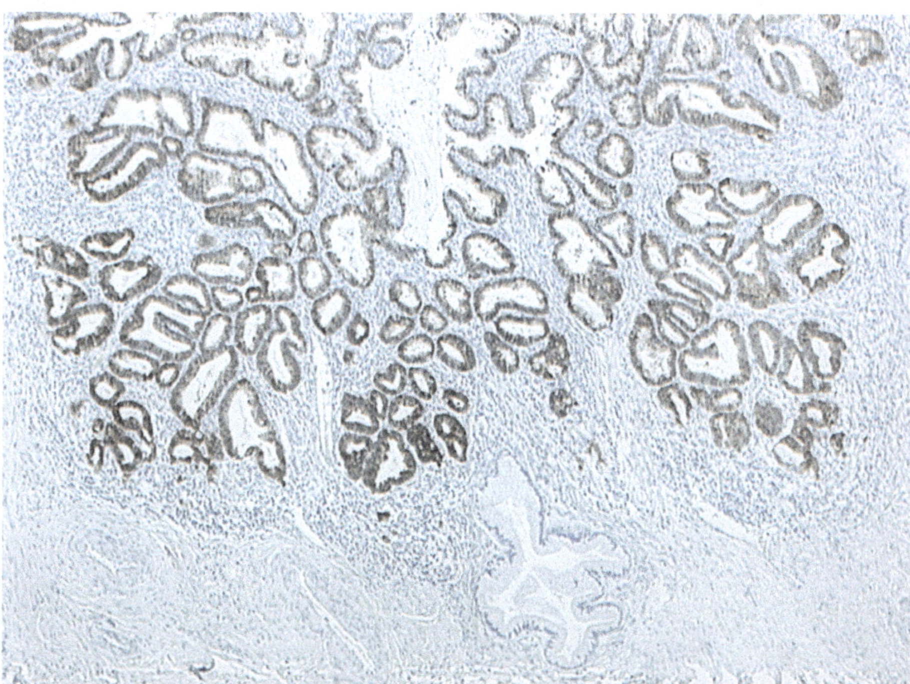

Fig. 183. Mucinous adenocarcinoma, grade 1 with surrounding inflammatory reaction. Diffuse, continuous positivity for p16^{INK4a} in atypical glands, negative reaction in normal endocervical glands. p16^{INK4a} immunostain

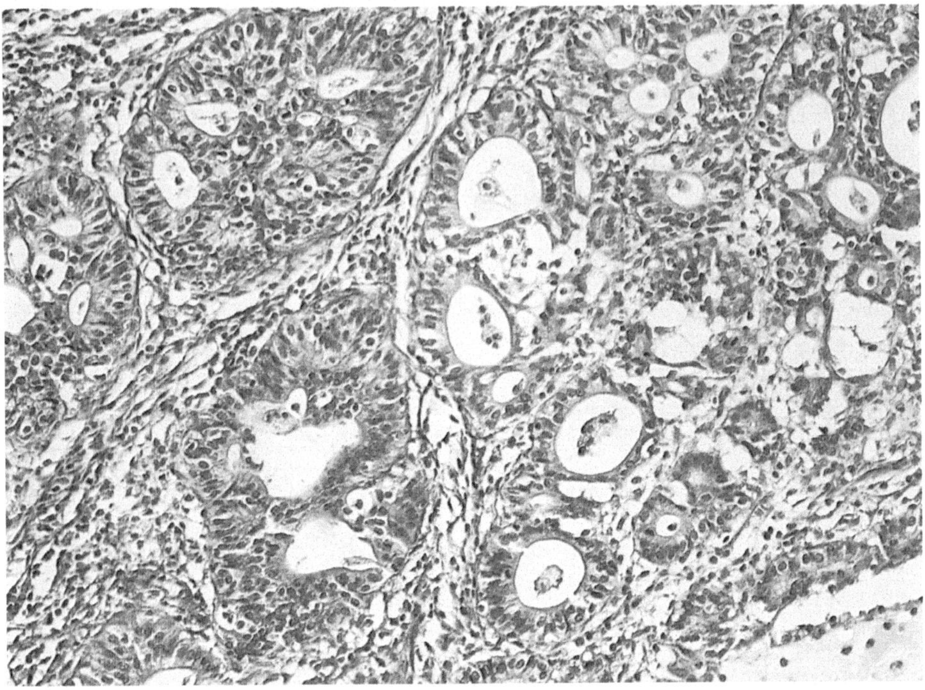

Fig. 184. Mucinous adenocarcinoma, grade 2. H&E

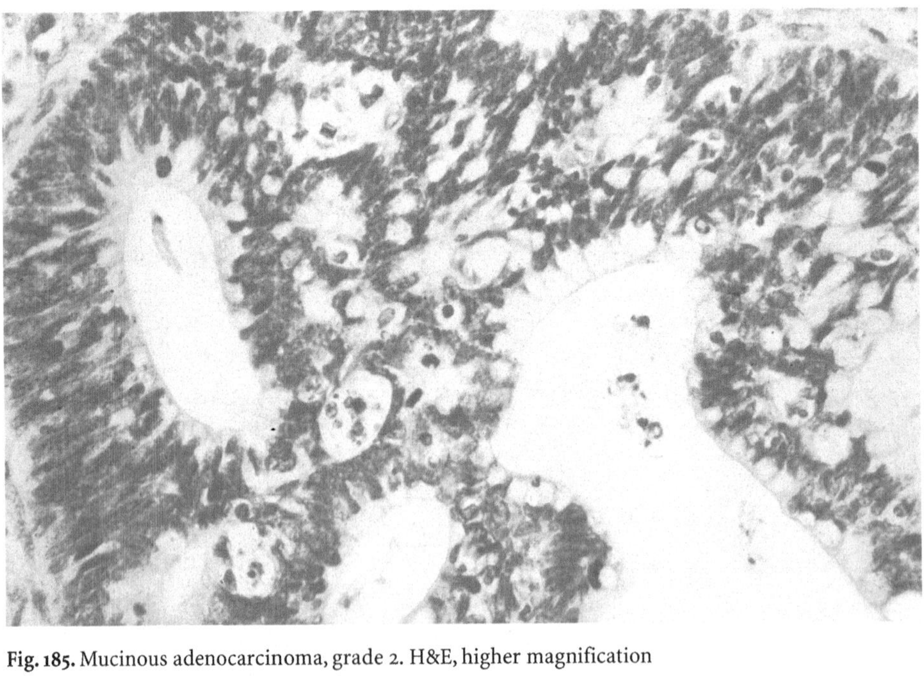

Fig. 185. Mucinous adenocarcinoma, grade 2. H&E, higher magnification

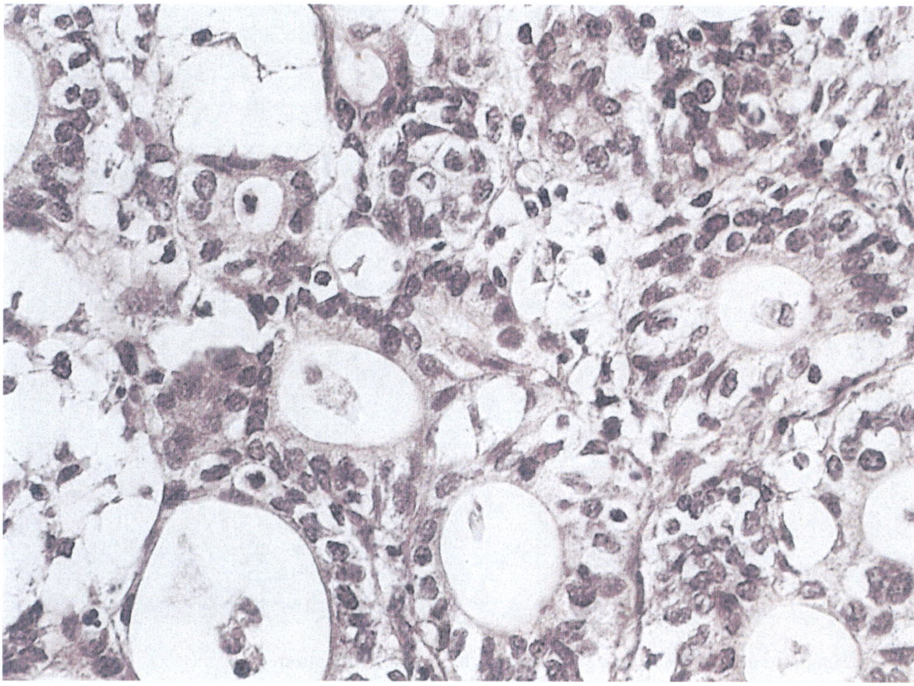

Fig. 186. Mucinous adenocarcinoma, grade 2–3. H&E

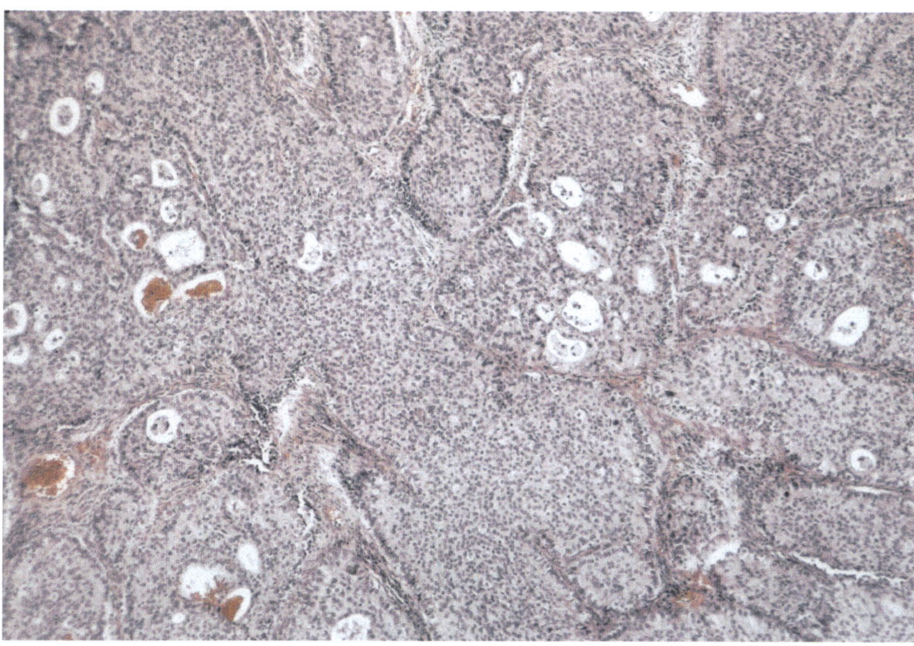

Fig. 187. Mucinous adenocarcinoma, grade 3. H&E

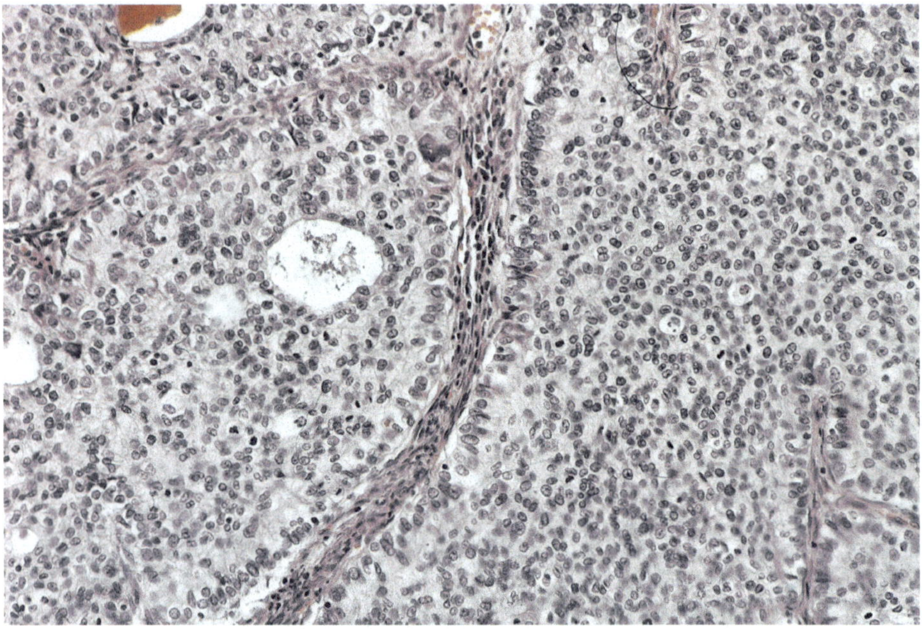

Fig. 188. Mucinous adenocarcinoma, grade 3. H&E, higher magnification

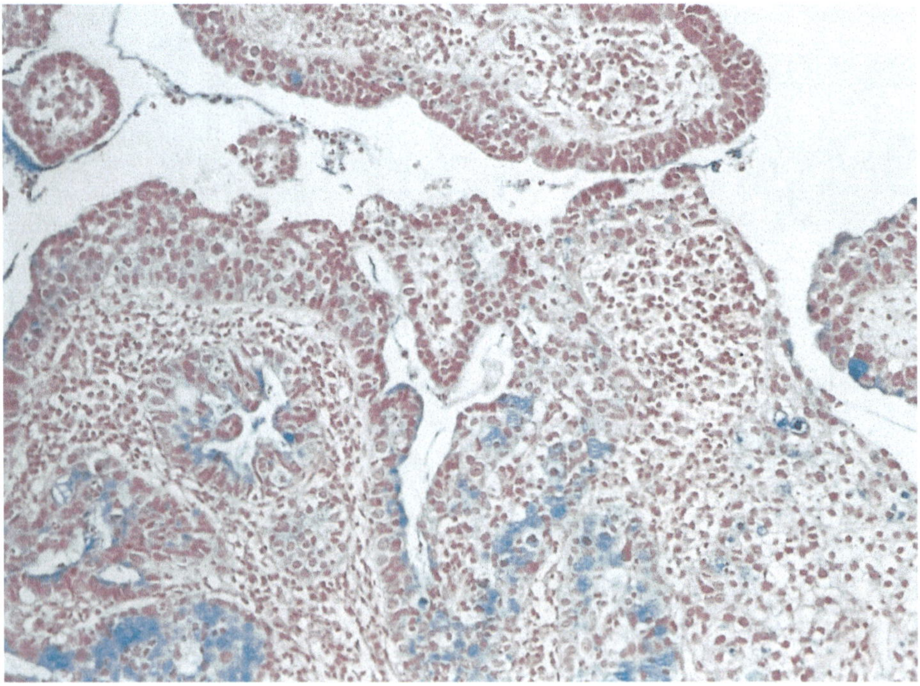

Fig. 189. Mucinous adenocarcinoma, grade 2. Alcian blue reaction

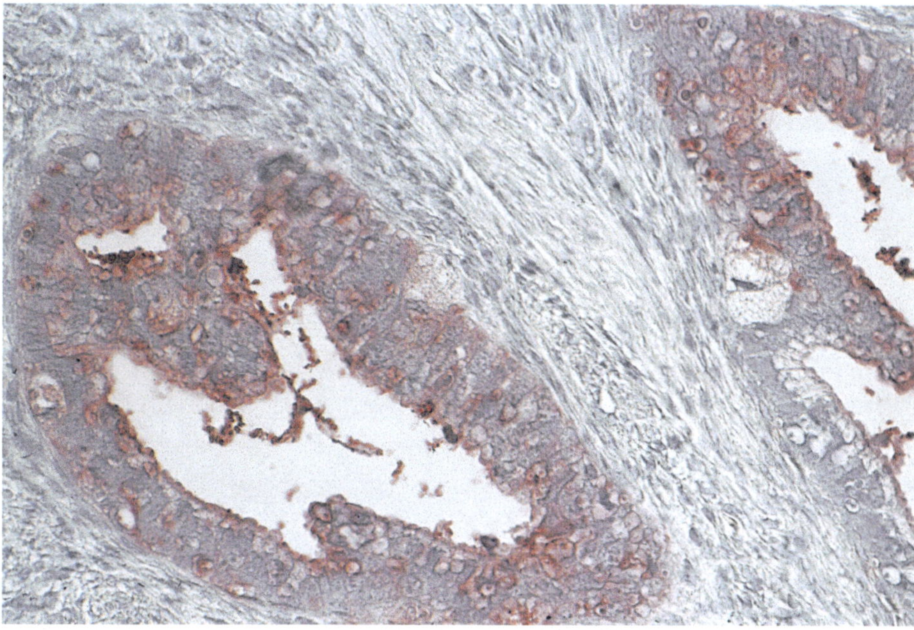

Fig. 190. Mucinous adenocarcinoma, grade 1. Immunohistochemical reaction for CEA

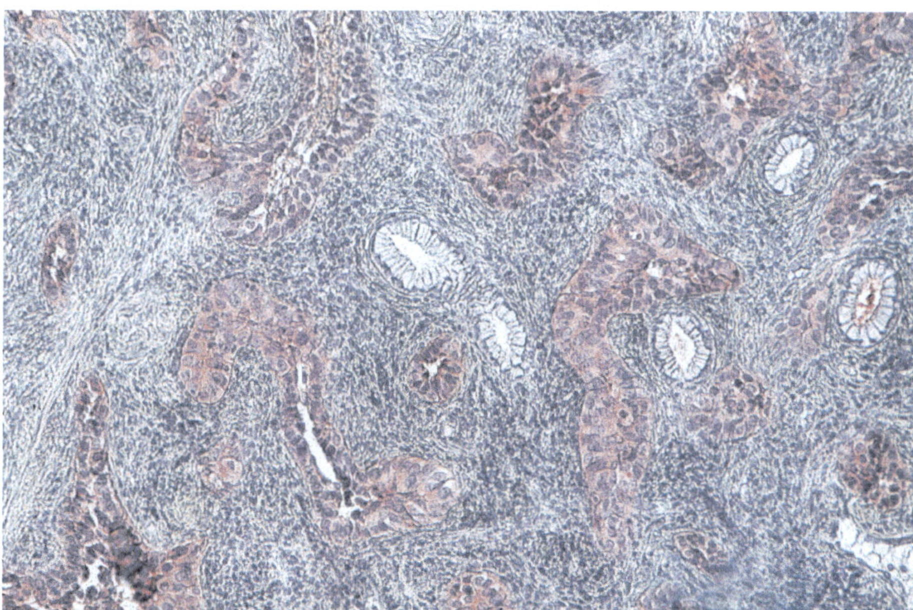

Fig. 191. Mucinous adenocarcinoma, grade 3. Immunohistochemical reaction for CEA (normal glands react negatively)

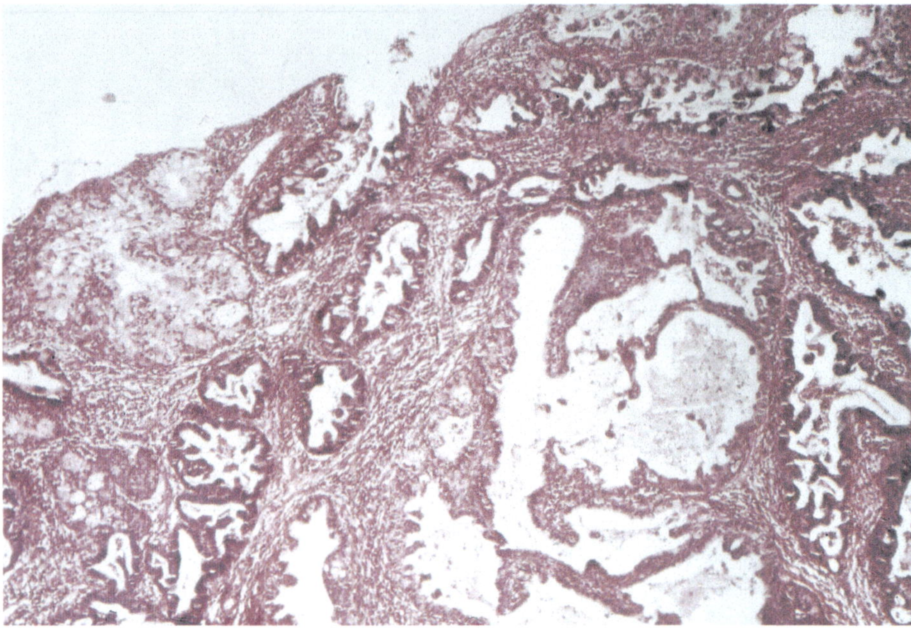

Fig. 192. Mucinous adenocarcinoma, grade 1, glandular-papillary. H&E

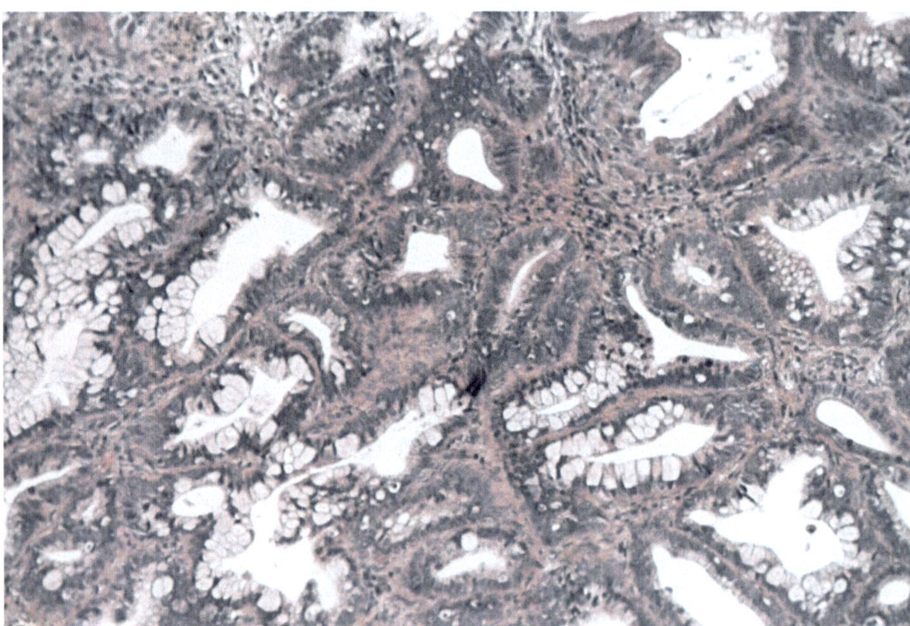

Fig. 193. Mucinous adenocarcinoma, intestinal type. H&E

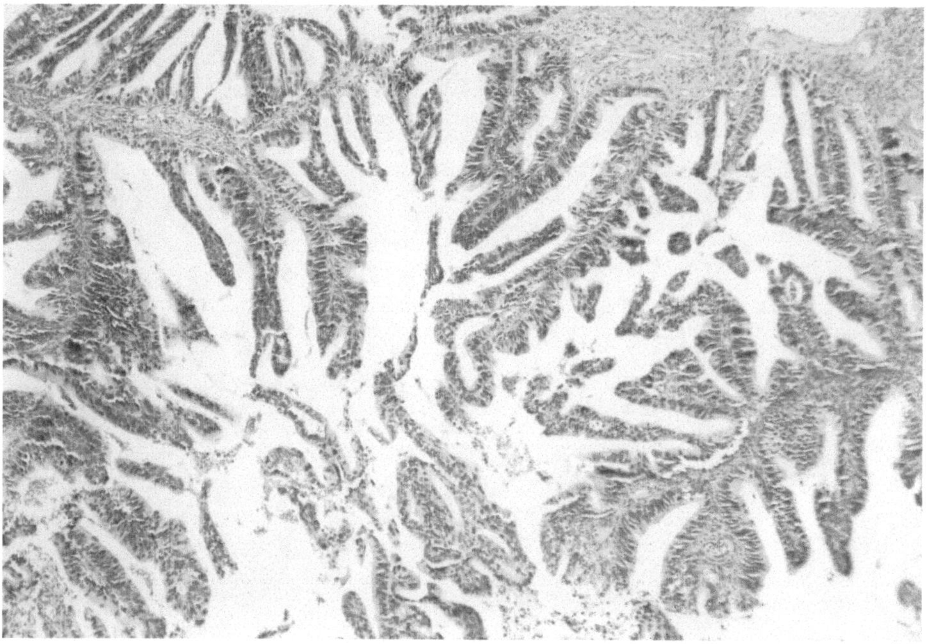

Fig. 194a. Mucinous adenocarcinoma, villoglandular type. **a** H&E

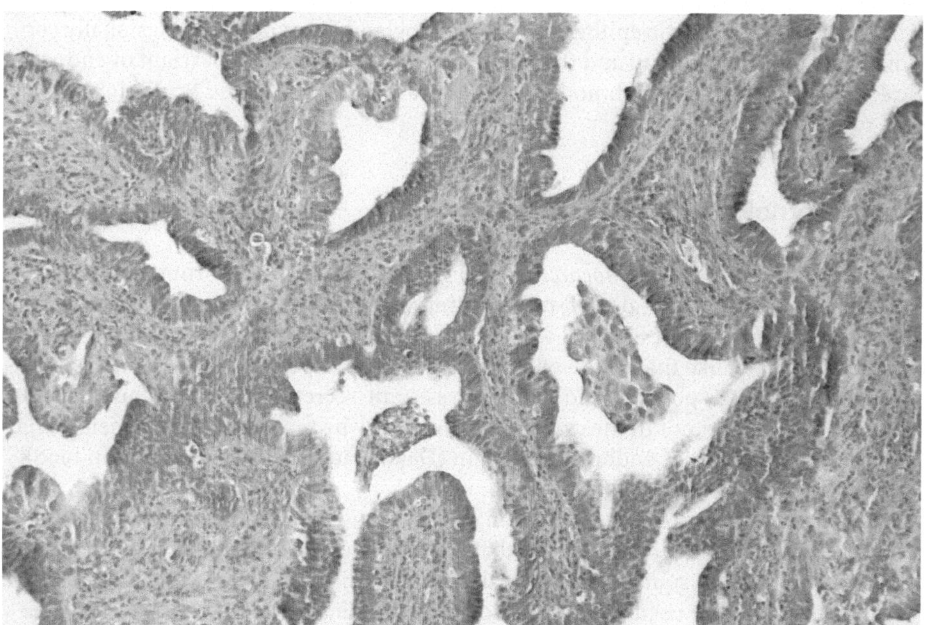

Fig. 194b. Mucinous adenocarcinoma, villoglandular type. **b** H&E

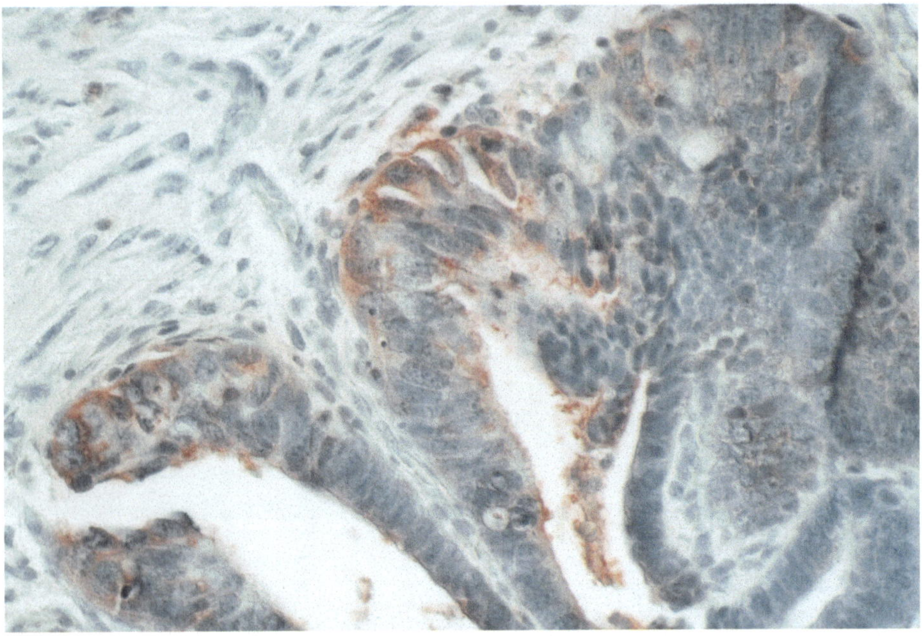

Fig. 194c. Mucinous adenocarcinoma, villoglandular type. **c** CEA

The *villoglandular type* [8262/3] (Fig. 194) shows a glandular-papillary surface involvement, but no extensive invasion, and therefore has a much better prognosis than the endometrioid type with deep invasion into the cervical wall. The well to moderately differentiated neoplastic epithelium of the villoglandular type may occasionally contain intracytoplasmic mucin and then be regarded as the mucinous variant of endocervical adenocarcinoma. Lymph node metastases are rare (Young and Scully 1989; Jones et al. 1993; Kaku et al. 1997).

Endometrioid Adenocarcinoma [8380/3]

The *endometrioid type of adenocarcinoma* (Figs. 195–197) may arise from metaplasia or from ectopic endometrial glands, representing embryological remnants displaced in the deeper portions of the cervical wall (Noda et al. 1983; Teshima et al. 1985). Its histological structure is like that of the endometrial-type adenocarcinoma arising from the corpus mucosa. PAS-positive and diastase-resistant secretions may be found in the glandular lumina, but not in the cytoplasm. There may be foci of squamous metaplasia, as in adenoacanthoma of endometrial origin (Dallenbach-Hellweg and Poulsen 1996).

■ **Differential Diagnosis.** Distinguishing an endometrioid type of adenocarcinoma from a primary endometrial adenocarcinoma that has extended or metastasized to the cervix may be impossible in routine histological examination of curettings or biopsies, even when mucin stains are used. Immunohistochemical stains, however, may help considerably (Cohen et al. 1982; Dabbs et al. 1986). Endometrioid type adenocarcinomas of endocervical origin, in contrast to primary endometrial carcinomas, are negative with vimentin (Fig. 196) and positive with CEA in most instances (Dallenbach-Hellweg and Lang 1991; Castrillon et al. 2002; McCluggage et al. 2002). $p16^{INK4a}$ immunostaining may also be helpful, since primary endocervical adenocarcinomas show a diffuse positivity, whereas endometrial adenocarcinomas display a focal pattern only (McCluggage and Jenkins 2003; Ansari-Lari et al. 2004) (see Figs. 197 and 198).

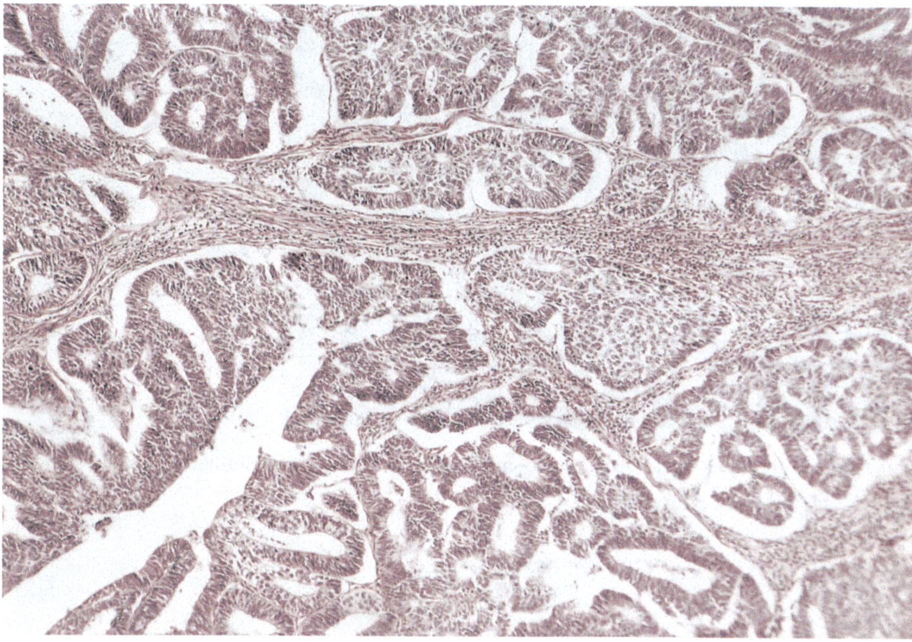

Fig. 195. Adenocarcinoma of endocervix, endometrioid type. H&E

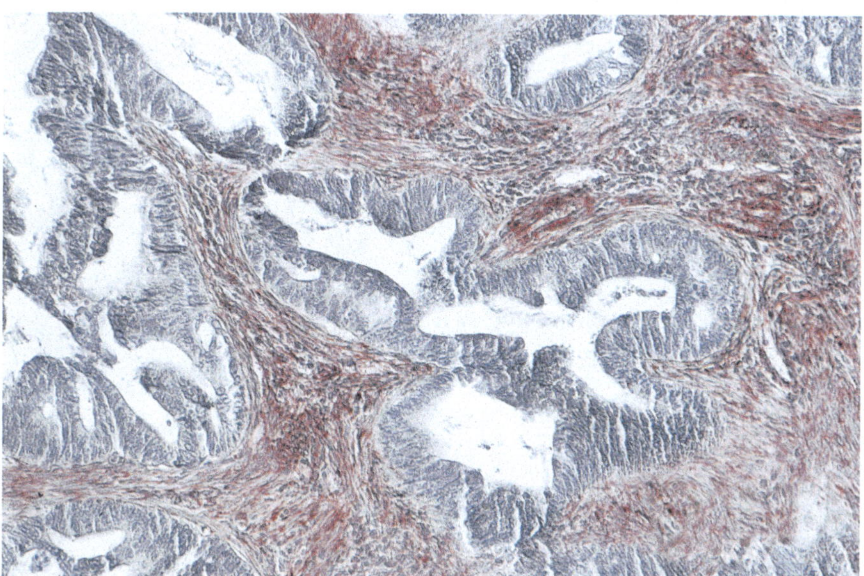

Fig. 196. Adenocarcinoma of endocervix, endometrioid type. Immunohistochemical reaction with antivimentin

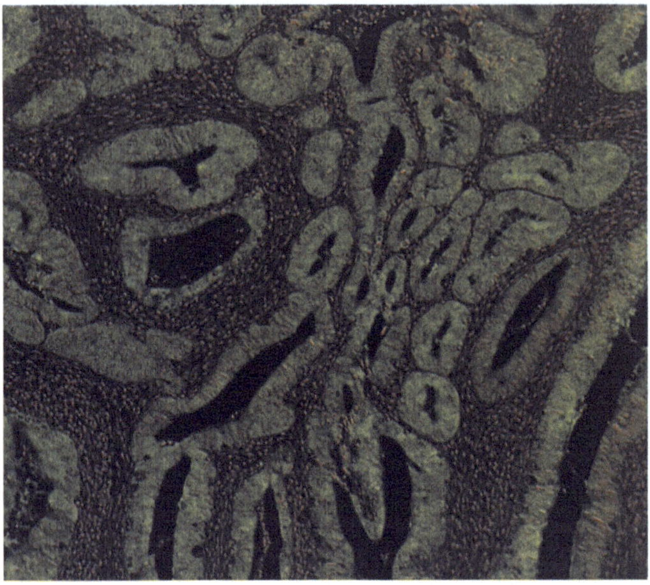

Fig 197. Adenocarcinoma of endocervix, endometrioid type. Diffuse and continuous positive staining reaction for $p16^{INK4a}$ in tumor cells. $p16^{INK4a}$ immunostain

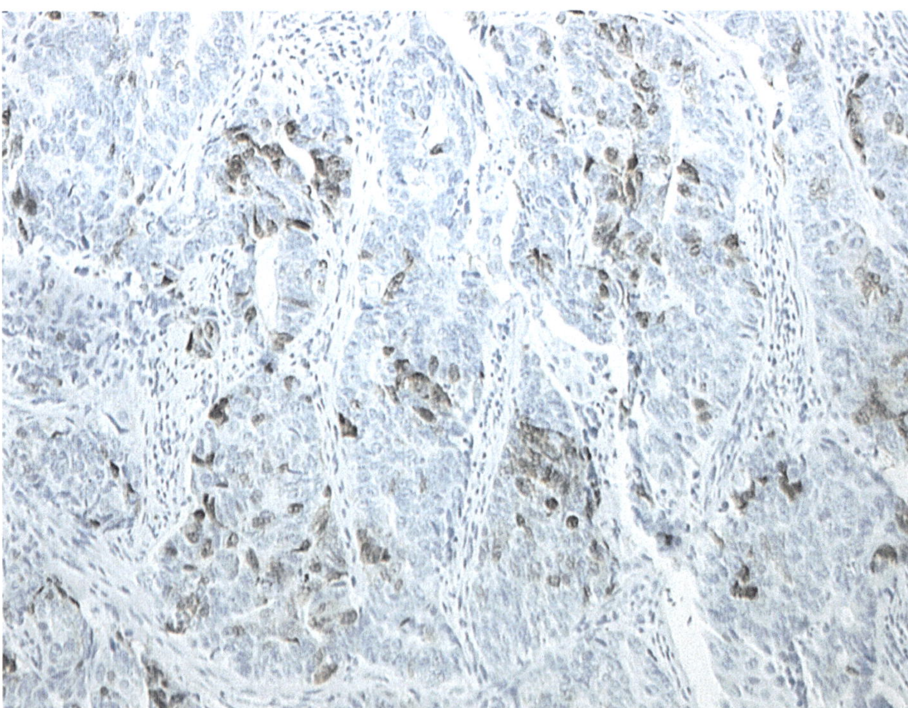

Fig 198. Adenocarcinoma of endometrium, endometrioid type. Scattered positive staining reaction for $p16^{INK4a}$. $p16^{INK4a}$ immunostain

Clear Cell Adenocarcinoma [8310/3]

The *clear cell adenocarcinoma* (Figs. 199–201) may be mainly solid (Fig. 201) or glandular (Fig. 199) with papillary protrusions (Fig. 200), hobnail cells, and a glycogen-rich cytoplasm (Fig. 199). It resembles closely the clear cell carcinomas of ovarian, endometrial, or vaginal origin. The endocervical clear cell adenocarcinomas most likely arise from reserve cells, which presumably through faulty differentiation remain at an intermediary stage of development between incomplete keratinization and the secretion of mucins (Dallenbach-Hellweg and Lang 1991).

Serous Adenocarcinoma [8441/3]

The *serous adenocarcinoma* (Figs. 202, 203), too, closely resembles those originating in the ovaries and endometrium (Dallenbach-Hellweg and Poulsen 1996). It may also contain psammoma bodies.

■ **Differential Diagnosis.** Clear cell and serous adenocarcinomas can be distinguished from atypical microglandular endocervical hyperplasia in most cases by showing their positive reaction with CEA; microglandular hyperplasia reacts negatively. Distinction from an Arias-Stella reaction should not be difficult, since that reaction is noninvasive and limited to the endocervical mucosa, and mitoses are rare or absent.

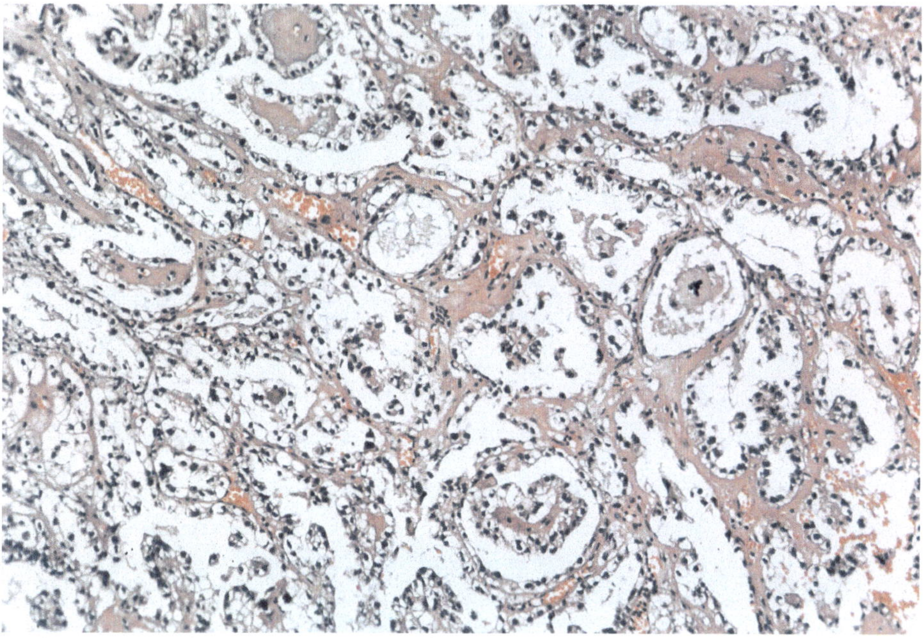

Fig. 199. Clear cell adenocarcinoma, glandular type. H&E

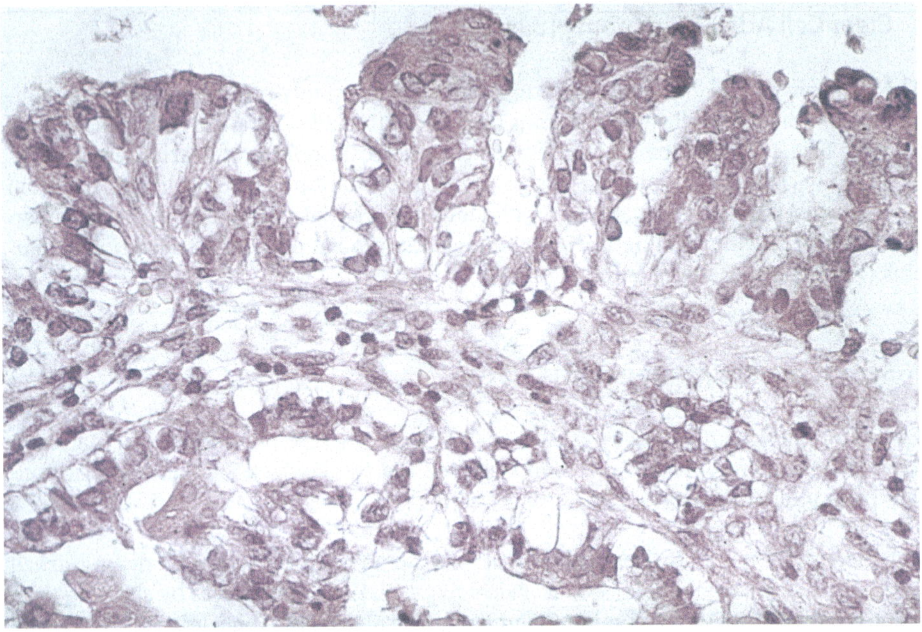

Fig. 200. Clear cell adenocarcinoma, glandular-papillary type. H&E

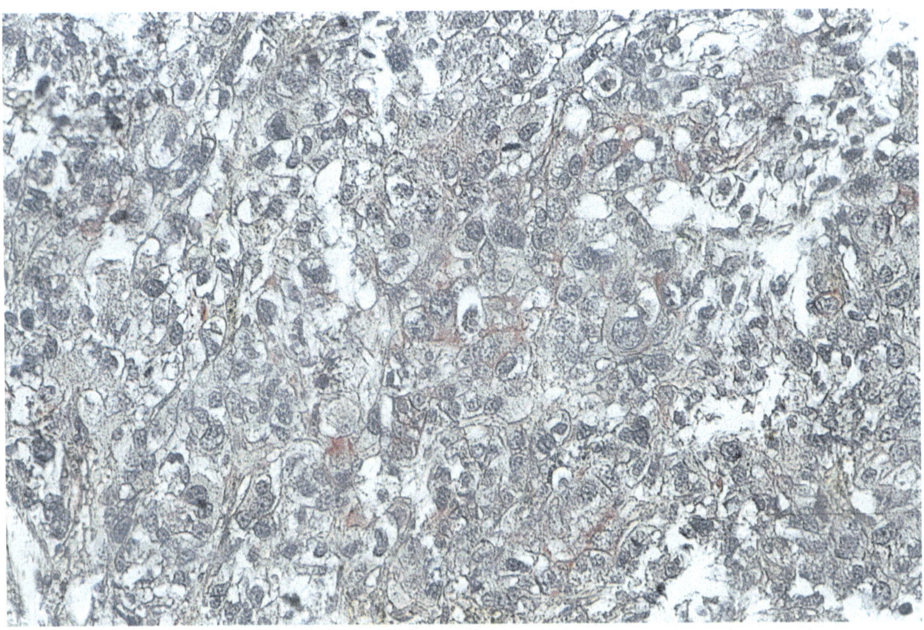

Fig. 201. Clear cell adenocarcinoma, solid type. Immunohistochemical reaction with cytokeratin 18

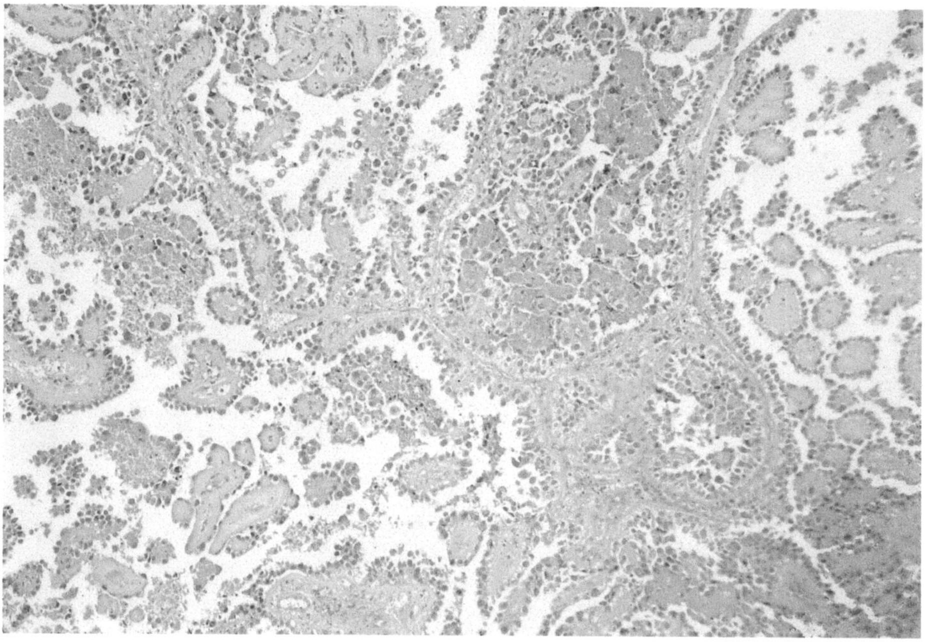

Fig. 202a. Serous adenocarcinoma. H&E

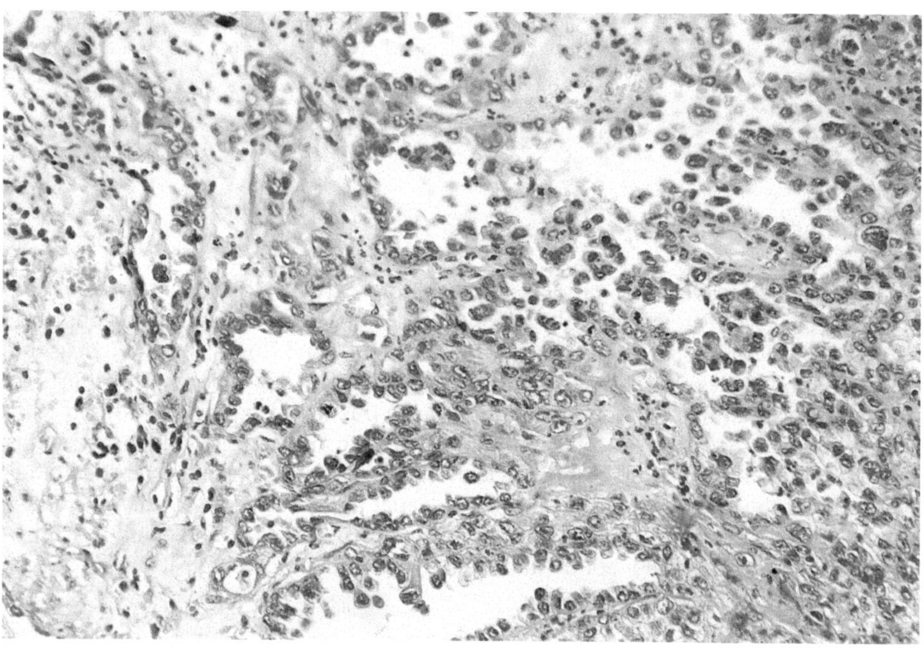

Fig. 202b. Serous adenocarcinoma. H&E, higher magnification

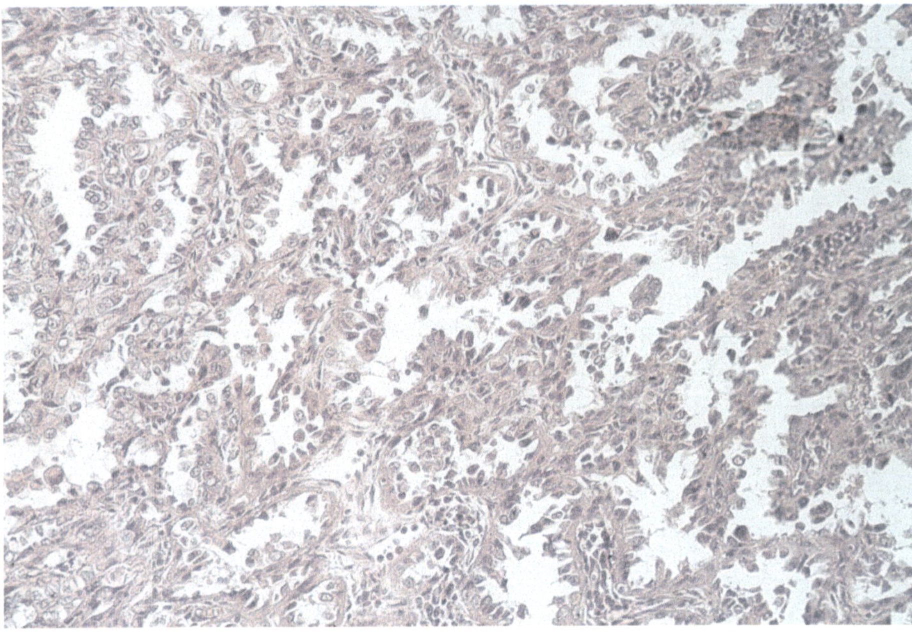

Fig. 203. Serous adenocarcinoma. H&E

Mesonephric Adenocarcinoma [9110/3]

The *mesonephric adenocarcinoma* (Figs. 204–208) is a rare cervical tumor (McGee et al. 1962; Buntine 1979; Ferry and Scully 1990; Clement et al. 1995), representing approximately 3% of the adenocarcinomas of this location (Hart and Norris 1972). Whereas the adenocarcinomas described above are of Müllerian origin, this type is not. Reports in the literature about incidence are conflicting, since this tumor has been confused with other types, mainly with clear cell carcinomas. The true mesonephric adenocarcinoma is a well-defined tumor, which originates from remnants of the mesonephric duct in the lateral wall of the cervix. Hence it is localized deeper in the cervical wall than the other types of adenocarcinoma. It consists of very characteristic small, round glandular lumina lined by a low cuboid epithelium usually devoid of cytological atypia (Figs. 204–206).

Mucin is absent in the sparse cytoplasm, but a small amount of PAS-positive material may be detected in the glandular lumina (Fig. 207). Solid strands of tumor cells may occasionally be seen between the small glands. Despite their bland appearance, the carcinomatous glands spread early and diffusely, invading all parts of the uterus. Both mesonephric hyperplasia and carcinoma have been observed more frequently during the past few years. They are often associated with microglandular hyperplasia of the endocervix or with in situ or invasive endocervical-type adenocarcinomas as well. Since the mesonephric ducts require testosterone for further development during ontogenesis, it has been suggested that an association exists between nortestosterone derivatives as components of oral contraceptives and an enhanced proliferation of mesonephric remnants in the cervix (Lang and Dallenbach-Hellweg 1990).

Differential Diagnosis. It is usually possible to distinguish mesonephric adenocarcinomas from endocervical and heterotopic Müllerian type adenocarcinomas by the characteristic histological appearances of their carcinomatous glands alone. Important and distinct differences in their immunohistochemical reactions, however, assist in the differentiation: the mesonephric adenocarcinoma reacts consistently negatively with CEA (Ayroud et al. 1985), but shows a positive reaction with CD 10 (Ordi et al. 2001), a weak expression of vimentin (Fig. 208) and a coexpression of cytokeratin 13, 7, 8 and 18 (Silver et al. 2001). Distinguishing it from florid mesonephric hyperplasia may be difficult, if not impossible, unless the whole uterus is available for examination (Fig. 209).

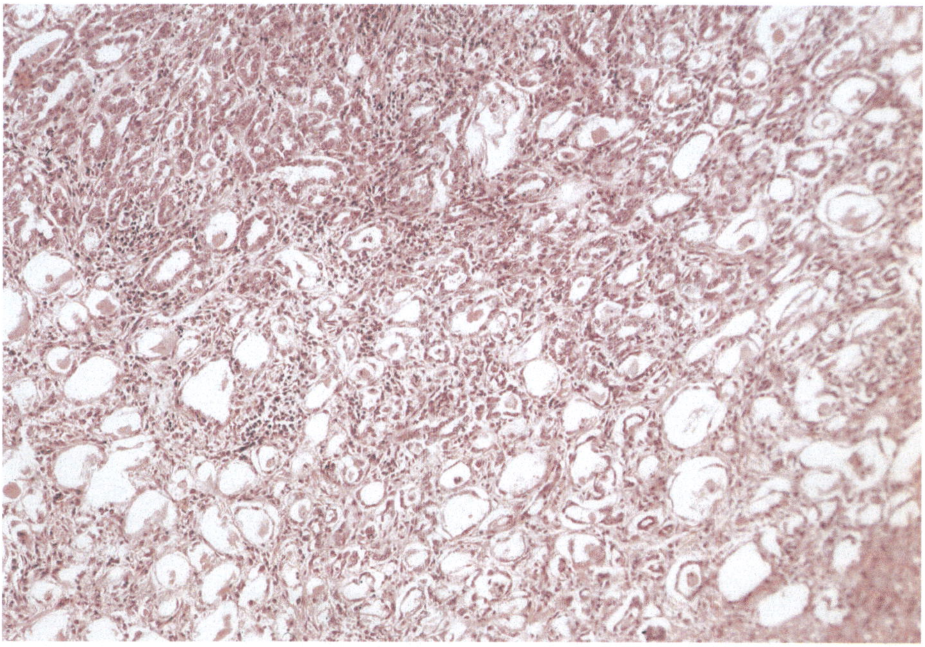

Fig. 204. Mesonephric adenocarcinoma. H&E

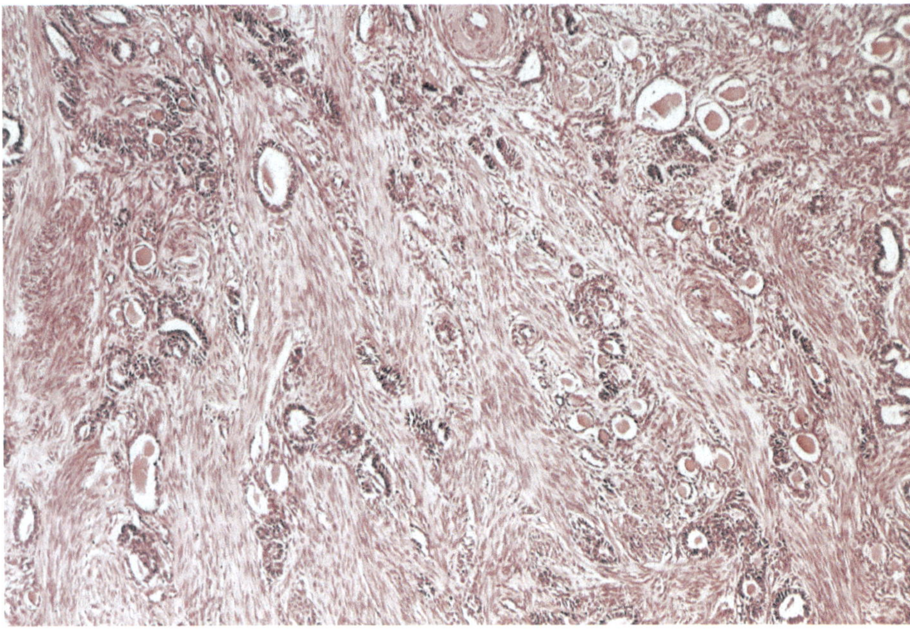

Fig. 205. Mesonephric adenocarcinoma. H&E

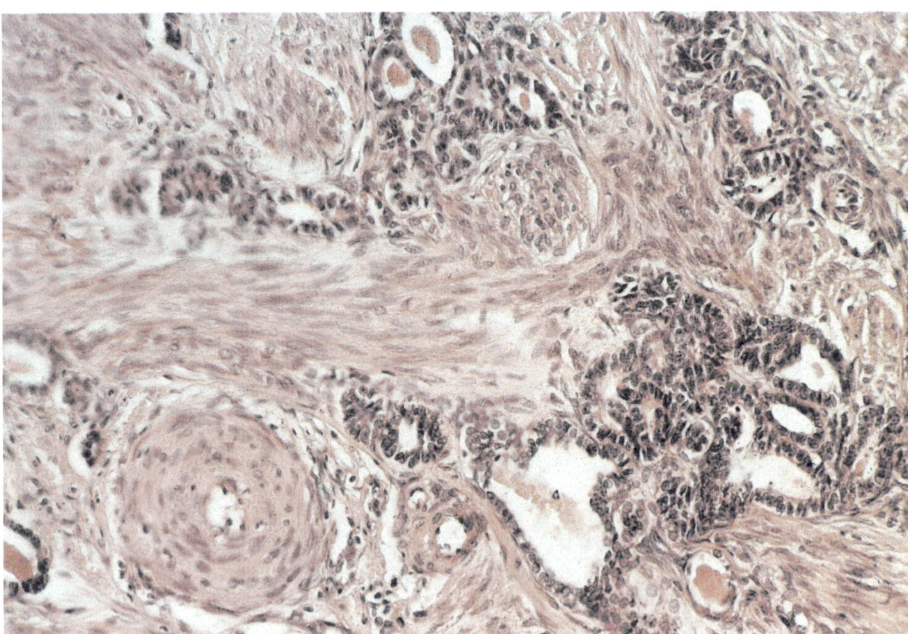

Fig. 206. Mesonephric adenocarcinoma. H&E, higher magnification

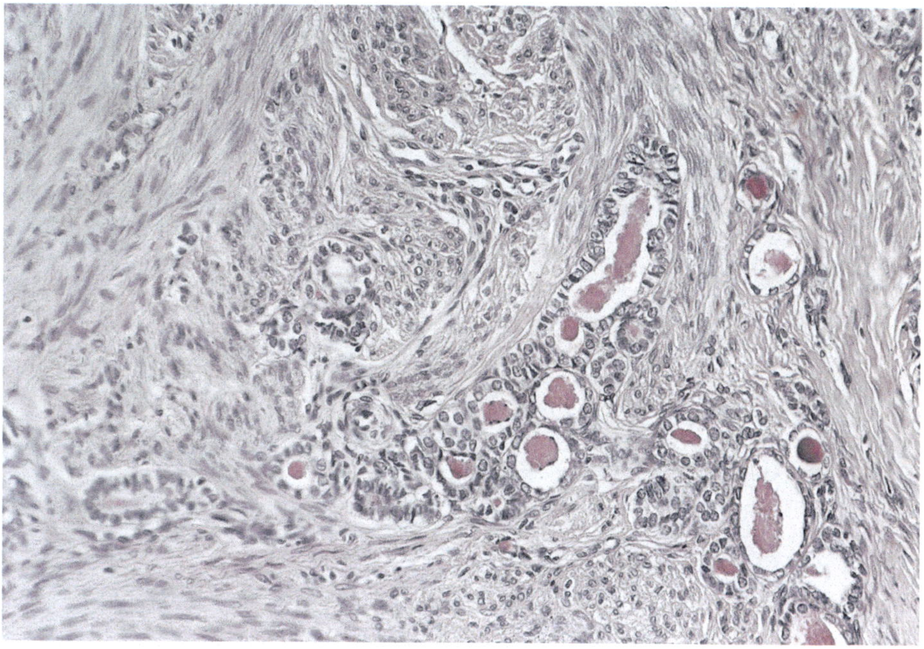

Fig. 207. Mesonephric adenocarcinoma. PAS reaction

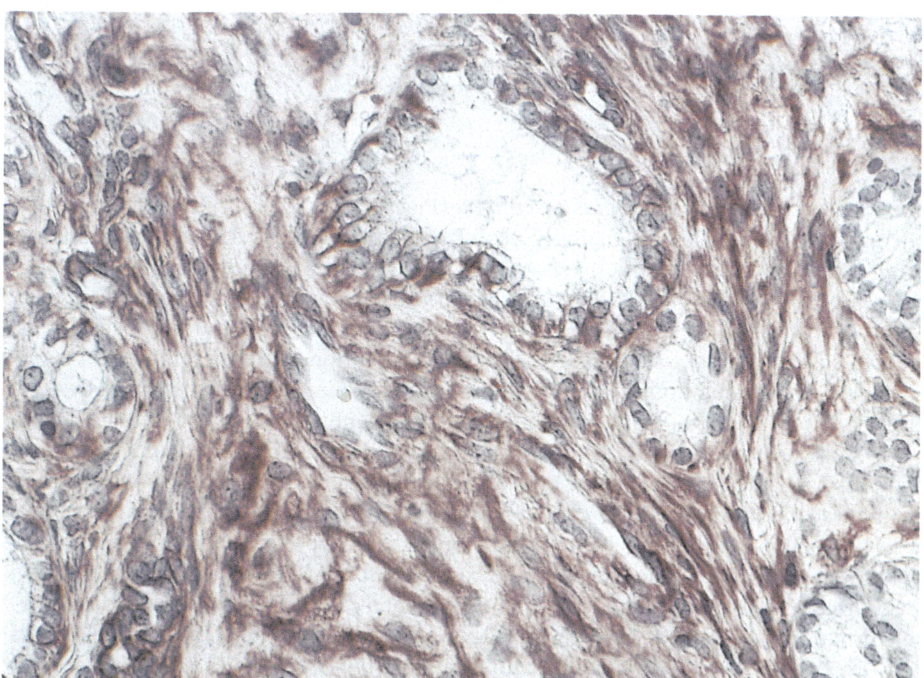

Fig. 208. Mesonephric adenocarcinoma. Immunohistochemical reaction with vimentin

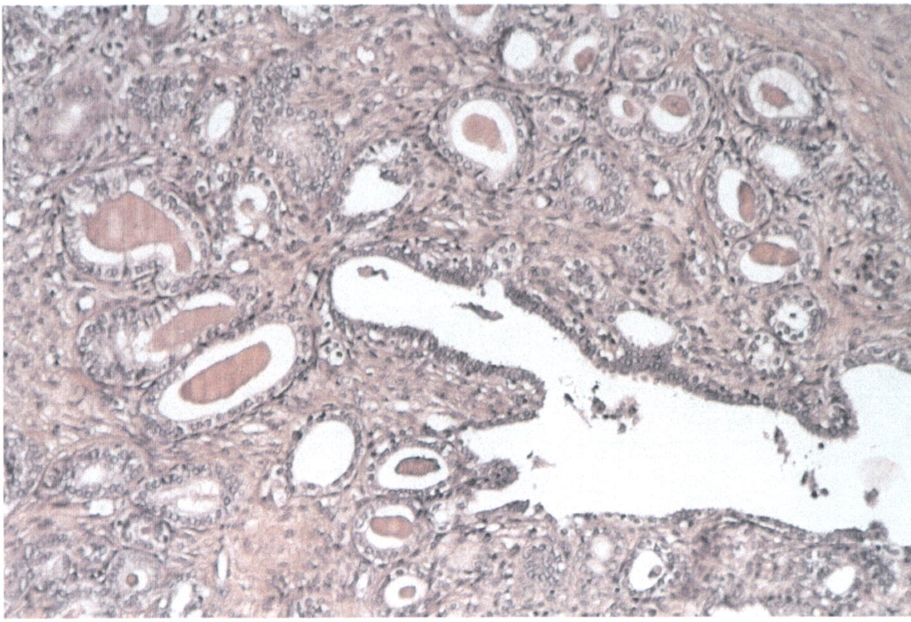

Fig. 209. Florid mesonephric hyperplasia. H&E

Mixed Type (Figs. 210–215)

Adenosquamous Carcinoma [8560/3]

The incidence of *adenosquamous carcinoma* (Figs. 210, 211) has significantly increased during the past decades, particularly in younger women (Adcock et al. 1982). Since it originates from the bipotential reserve cells, and since it is frequently associated with HPV infection type 18 (Smotkin et al. 1986) or the equally frequent type 16 (Tase et al. 1988), this increase is explainable by hormonal overstimulation and the resulting increased susceptibility of the reserve cells already mentioned. Besides, the endogenous hormonal overstimulation during pregnancy may explain why 50% of all invasive cervical carcinomas in pregnant women are of the adenosquamous type (Glücksmann 1957). Furthermore, refined histological, immunohistochemical, and ultrastructural methods have helped to recognize mixed epithelial patterns more readily. For instance, using these methods, *glassy cell carcinomas of the endocervix* [8015/3], characterized by large cells with abundant finely granular, ground-glass-type cytoplasm, prominent nuclei and lack of intercellular bridges and resembling clear cell carcinomas, have been recognized as poorly differentiated adenosquamous carcinomas with a very unfavorable prognosis (Richard et al. 1981; Ulbright and Gersell 1983; Tanaka et al. 1984; Wells and Brown 1986). In the moderately differentiated types of adenosquamous carcinomas, both glandular and squamous elements are either intimately mixed (Fig. 211) or more or less sharply demarcated from each other according to the reserve cell potential for either squamous epithelium or glands. Either keratinization (Fig. 210) or mucin formation (Fig. 211) may predominate.

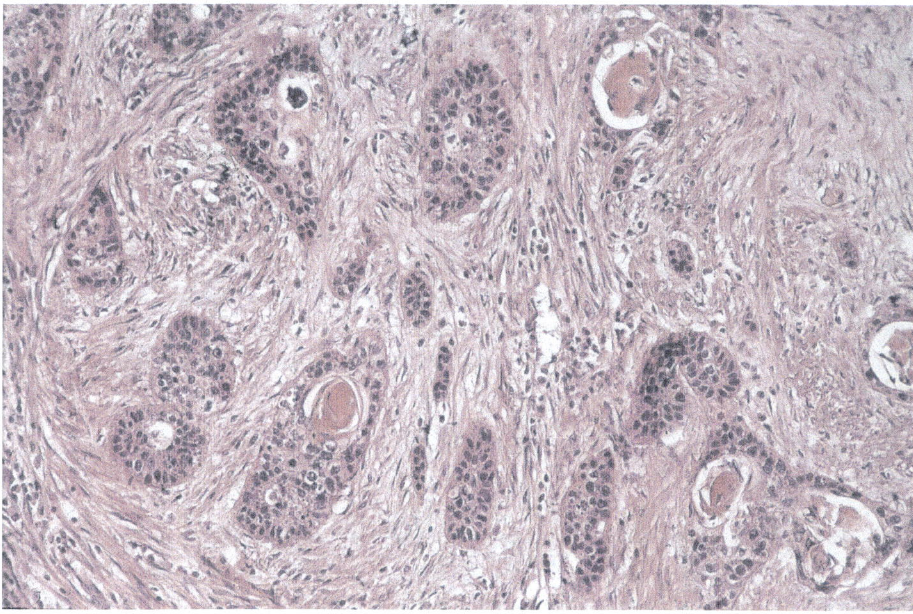

Fig. 210. Adenosquamous carcinoma, with formation of keratin pearls. H&E

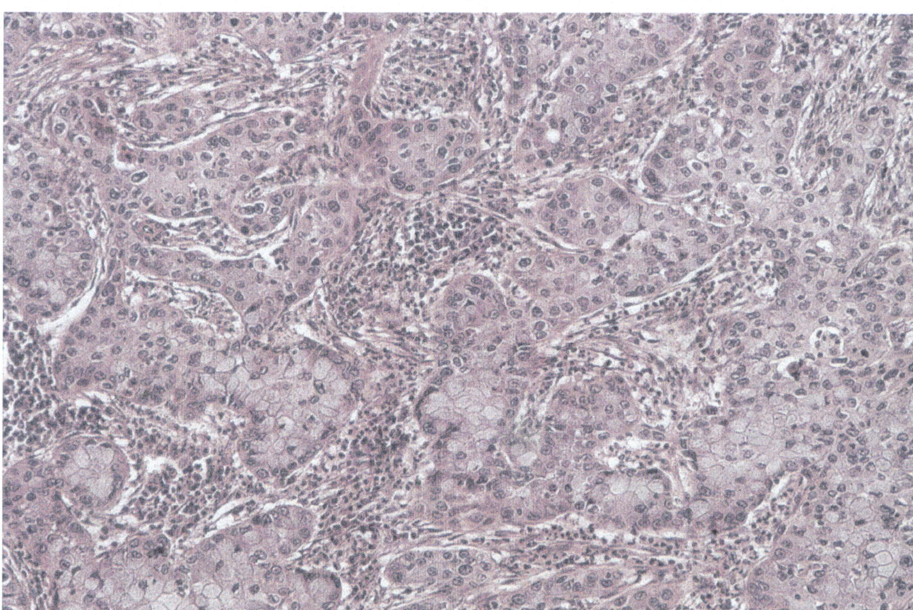

Fig. 211. Adenosquamous carcinoma, with predominant mucinous differentiation. H&E

■ **Differential Diagnosis.** Distinguishing an endocervical carcinoma from a primary adenosquamous carcinoma or adenoacanthoma of the endometrium is possible immunohistochemically. The endocervical carcinomas are nearly always positive for CEA and always negative for vimentin, and most of them are HPV-positive.

Mucoepidermoid Carcinoma [8560/3]

The *mucoepidermoid carcinoma* (Figs. 212–215) differs from the adenosquamous carcinoma by its mono- or multicellular production of mucin within solid strands of squamoid cells. Mono- or multicellular keratinization is often evident in cells neighboring mucin-secreting cells (Figs. 214, 215). Histogenetically, these carcinomas also originate from bipotential reserve cells that are intermixed (Figs. 212, 213). In poorly differentiated forms of mucoepidermoid carcinoma, mucin production may be discrete and only detectable when a PAS reaction is used. With this stain, it readily becomes apparent that the percentage of mucin-secreting squamous carcinomas is surprisingly high (Hellweg 1957; Benda et al. 1985).

■ **Differential Diagnosis.** The distinction between mucoepidermoid (mixed) and squamous carcinomas is of clinical importance, since mixed carcinomas metastasize to pelvic lymph nodes in 30% of the patients compared with 7% in nonmucin-producing carcinomas (Benda et al. 1985). In comparison, the metastatic rate to pelvic lymph nodes of pure adenocarcinomas is said to be about 15%. In spite of this, the prognosis in patients with adenocarcinomas is even worse than in those with mixed mucin-producing tumors, apparently because of the early vascular invasion of the adenocarcinomas.

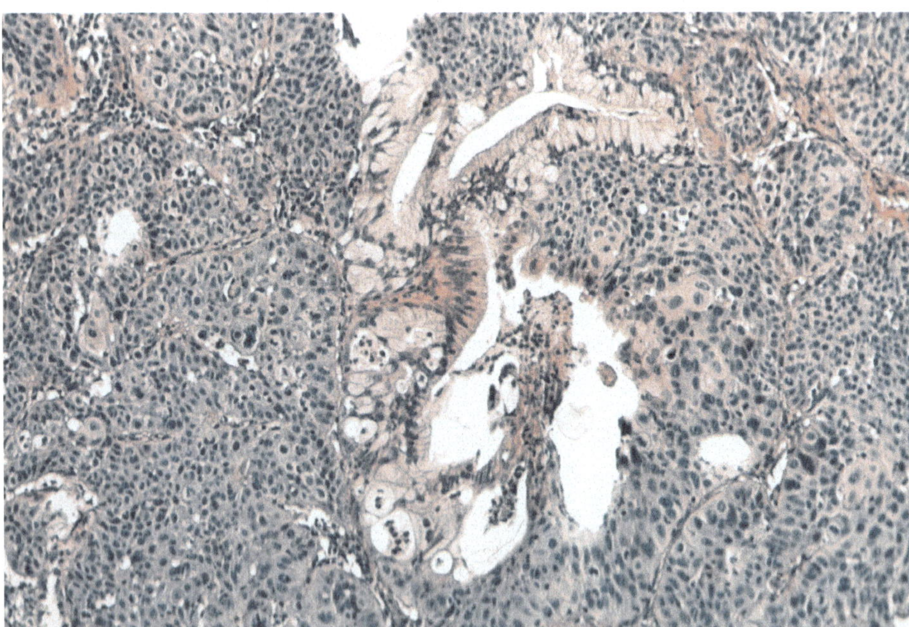

Fig. 212. Mucoepidermoid carcinoma. H&E

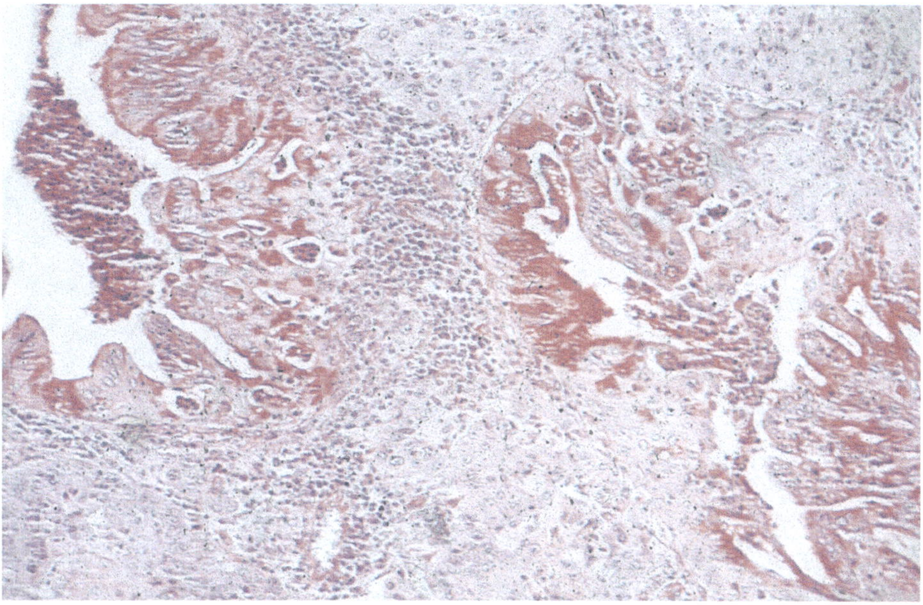

Fig. 213. Mucoepidermoid carcinoma. PAS reaction

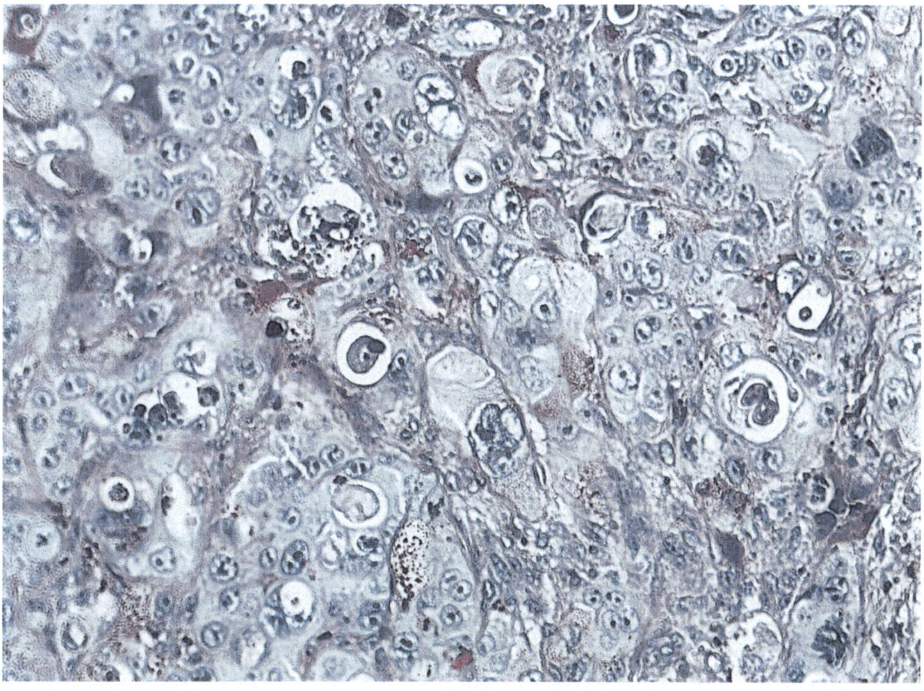

Fig. 214. Mucoepidermoid carcinoma, monocellular mucin formation. PAS reaction

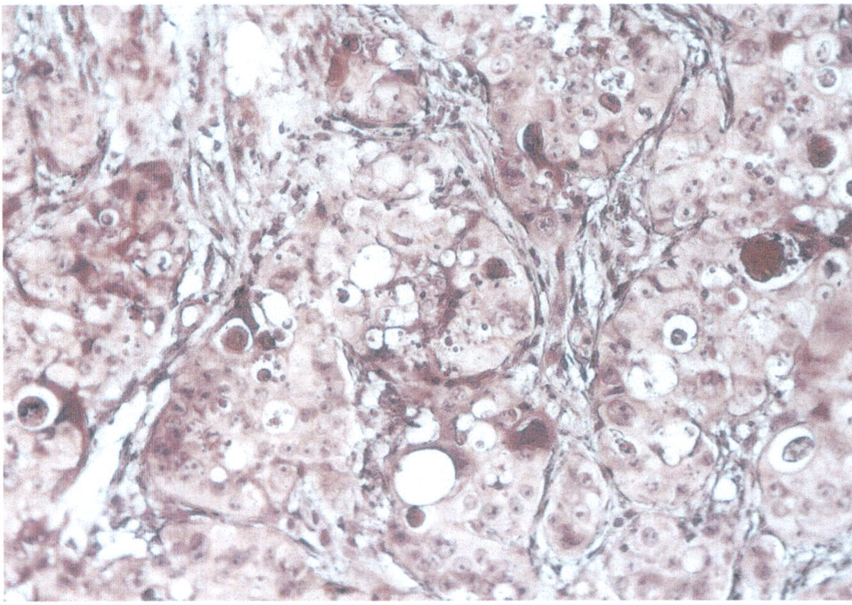

Fig. 215. Mucoepidermoid carcinoma, monocellular keratinization. Phloxine-tartrazine stain

Adenoid Type (Figs. 216–219)

Adenoid Cystic Carcinoma [8200/3]

The *adenoid cystic carcinoma* (Figs. 216–218) is characterized by a cribriform or cylindromatous pattern. It is composed of fairly uniform, small basaloid cells with scanty cytoplasm and rounded or angulated hyperchromatic nuclei. These cells form small branching (Fig. 216) or larger strands (Fig. 218), surround small or larger cysts (Fig. 217), or form small acini filled with a hyaline or basement membrane-like material rich in acid mucopolysaccharides. This tumor is often associated with foci of squamous cell or adenocarcinoma. Adenoid cystic carcinomas show early lymphatic invasion and are more aggressive than most cervical adenocarcinomas (Hoskins et al. 1979; Ferry and Scully 1988; Grayson et al. 1999).

Adenoid Basal Carcinoma [8092/3]

The *adenoid basal carcinoma* (Fig. 219) must be differentiated from the adenoid cystic carcinoma because of its much better prognosis (Hart 2002). It consists of small, round to oval branching nests of cells, resembling those of basal cell carcinoma of the skin, with palisading of the peripheral cell layers. There are no or only rare cystic pseudoglands. The tumor cells are small and uniform, with rounded hyperchromatic nuclei in scanty cytoplasm. Mitoses are infrequent.

Adenoid cystic and adenoid basal carcinoma have a similar cytoskeleton of intermediate filaments, which indicates they apparently arise from pluripotent reserve cells of the endocervix (Ferry and Scully 1988; Grayson et al. 1999).

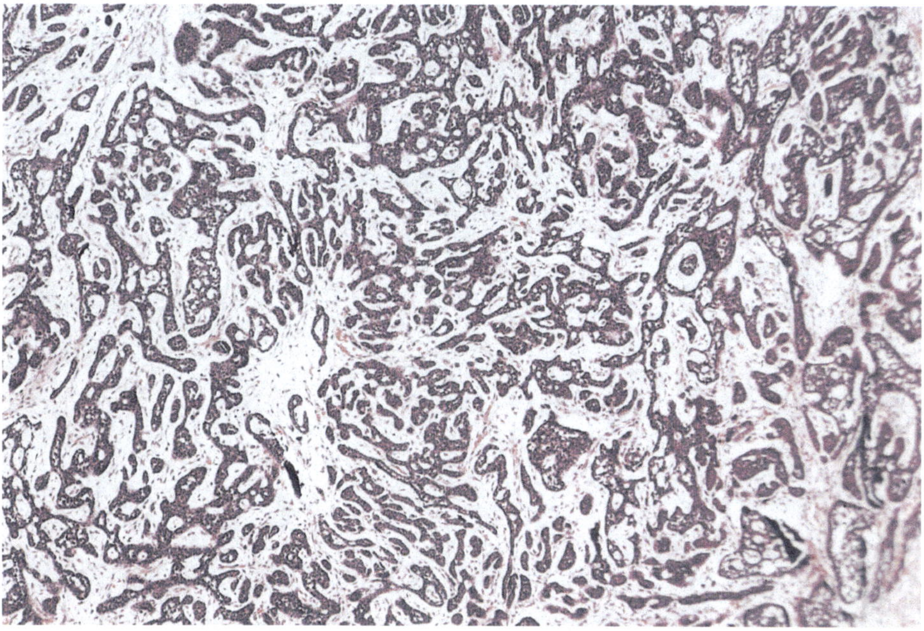

Fig. 216. Adenoid cystic carcinoma. H&E

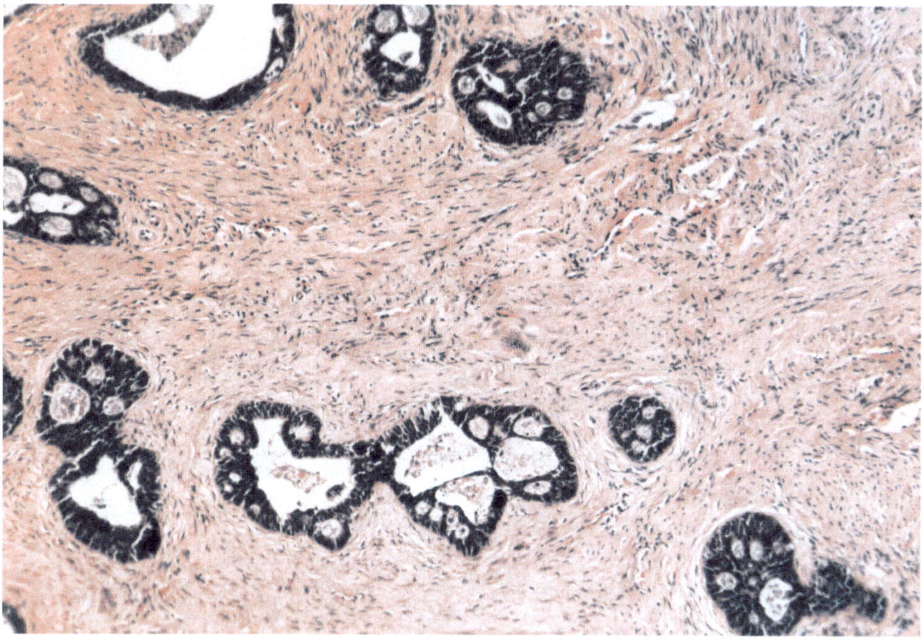

Fig. 217. Adenoid cystic carcinoma. H&E, higher magnification

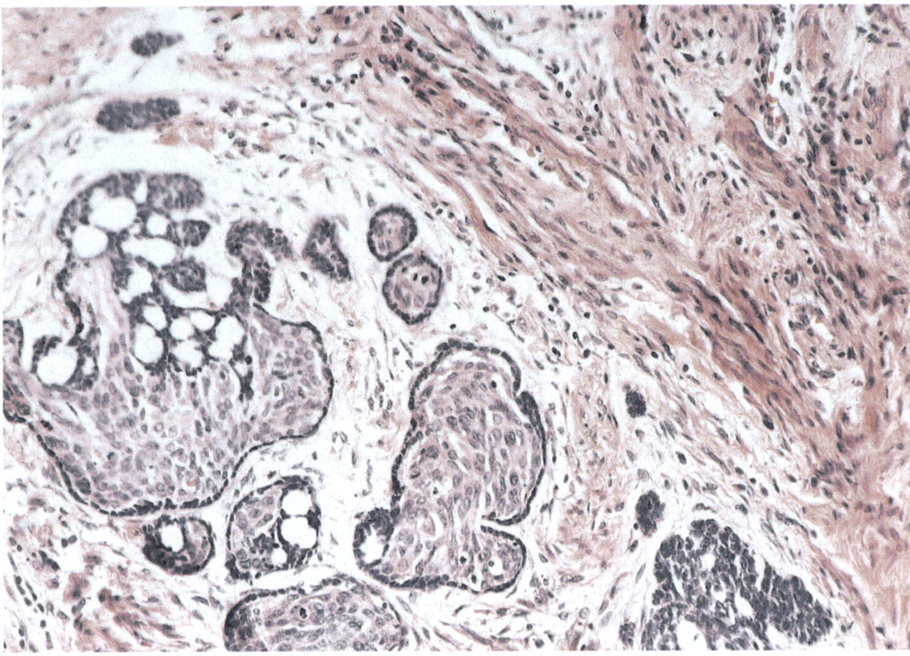

Fig. 218. Adenoid cystic carcinoma, with foci of squamoid differentiation. H&E, higher magnification

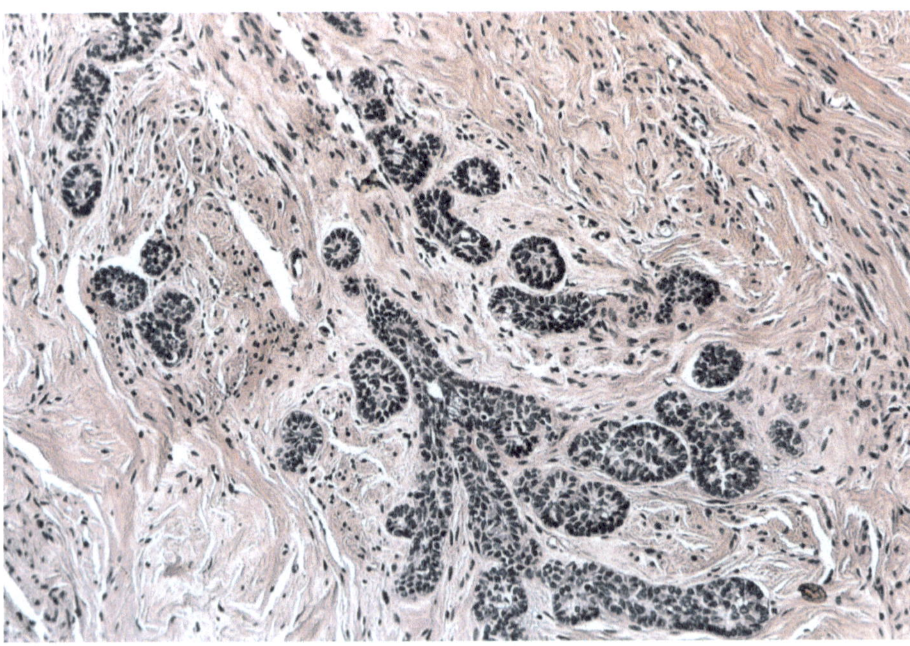

Fig. 219. Adenoid basal carcinoma. H&E

Differential Diagnosis. It is important to distinguish adenoid basal from adenoid cystic carcinoma because a patient with adenoid basal carcinoma has a much more favorable prognosis; only a simple hysterectomy is required (van Dinh and Woodruff 1985). Histological differentiation is possible by applying the different architectural and cytological features described above.

Neuroendocrine Type (Fig. 220)

This group includes carcinoids, atypical carcinoids, and small cell and large cell neuroendocrine carcinomas (Albores-Saavedra et al. 1997; Straughn et al. 2001). Neuroendocrine carcinomas most likely develop from neuroendocrine cells occurring in the normal endocervix (Scully et al. 1984; Fetissof et al. 1985), or from stimulated multipotential reserve cells of the endocervical epithelium undergoing neuroendocrine metaplasia and hyperplasia (Chan et al. 1989). They may be fairly well differentiated (carcinoids) or poorly differentiated (small cell carcinomas).

Carcinoid tumors [8240/3] of the cervix are thought to originate from endocervical argyrophil cells. The tumors consist of rather uniform, small, round or ovoid cells growing in solid sheets, small lobules, or trabeculae. They are usually benign. Occasionally, flattened cells line glandlike, mucin-containing microcysts. The slightly elongated nuclei of the tumor cells have a coarse chromatin pattern. Atypical carcinoids [8249/3] show cytologic atypia and contain foci of necrosis. Mitoses are frequent. Vascular invasion is often obvious, giving evidence of the malignant behavior of these tumors.

Small cell carcinomas of neuroendocrine origin [8041/3] (Fig. 220) are considered to be the poorly differentiated variety of carcinoid tumors, resembling small cell carcino-

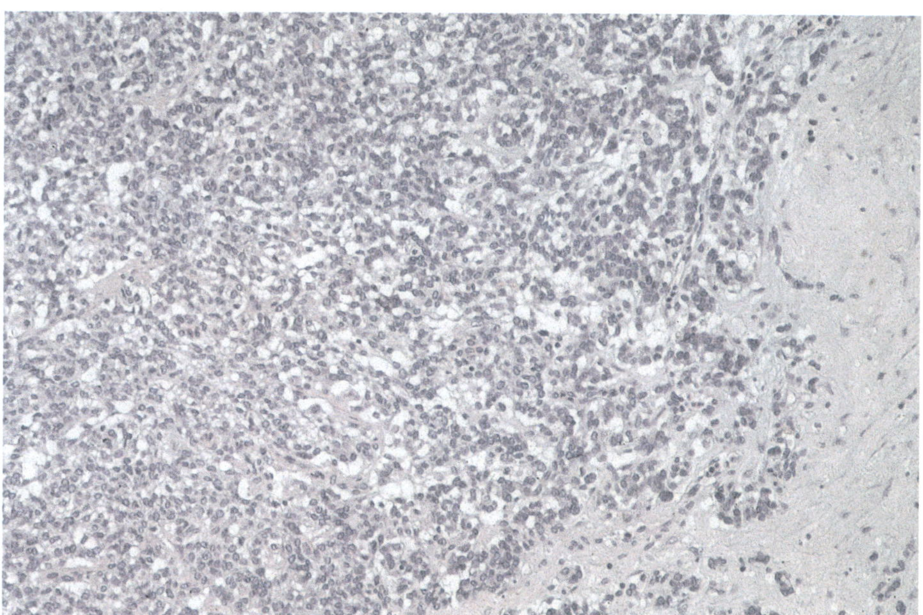

Fig. 220. Neuroendocrine (small cell) carcinoma. H&E

mas of the lung (Abeler et al. 1994; Bermudez et al. 2001), although mutations of p53 and LOH are less common in the cervical tumor. Almost all neuroendocrine carcinomas of the cervix are associated with HPV 18 (Stoler et al. 1991; Ishida et al. 2004) or seldom HPV 16. Squamous or glandular differentiation may be present (Mannion et al. 1998). The cells of these tumors are spindle shaped. Mitoses are numerous. Their scanty cytoplasm contains argyrophilic neurosecretory granules, demonstrable by the Grimelius stain (Yamasaki et al. 1984), S100, or by specific neuroendocrine markers such as NSE, chromogranin A, and synaptophysin (Hachitanda et al. 1989). Among these, CD 56, a neural cell adhesion molecule, appears to be the most sensitive marker (Albores-Saavedra et al. 2005).

■ **Large cell neuroendocrine carcinomas** [8013/3] are very rare. Their cells contain large nuclei with prominent nucleoli in abundant cytoplasm. Mitoses are very frequent. The cells are positive for cytokeratin, chromogranin and focally contain mucin. Most of these tumors contain foci of in situ or invasive adenocarcinoma (Gilks et al. 1997). Since both tumor components are positive for chromogranin, they are most likely of common origin with divergent differentiation (Cui et al. 2001).

Neuroectodermal Type (Figs. 221–223)

Primitive neuroectodermal tumors (PNET) of the cervix are very rare. We observed a very undifferentiated cervical tumor in a 29-year-old woman. The solid, round, and small-celled tumor was negative with most of the markers for intracytoplasmatic intermediate filaments, including cytokeratins, S100, and CEA, but showed a distinct immunohistochemical reaction for NSE.

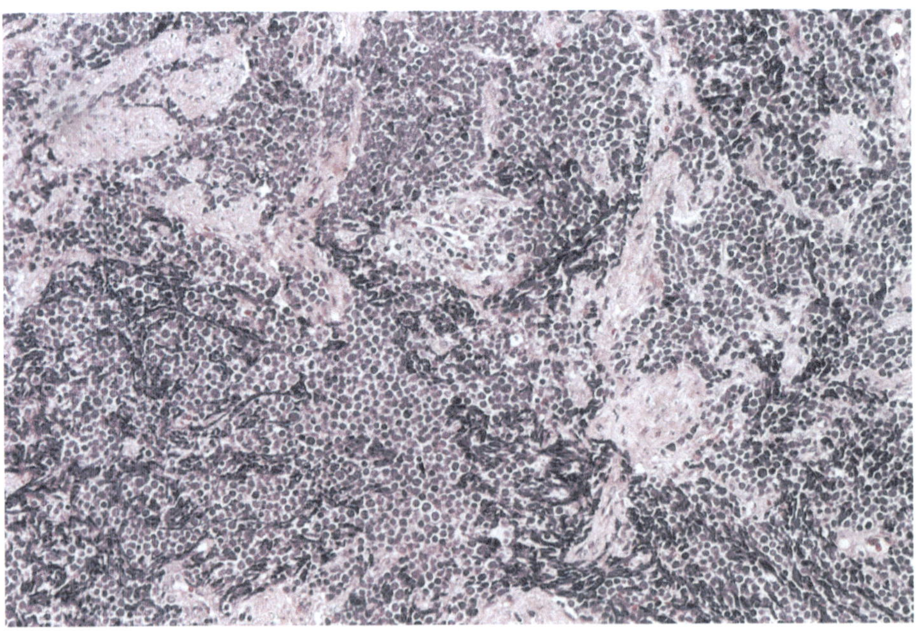

Fig. 221. Primitive neuroectodermal tumor. H&E

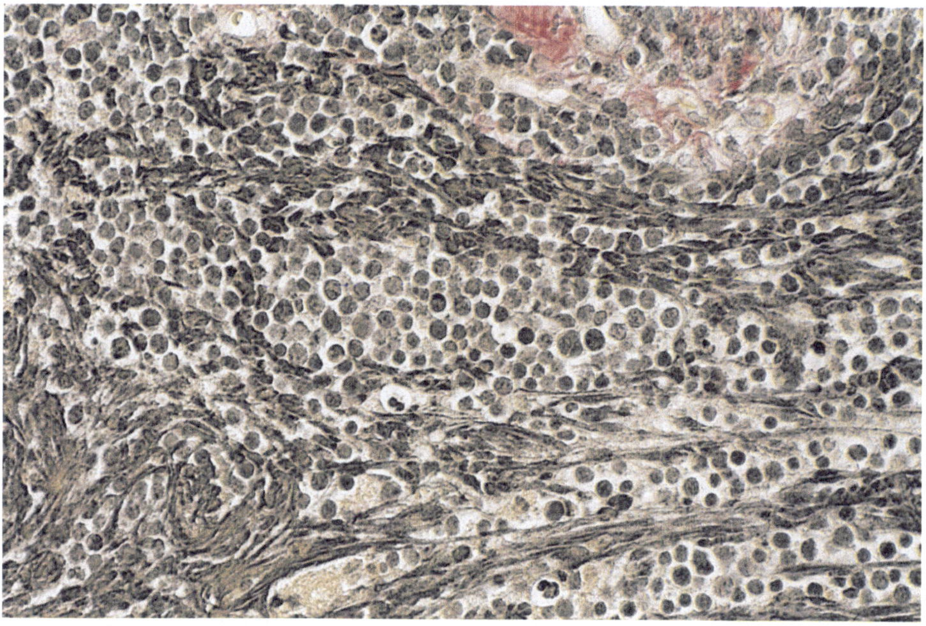

Fig. 222. Primitive neuroectodermal tumor. Van Gieson's stain

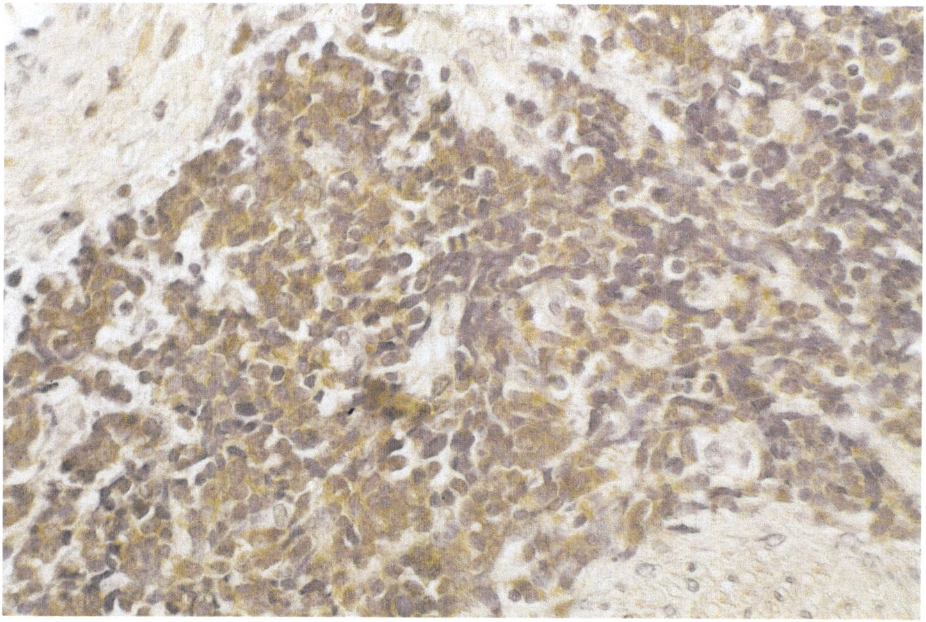

Fig. 223. Primitive neuroectodermal tumor. Immunohistochemical reaction with NSE

Differential Diagnosis. Carcinoid tumors can be distinguished from adenosquamous carcinomas by detecting neuroendocrine granules in the carcinoid cells (Grimelius stain). Small cell neuroendocrine carcinomas must be differentiated from nonendocrine, poorly differentiated small cell carcinomas of the reserve cell type, with which they have often been confused (Groben et al. 1985), although the small cell carcinomas lack neuroendocrine differentiation (Fujii et al. 1986). With the aid of immunohistochemistry, it has become obvious that not all small cell carcinomas of the cervix are of neuroendocrine origin (Ulich et al. 1986; Ueda et al. 1989). Since most neuroendocrine carcinomas are also positive for CEA and cytokeratin (Gersell et al. 1988), a distinction from undifferentiated reserve cell carcinomas is only possible with markers for neurosecretory granules.

Primitive neuroectodermal tumors can be distinguished from small cell carcinomas and from neuroendocrine tumors by their negative reaction for cytokeratins, CEA, and S-100. Hence, one should not be satisfied in saying an undifferentiated tumor is unclassifiable before attempting to detect specific intermediate filaments with immunohistochemical methods.

In general, patients with neuroendocrine tumors of the cervix seem to have a poor prognosis, regardless of type (Walker et al. 1988). According to recent observations, however, patients with tumors of neural crest origin (neuroendocrine carcinomas), which reacted positively with S-100 had a much more favorable prognosis than those with S-100-negative neuroblastic tumors (Aoyama et al. 1990). By collecting such observations, differences in clinical behavior between small cell carcinomas of neuroendocrine or reserve cell origin may become obvious.

Mesenchymal Tumors (Figs. 224, 225)

Primary mesenchymal tumors of the cervix are rare compared with their counterparts in the uterine corpus, to which they are structurally identical. *Leiomyosarcomas* [8890/3] (Fig. 224) consist of pleomorphic myoblasts with polyploid nuclei. *Endometrial stromal sarcomas* [8931/3] resemble endometrial stromal cells. *Rhabdomyosarcomas* and *chondrosarcomas* (Fig. 225) may occur in adults in the pure form or as part of a *mesodermal mixed tumor* (Fig. 228, 229). The same holds true for *osteosarcoma* (Bloch et al. 1988) and *angiosarcoma* [9120/3]. The primary occurrence of an *alveolar soft part sarcoma* [9581/3] in the uterine cervix is extremely rare (Flint et al. 1985). They are histologically similar to those in other sites, but appear to have a better prognosis (Nielsen et al. 1995).

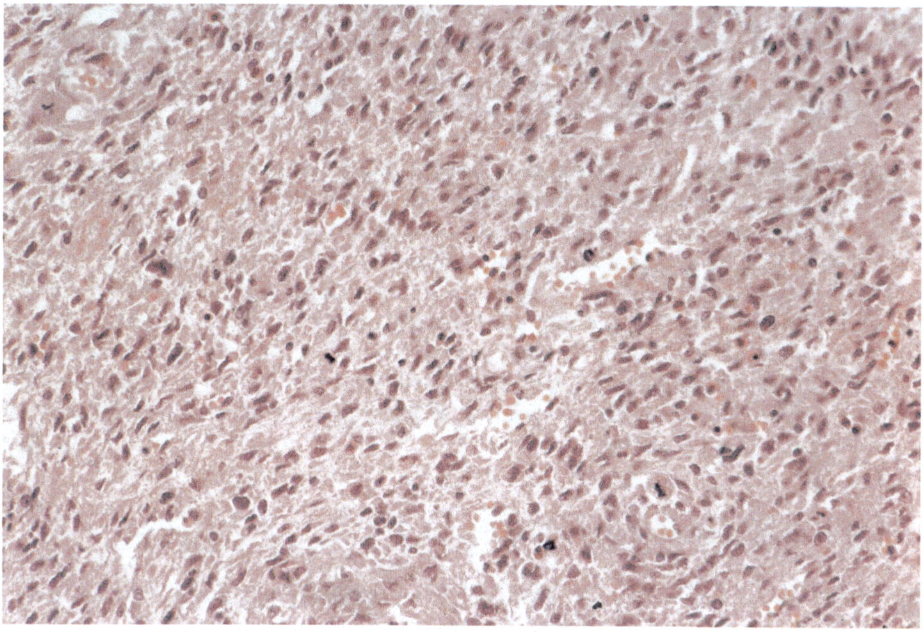

Fig. 224. Leiomyosarcoma. H&E

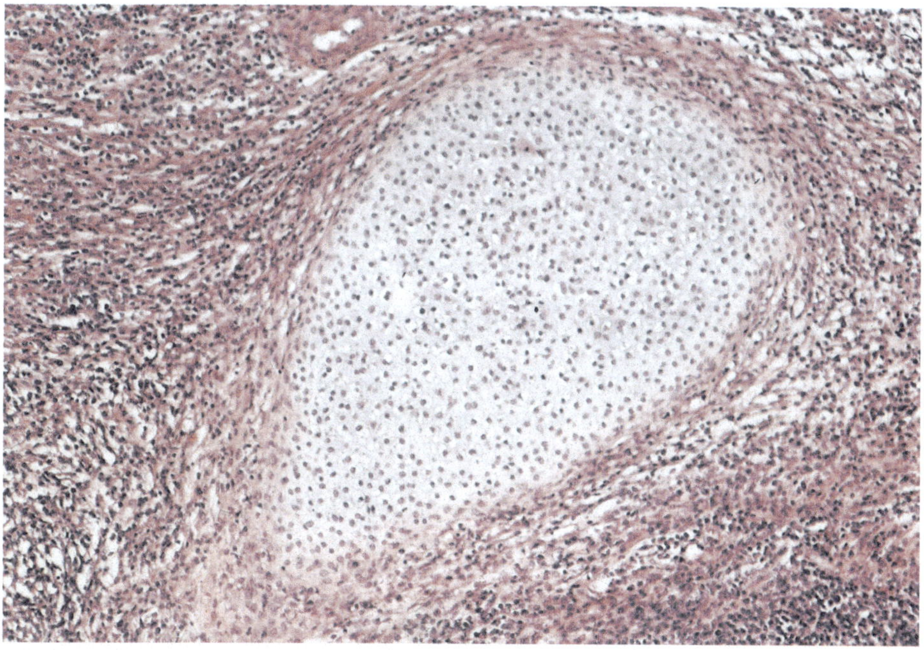

Fig. 225. Chondrosarcoma. H&E

Mixed Epithelial and Mesenchymal Tumors (Figs. 226–235)

Carcinosarcoma

Carcinosarcomas (Figs. 226, 227) and *malignant Müllerian mixed tumors* [8980/3] (-Figs. 228–230) are identical to and often part of the corresponding tumors of the uterine corpus. Carcinosarcomas consist of carcinomatous glands of endometrial, mucinous, or occasionally clear cell type, and sarcomatous fibroblasts or stromal cells. The malignant Müllerian mixed tumors, on the other hand, are composed of heterologous epithelial and mesenchymal elements, and may show a great variety of structures. The sarcomatous component, in particular, may be very pleomorphic, forming rhabdomyoblasts (Fig. 228), chondroblasts (Fig. 229), or osteoblasts (Fig. 230). When large enough sections are available for study, the recognition of a malignant Müllerian mixed tumor is no problem (Clement et al. 1998).

Müllerian Adenosarcoma [8933/3] (Figs. 231, 232)

The *Müllerian adenosarcoma* usually arises from the endometrium, but occasionally from the endocervix. It consists of sarcomatous endocervical stromal cells and fibroblasts focally intermingled with rhabdomyoblasts. The mitotic activity is moderate (Clement and Scully 1974; Zaloudek and Norris 1981). Round concentric hypercellular foci form perivascular nodules and periglandular cuffs (Fig. 231, 232). A few slitlike remnants of benign endocervical glands may be found surrounded by compact sarcoma cells. Long invaginations of the endocervical surface epithelium may produce fingerlike protrusions at the tumor periphery. Adult women with adenosarcoma have a more favorable prognosis than those with other types of sarcoma.

■ **Differential Diagnosis.** Distinguishing carcinosarcoma from malignant Müllerian mixed tumor is possible by carefully evaluating the epithelial components. In the Müllerian adenosarcoma, there are no carcinomatous cells; only benign glandular structures may be seen.

Embryonal Rhabdomyosarcoma [8910/3] (Figs. 233–235)

The *embryonal rhabdomyosarcoma* [8910/3] (sarcoma botryoides; Figs. 233–235) has its peak incidence in young girls and adolescents (Brand et al. 1987; Daya and Scully 1988). Chromosomal abnormalities have been detected in isolated cases (Palazzo et al. 1993; Semczuk et al. 1999). On gross examination, its grapelike protrusions may grow beyond the external cervical os and protrude into the vagina. Microscopically, it consists of immature rhabdomyoblasts of the embryonal type, which occasionally may be mature enough to form cross striations (Fig. 235). Cords of glandlike structures of carcinomatous cells may be found among the sarcomatous elements; mitoses are frequent. Prognosis is much less favorable than it is for adult women with adenosarcoma.

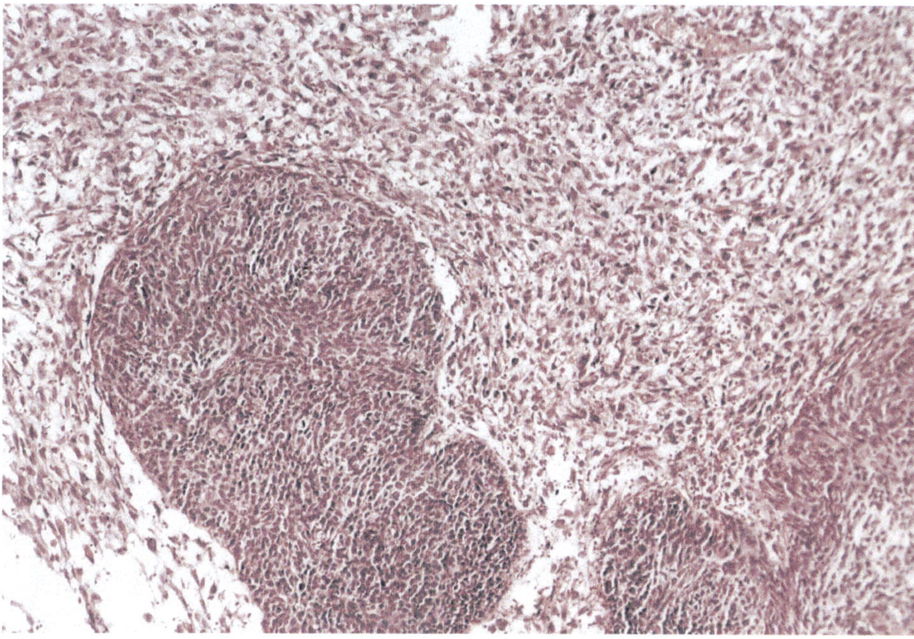

Fig. 226. Carcinosarcoma with solid epithelial nests. H&E

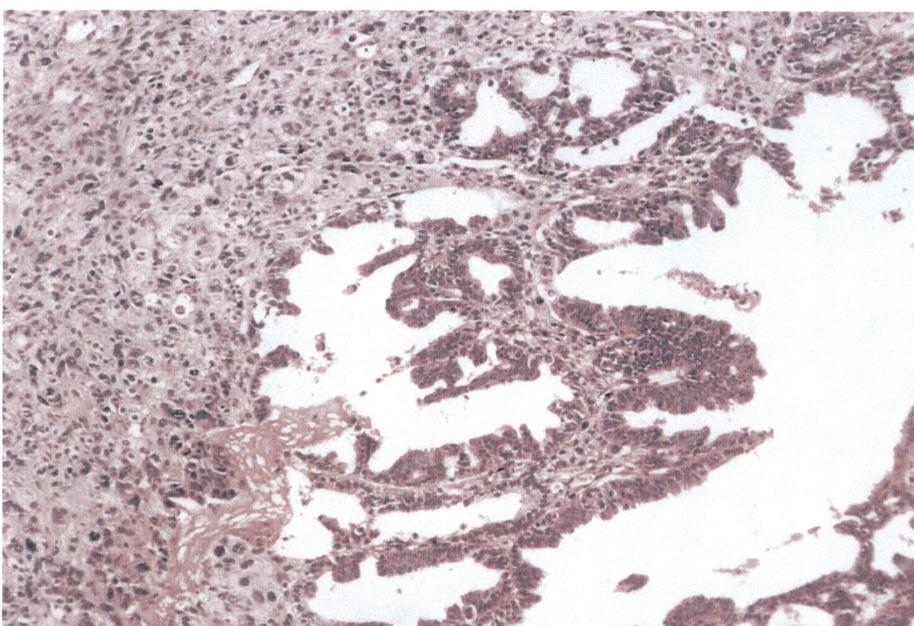

Fig. 227. Carcinosarcoma with gland formation. H&E

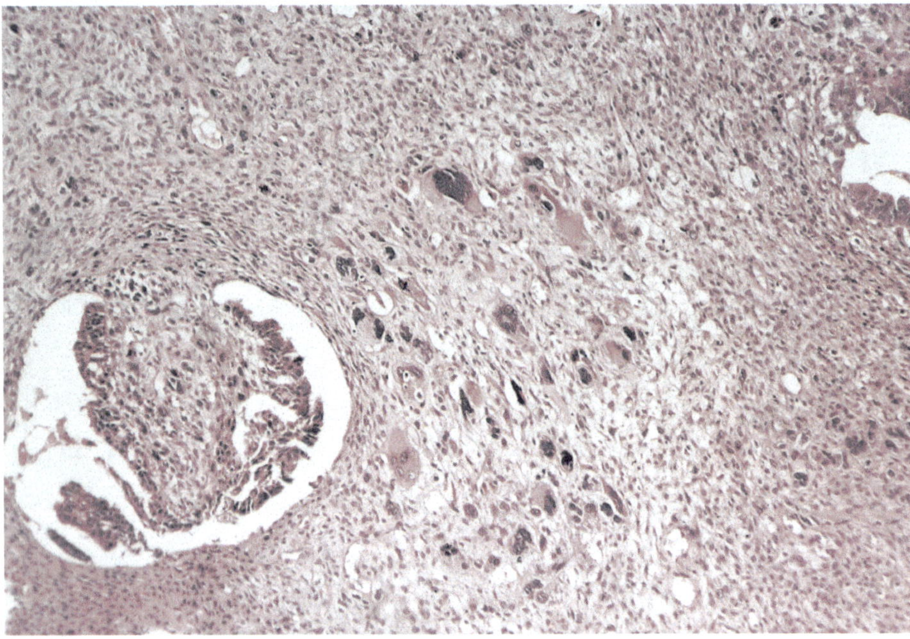

Fig. 228. Malignant Müllerian mixed tumor, with rhabdomyoblasts. H&E

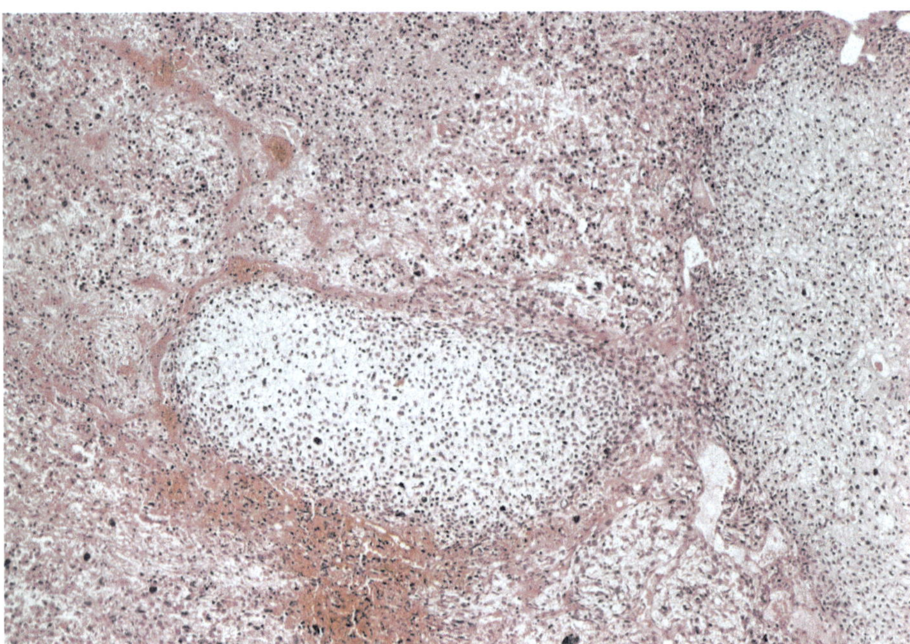

Fig. 229. Malignant Müllerian mixed tumor, with chondroblasts. H&E

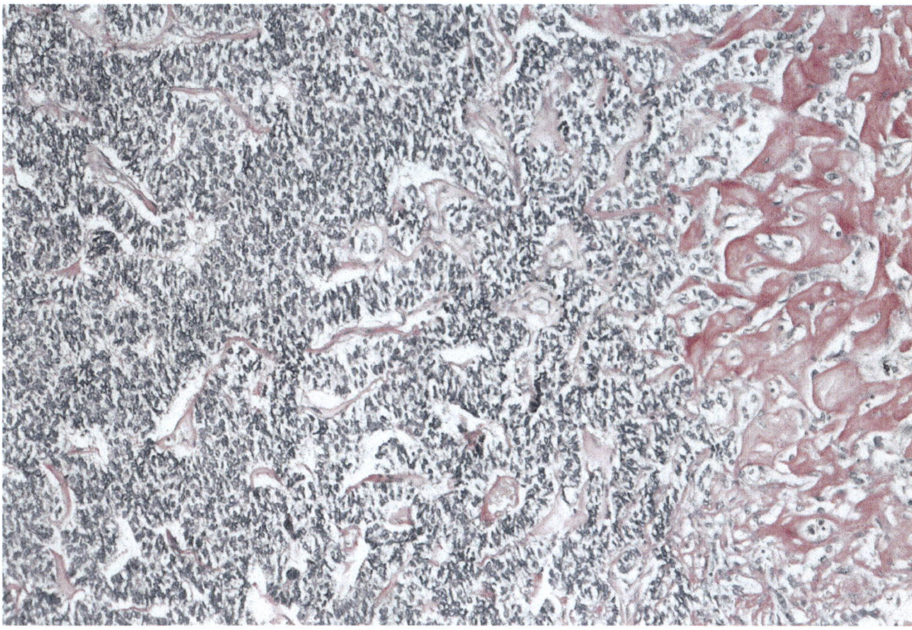

Fig. 230. Malignant Müllerian mixed tumor, with osteoblasts. H&E

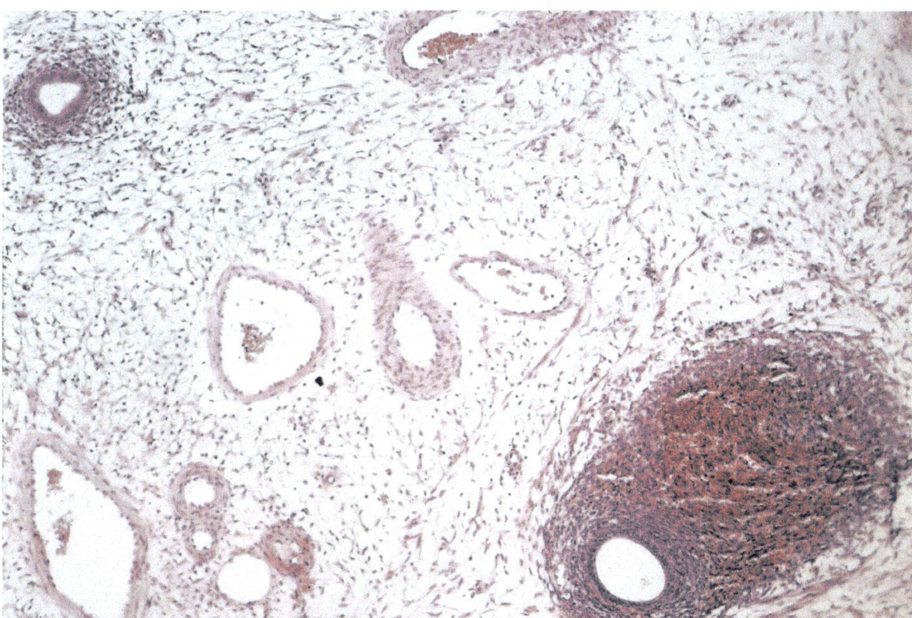

Fig. 231. Müllerian adenosarcoma. H&E

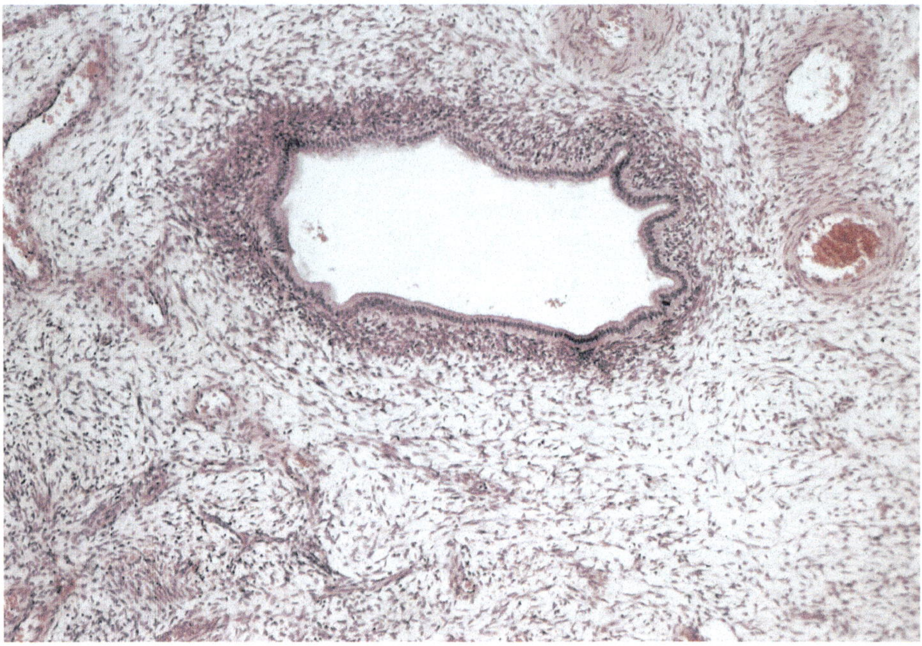

Fig. 232. Müllerian adenosarcoma. H&E

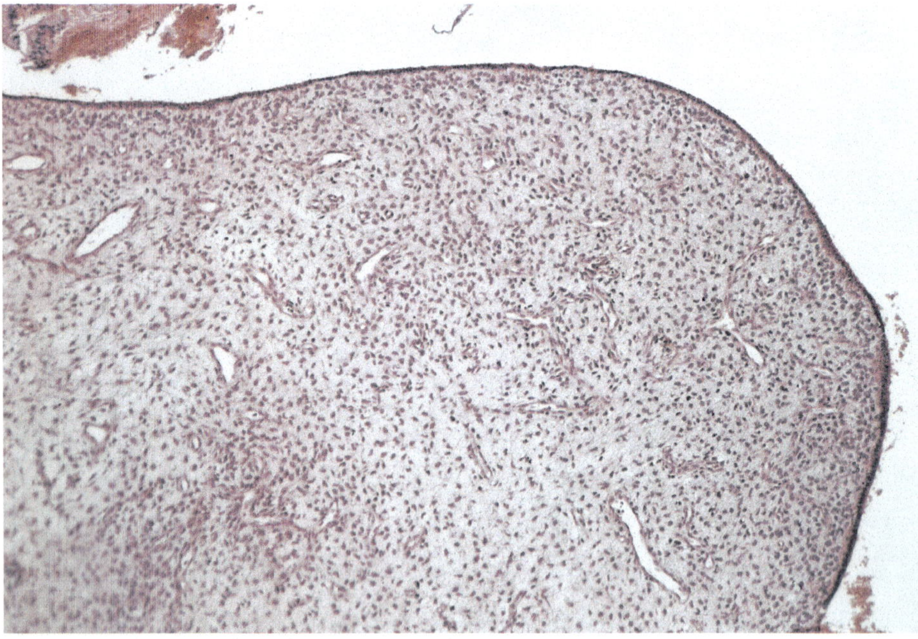

Fig. 233. Embryonal rhabdomyosarcoma. H&E

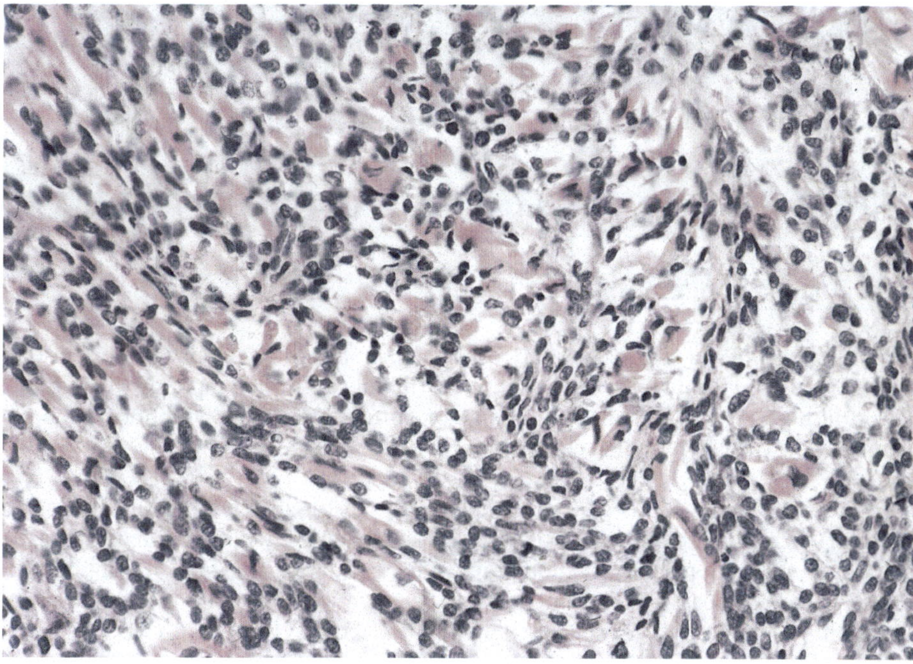

Fig. 234. Embryonal rhabdomyosarcoma. H&E, higher magnification

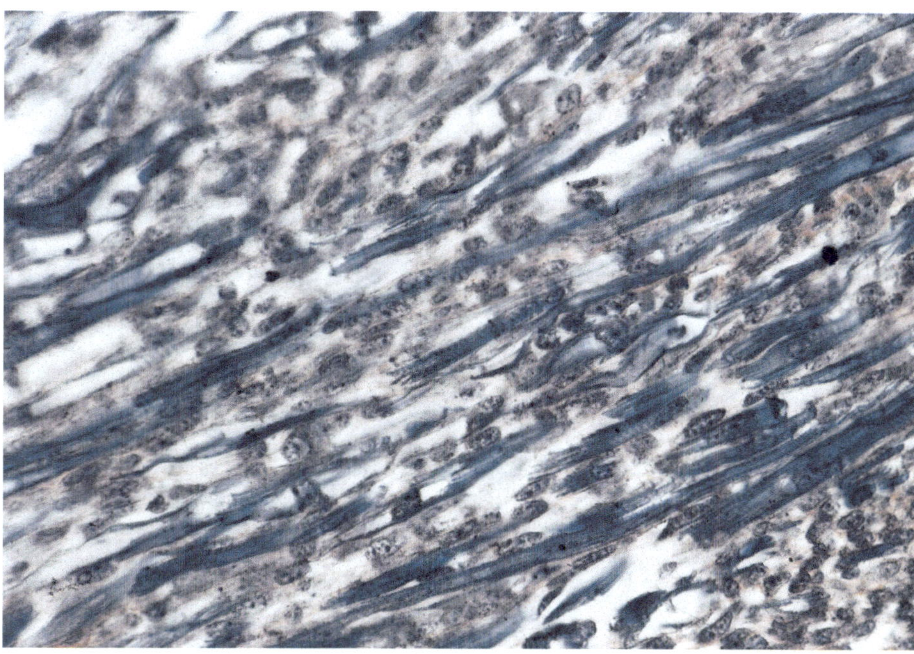

Fig. 235. Embryonal rhabdomyosarcoma. PTAH stain

Wilms Tumor [8960/3]

Only occasional cases of *Wilms tumor* [8960/3] arising in the cervix have been described, resembling that of the kidney (Babin et al. 2000)

Miscellaneous Tumors

Malignant Lymphomas (Figs. 236, 237)

Malignant lymphomas (Fig. 236) rarely occur as primary or secondary tumors in the cervix (Harris and Scully 1984; Vang et al. 2000), mainly as B-cell lymphomas with nodular or diffuse pattern (follicular lymphoma or diffuse large B-cell lymphoma according to the new WHO lymphoma classification (Stein 2000)).

■ **Differential Diagnosis.** It is clinically important to distinguish lymphomas from undifferentiated small or large cell carcinomas, since malignant lymphomas may be treated successfully with specific chemotherapy. Further subclassification of lymphomas permits even more precise recommendations for therapy. This distinction is possible immunohistochemically with specific markers, e.g., CD 20 (L26) for B-cells (Fig. 237) and Ki-67 for determining the growth fraction (Dallenbach et al. 2000). Marginal zone B-cell lymphomas of MALT type (CD 20-negative, but IgM-positive) are extremely rare in the cervix (Dallenbach et al. 2000). They may grossly resemble an endocervical polyp (Rossi et al. 2001). Secondary involvement of the cervix by a systemic lymphoma must

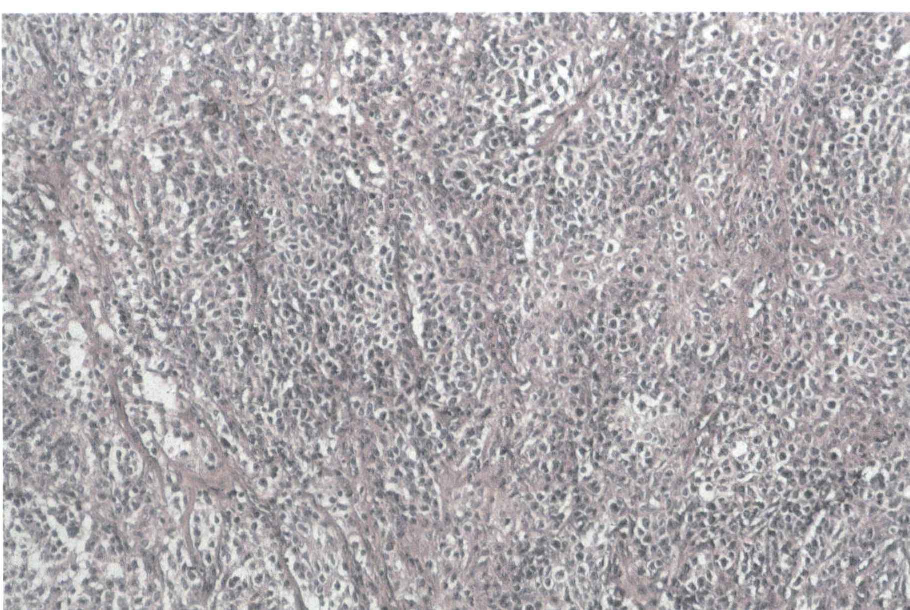

Fig. 236. Diffuse large B-cell lymphoma, multilobulated centroblastic type. H&E

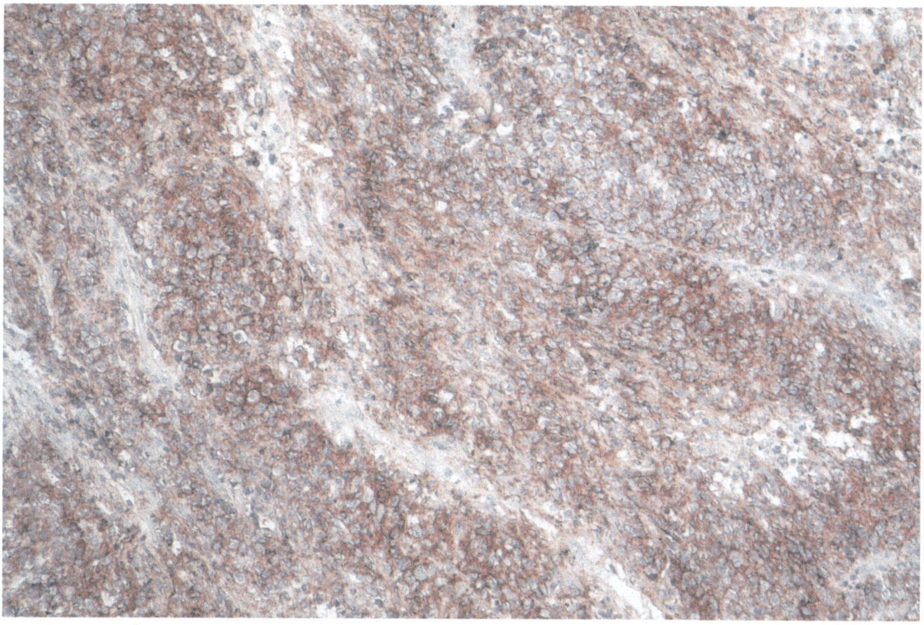

Fig. 237. Diffuse large B-cell lymphoma. Immunohistochemical reaction with CD 20 (L 26)

always be considered, but can only be distinguished clinically. Discriminating malignant lymphoma from benign lymphoma-like lesions may be difficult (Young et al. 1985). Surface ulcerations and mixed infiltrates of acute inflammatory cells and plasma cells are rarely seen in lymphomas, whereas deep extension into the cervix and cellular monomorphism are usually absent in benign inflammatory conditions.

Granulocytic Sarcoma

Granulocytic sarcoma of the cervix is an extremely rare local tumorous manifestation and precursor of myelogenous leukemia (Abeler et al. 1983; Banik et al. 1989). Its differentiation from malignant lymphoma or small cell carcinoma may be impossible in routine histological sections. Special stains, like the immunohistochemical detection of lysozyme, are useful. Granulocytic sarcoma also express CD43 and CD68, but are negative for CD20 (Oliva et al. 1997).

Malignant Melanoma [8720/3] (Fig. 238)

It is extremely rare for the cervix to be the primary tumor site for *malignant melanoma* (Fig. 238). Only a few cases have been reported in the literature (Hall et al. 1980) and recently summarized (Holmquist and Torres 1988; Cantuaria et al. 1999). Histogenetically, the tumor is of melanocytic origin. Occasional melanocytes can be found in the normal ectocervical epithelium (Stegner 1959). As in the skin, or elsewhere, the tumor is composed of pleomorphic round to spindle-shaped cells containing varying amounts of

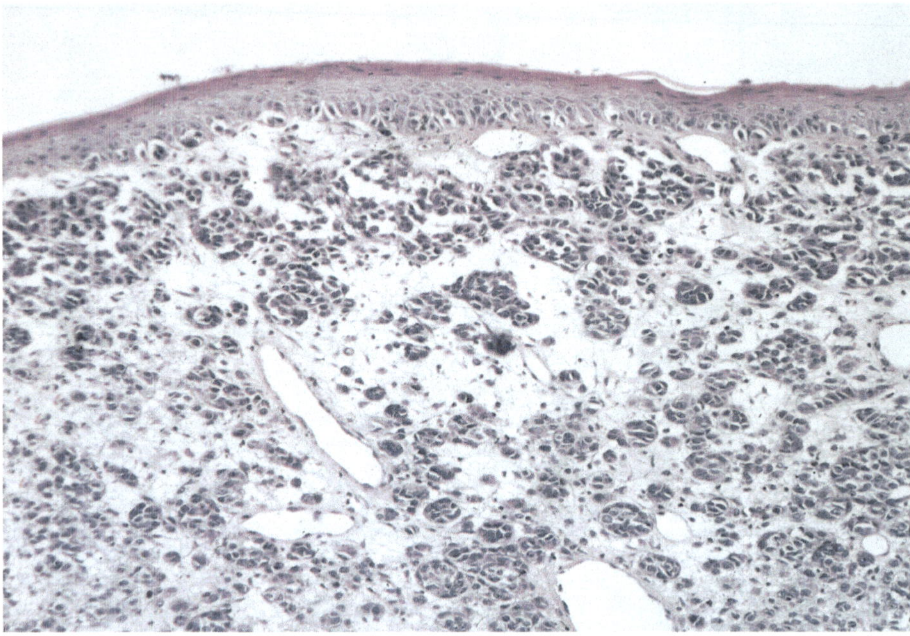

Fig. 238. Malignant melanoma. H&E

fine melanin pigment (Fig. 238). The tumor cells spread diffusely throughout the cervix, while the covering ectocervical epithelium usually remains intact. When melanin pigment is absent or very scanty, it is possible to distinguish the melanoma from undifferentiated carcinomas or sarcomas with the S-100 reaction, which is consistently positive in malignant melanoma.

Endodermal Sinus (Yolk Sac) Tumor [9071/3]

Endodermal sinus (yolk sac) tumor [9071/3] may also arise within the cervix (Copeland et al. 1985).

Secondary Tumors (Fig. 239)

Pelvic carcinomas, mainly those arising in the endometrium, ovary, rectum, and bladder, may extend into the cervix (Lemoine and Hall 1986; Mulvany et al. 1996). Distinguishing metastatic tumors from primary endocervical adenocarcinoma is often possible immunohistochemically (see p. 11, 148). Metastases from distant primary tumors are rare. If they occur, the primary site most likely will be the breast (Fig. 239) or the gastrointestinal tract (Zhang et al. 1983).

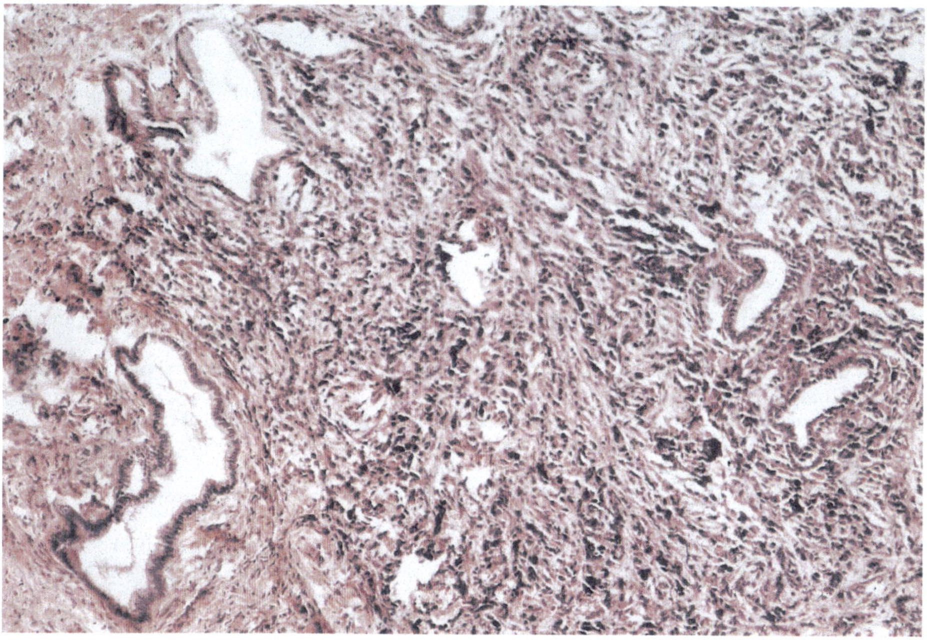

Fig. 239. Metastatic carcinoma from primary breast carcinoma. H&E

References

Abeler V, Kjorstad KE, Langholm R, Marton PF (1983) Granulocytic sarcoma (chloroma) of the uterine cervix: report of two cases. Int J Gynecol Pathol 2: 88–92

Abeler VM, Holm R, Nesland JM, Kjorstad KE (1994) Small cell carcinoma of the cervix. A clinicopathologic study of 26 patients. Cancer 73: 672–677

Abell MR (1971) Papillary adenofibroma of the uterine cervix. Am J Obstet Gynecol 110: 990–993

Abell MR, Gosling JR (1962) Gland cell carcinoma (adenocarcinoma) of the uterine cervix. Am J Obstet Gynecol 83: 729–755

Adcock LL, Julian TM, Okagaki T, Jones TK, Prem KA, Twiggs LB, Potish RA, Phillips GL (1982) Carcinoma of the uterine cervix FIGO Stage I-B. Gynecol Oncol 14: 199–208

al-Saleh W, Delvenne P, Greimers R, Fridman V, Doyen J, Boniver J (1995) Assessment of Ki-67 antigen immunostaining in squamous intraepithelial lesions of the uterine cervix. Correlation with the histologic grade and human papillomavirus type. Am J Clin Pathol 104: 154–160

Albores-Saavedra J, Gersell D, Gilks CB, Henson DE, Lindberg G, Santiago H, Scully RE, Silva E, Sobin LH, Tavassoli FJ, Travis WD, Woodruff JM (1997) Terminology of endocrine tumors of the uterine cervix: results of a workshop sponsored by the College of American Pathologists and the National Cancer Institute. Arch Pathol Lab Med 121: 34–39

Albores-Saavedra J, Latif S, Carrick KS, Alvaarado-Cabrerol, Fowler MR (2005) CD 56 reactivity in small cell carcinoma of the uterine cervix. Int J Gynecol Pathol 24: 113–117

Albores-Saavedra J, Young RH (1995) Transitional cell neoplasms (carcinomas and inverted papillomas) of the uterine cervix. A report of five cases. Am J Surg Pathol 19: 1138–1145

Alfsen GC, Kristensen GB, Skovlund E, Pettersen EO, Abeler VM (2001) Histologic subtype has minor importance for overall survival in patients with adenocarcinoma of the uterine cervix: a population-based study of prognostic factors in 505 patients with nonsquamous cell carcinomas of the cervix. Cancer 92: 2471–2483

Alkushi A, Irving J, Hsu F, Dupuis B, Liu CL, Rijn M, Gilks CB (2003) Immunoprofile of cervical and endometrial adenocarcinomas using a tissue microarray. Virchows Arch 442: 271–277

Alva J, Lauchlan SC (1975) The histogenesis of mixed cervical carcinomas. The concept of endocervical columnar-cell dysplasia. Am J Clin Pathol 64: 20–25

Ambros RA, Park JS, Shah KV, Kurman RJ (1991) Evaluation of histologic, morphometric, and immunohistochemical criteria in the differential diagnosis of small cell carcinomas of the cervix with particular reference to human papillomavirus types 16 and 18. Mod Pathol 4: 586–593

Ansari-Lari MA, Staebler A, Zaino RJ, Shah KV, Ronnett BM (2004) Distinction of endocervical and endometrial adenocarcinomas: immunohistochemical p16 expression correlated with human papillomavirus (HPV) DNA detection. Am J Surg Pathol 28: 160–167

Aoyama C, Qualman SJ, Regan M, Shimada H (1990) Histopathologic features of composite ganglioneuroblastoma. Immunohistochemical distinction of the stromal component is related to prognosis. Cancer 65: 255–264

Ayroud Y, Gelfand MM, Ferenczy A (1985) Florid mesonephric hyperplasia of the cervix: a report of a case with review of the literature. Int J Gynecol Pathol 4: 245–254

Babin EA, Davis JR, Hatch KD, Hallum AV 3rd (2000) Wilms' tumor of the cervix: a case report and review of the literature. Gynecol Oncol 76: 107–111

Banik S, Grech AB, Eyden BP (1989) Granulocytic sarcoma of the cervix: an immunohistochemical, histochemical, and ultrastructural study. J Clin Pathol 42: 483–488

Barker B, Garcia FA, Warner J, Lozerski J, Hatch K (2002) Baseline inaccuracy rates for the comparison of cervical biopsy to loop electrosurgical excision histopathologic diagnoses. Am J Obstet Gynecol 187: 349–352

Barter RA, Waters ED (1970) Cyto- and histo-morphology of cervical adenocarcinoma in situ. Pathology 2: 33–40
Beecham JB, Halvorsen T, Kolbenstvedt A (1978) Histologic classification, lymph node metastases, and patient survival in stage IB cervical carcinoma: an analysis of 245 uniformly treated cases. Gynecol Oncol 6: 95–105
Benda JA (1996) Histopathologic prognostic factors in early stage cervical carcinoma. J Natl Cancer Inst Monogr: 27–34
Benda JA, Platz CE, Buchsbaum H, Lifshitz S (1985) Mucin production in defining mixed carcinoma of the uterine cervix: a clinicopathologic study. Int J Gynecol Pathol 4: 314–327
Berdichevsky L, Karmin R, Chuang L (2004) Treatment of high-grade squamous intraepithelial lesions: a 2- versus 3-step approach. Am J Obstet Gynecol 190: 1424–1426
Bermudez A, Vighi S, Garcia A, Sardi J (2001) Neuroendocrine cervical carcinoma: a diagnostic and therapeutic challenge. Gynecol Oncol 82: 32–39
Bloch T, Roth LM, Stehman FB, Hull MT, Schwenk GR Jr. (1988) Osteosarcoma of the uterine cervix associated with hyperplastic and atypical mesonephric rests. Cancer 62: 1594–1600
Boon ME, Baak JP, Kurver PJ, Overdiep SH, Verdonk GW (1981) Adenocarcinoma in situ of the cervix: an underdiagnosed lesion. Cancer 48: 768–773
Boon ME, Kirk RS, Rietveld-Scheffers PE (1981) The morphogenesis of adenocarcinoma of the cervix – a complex pathological entity. Histopathology 5: 565–577
Bosch FX, Lörincz A, Munoz N, Meijer CJ, Shah KV (2002) The causal relation between human papillomavirus and cervical cancer. J Clin Pathol 55: 244–265
Boyes DA, Worth AJ, Fidler HK (1970) The results of treatment of 4389 cases of preclinical cervical squamous carcinoma. J Obstet Gynaecol Br Commonw 77: 769–780
Brand E, Berek JS, Nieberg RK, Hacker NF (1987) Rhabdomyosarcoma of the uterine cervix. Sarcoma botryoides. Cancer 60: 1552–1560
Brinck U, Jakob C, Bau O, Fuzesi L (2000) Papillary squamous cell carcinoma of the uterine cervix: report of three cases and a review of its classification. Int J Gynecol Pathol 19: 231–235
Brinton LA, Huggins GR, Lehman HF, Mallin K, Savitz DA, Trapido E, Rosenthal J, Hoover R (1986) Long-term use of oral contraceptives and risk of invasive cervical cancer. Int J Cancer 38: 339–344
Bulk S, Visser O, Rozendaal L, Verheijen RH, Meijer CJ (2005) Cervical cancer in the Netherlands 1989–1998: Decrease of squamous cell carcinoma in older women, increase of adenocarcinoma in younger women. Int J Cancer 113: 1005–1009
Bulten J, van der Laak JA, Gemmink JH, Pahlplatz MM, de Wilde PC, Hanselaar AG (1996) MIB1, a promising marker for the classification of cervical intraepithelial neoplasia. J Pathol 178: 268–273
Buntine DW (1979) Adenocarcinoma of the uterine cervix of probable Wolffian origin. Pathology 11: 713–718
Burd EM (2003) Human papillomavirus and cervical cancer. Clin Microbiol Rev 16: 1–17
Burger RA, Monk BJ, Kurosaki T, Anton-Culver H, Vasilev SA, Berman ML, Wilczynski SP (1996) Human papillomavirus type 18: association with poor prognosis in early stage cervical cancer. J Natl Cancer Inst 88: 1361–1368
Burkman RT, Damewood MT (1985) Actinomyces and the intrauterine conceptive device. In: Zatuchni GI, Goldsmith A, Sciarra J (eds) Intrauterine conception. Advances and future prospects. Harper and Row, New York, pp 427–437
Cameron RI, Maxwell P, Jenkins D, McCluggage WG (2002) Immunohistochemical staining with MIB1, bcl2 and p16 assists in the distinction of cervical glandular intraepithelial neoplasia from tubo-endometrial metaplasia, endometriosis and microglandular hyperplasia. Histopathology 41: 313–321
Campion MJ, McCance DJ, Cuzick J, Singer A (1986) Progressive potential of mild cervical atypia: prospective cytological, colposcopic, and virological study. Lancet 2: 237–240
Candy J, Abell MR (1968) Progesterone-induced adenomatous hyperplasia of the uterine cervix. JAMA 203: 323–326
Cantuaria G, Angioli R, Nahmias J, Estape R, Penalver M (1999) Primary malignant melanoma of the uterine cervix: case report and review of the literature. Gynecol Oncol 75: 170–174
Castellsague X, Munoz N (2003) Chapter 3: Cofactors in human papillomavirus carcinogenesis – role of parity, oral contraceptives, and tobacco smoking. J Natl Cancer Inst Monogr: 20–28
Castrillon DH, Lee KR, Nucci MR (2002) Distinction between endometrial and endocervical adenocarcinoma: an immunohistochemical study. Int J Gynecol Pathol 21: 4–10
Chan JK, Tsui WM, Tung SY, Ching RC (1989) Endocrine cell hyperplasia of the uterine cervix. A precursor of neuroendocrine carcinoma of the cervix? Am J Clin Pathol 92: 825–830

Christopherson WM, Nealon N, Gray LA Sr. (1979) Noninvasive precursor lesions of adenocarcinoma and mixed adenosquamous carcinoma of the cervix uteri. Cancer 44: 975–983
Cina SJ, Richardson MS, Austin RM, Kurman RJ (1997) Immunohistochemical staining for Ki-67 antigen, carcinoembryonic antigen, and p53 in the differential diagnosis of glandular lesions of the cervix. Mod Pathol 10: 176–180
Clement PB, Scully RE (1974) Mullerian adenosarcoma of the uterus. A clinicopathologic analysis of ten cases of a distinctive type of mullerian mixed tumor. Cancer 34: 1138–1149
Clement PB, Scully RE (1982) Carcinoma of the cervix: histologic types. Semin Oncol 9: 251–264
Clement PB, Young RH, Keh P, Östör AG, Scully RE (1995) Malignant mesonephric neoplasms of the uterine cervix. A report of eight cases, including four with a malignant spindle cell component. Am J Surg Pathol 19: 1158–1171
Clement PB, Zubovits JT, Young RH, Scully RE (1998) Malignant mullerian mixed tumors of the uterine cervix: a report of nine cases of a neoplasm with morphology often different from its counterpart in the corpus. Int J Gynecol Pathol 17: 211–222
Cohen C, Shulman G, Budgeon LR (1982) Endocervical and endometrial adenocarcinoma: an immunoperoxidase and histochemical study. Am J Surg Pathol 6: 151–157
Colgan TJ, Percy ME, Suri M, Shier RM, Andrews DF, Lickrish GM (1989) Human papillomavirus infection of morphologically normal cervical epithelium adjacent to squamous dysplasia and invasive carcinoma. Hum Pathol 20: 316–319
Copeland LJ, Sneige N, Ordonez NG, Hancock KC, Gershenson DM, Saul PB, Kavanagh JJ (1985) Endodermal sinus tumor of the vagina and cervix. Cancer 55: 2558–2565
Corey L (1984) Genital herpes. In: Holmes KK, Mardh PA, Sparling PF, Wiesner PJ (eds) Sexually transmitted diseases. McGraw-Hill, New York, pp 449–474
Crissman JD, Budhraja M, Aron BS, Cummings G (1987) Histopathologic prognostic factors in stage II and III squamous cell carcinoma of the uterine cervix. An evaluation of 91 patients treated primarily with radiation therapy. Int J Gynecol Pathol 6: 97–103
Crum CP (2003) Symposium part 1: Should the Bethesda System terminology be used in diagnostic surgical pathology? Point. Int J Gynecol Pathol 22: 5–12
Crum CP, Ikenberg H, Richart RM, Gissman L (1984) Human papillomavirus type 16 and early cervical neoplasia. N Engl J Med 310: 880–883
Crum CP, Nagai N, Mitao M, Levine RU, Silverstein S (1985) Histological and molecular analysis of early cervical neoplasia. J Cell Biochem 9 Suppl: 70
Cui S, Lespinasse P, Cracchiolo B, Sama J, Kreitzer MS, Heller DS (2001) Large cell neuroendocrine carcinoma of the cervix associated with adenocarcinoma in situ: evidence of a common origin. Int J Gynecol Pathol 20: 311–312
Czernobilsky B, Moll R, Franke WW, Dallenbach-Hellweg G, Hohlweg-Majert P (1984) Intermediate filaments of normal and neoplastic tissues of the female genital tract with emphasis on problems of differential tumor diagnosis. Pathol Res Pract 179: 31–37
Dabbs DJ, Geisinger KR, Norris HT (1986) Intermediate filaments in endometrial and endocervical carcinomas. The diagnostic utility of vimentin patterns. Am J Surg Pathol 10: 568–576
Dallenbach FE, Coupland SE, Stein H (2000) [Marginal zone lymphomas: extranodal MALT type, nodal and splenic]. Pathologe 21: 162–177
Dallenbach-Hellweg G (1981) Structural variations of cervical cancer and its precursors under the influence of exogenous hormones. In: Dallenbach-Hellweg G (ed) Cervical cancer. Springer, Berlin Heidelberg New York, pp 143–170
Dallenbach-Hellweg G (1984) On the origin and histological structure of adenocarcinoma of the endocervix in women under 50 years of age. Pathol Res Pract 179: 38–50
Dallenbach-Hellweg G (1985) Probleme der histopathologischen Untersuchung weiblicher Genitaltumoren. In: Wulf KH, Schmidt-Matthiesen H (eds) Klinik der Frauenheilkunde und Geburtshilfe, vol 10. Urban und Schwarzenberg, München, pp 87–98
Dallenbach-Hellweg G, Lang G (1991) Immunohistochemical studies on uterine tumors. I. Invasive squamous cell carcinomas of the cervix and their precursors. Pathol Res Pract 187: 36–43
Dallenbach-Hellweg G, Poulsen H (1996) Atlas of endometrial Histopathology. Springer, Berlin, Heidelberg, New York
Daya DA, Scully RE (1988) Sarcoma botryoides of the uterine cervix in young women: a clinicopathological study of 13 cases. Gynecol Oncol 29: 290–304
de Villiers EM, Fauquet C, Broker TR, Bernard HU, zur Hausen H (2004) Classification of papillomaviruses. Virology 324: 17–27

de Villiers EM, Wagner D, Schneider A, Wesch H, Miklaw H, Wahrendorf J, Papendick U, zur Hausen H (1987) Human papillomavirus infections in women with and without abnormal cervical cytology. Lancet 2: 703–706
Dodson MK, Sharp HT (1999) Uses and abuses of the loop electrosurgical excision procedure (LEEP). Clin Obstet Gynecol 42: 916–921
Dougherty CM, Moore WR, Cotten N (1962) Histologic diagnosis and clinical significance of benign lesions of the nonpregnant cervix. Ann NY Acad Sci 97: 683
Duensing S, Münger K (2004) Mechanisms of genomic instability in human cancer: insights from studies with human papillomavirus oncoproteins. Int J Cancer 109: 157–162
Eide TJ (1987) Cancer of the uterine cervix in Norway by histologic type, 1970–84. J Natl Cancer Inst 79: 199–205
Elson DA, Riley RR, Lacey A, Thordarson G, Talamantes FJ, Arbeit JM (2000) Sensitivity of the cervical transformation zone to estrogen-induced squamous carcinogenesis. Cancer Res 60: 1267–1275
Fanning J, Padratzik J (2002) Cold knife conization vs. LEEP. Are they the same procedure? J Reprod Med 47: 33–35
Farnsworth A, Laverty C, Stoler MH (1989) Human papillomavirus messenger RNA expression in adenocarcinoma in situ of the uterine cervix. Int J Gynecol Pathol 8: 321–330
Ferenczy A, Winkler B (1987) Carcinoma and metastatic tumors of the cervix. In: Kurman RJ (ed) Blaustein's pathology of the female genital tract. Springer, Berlin Heidelberg New York, pp 218–256
Ferenczy A, Wright T (1993) Managing abnormal Papanicolaou findings: large-loop excision of the transformation zone. The Female Patient 18: 37–44
Ferry JA, Scully RE (1988) "Adenoid cystic" carcinoma and adenoid basal carcinoma of the uterine cervix. A study of 28 cases. Am J Surg Pathol 12: 134–144
Ferry JA, Scully RE (1990) Mesonephric remnants, hyperplasia, and neoplasia in the uterine cervix. A study of 49 cases. Am J Surg Pathol 14: 1100–1111
Fetissof F, Berger G, Dubois MP, Arbeille-Brassart B, Lansac J, Sam-Giao M, Jobard P (1985) Endocrine cells in the female genital tract. Histopathology 9: 133–145
Flint A, Gikas PW, Roberts JA (1985) Alveolar soft part sarcoma of the uterine cervix. Gynecol Oncol 22: 263–267
Franke WW, Moll R, Achtstaetter T, Kuhn C (1986) Cell typing of epithelia and carcinomas of the female genital tract using cytoskeletal proteins as markers. In: Peto R, zur Hausen H (eds) Viral etiology of cervical cancer. Cold Spring Harbor Laboratory, Cold Spring Harbor, pp 121–148
Friedell GH, Mc KD (1953) Adenocarcinoma in situ of the endocervix. Cancer 6: 887–897
Frisch M, Biggar RJ, Goedert JJ (2000) Human papillomavirus-associated cancers in patients with human immunodeficiency virus infection and acquired immunodeficiency syndrome. J Natl Cancer Inst 92: 1500–1510
Fu YS, Reagan JW, Fu AS, Janiga KE (1982) Adenocarcinoma and mixed carcinoma of the uterine cervix. II. Prognostic value of nuclear DNA analysis. Cancer 49: 2571–2577
Fu YS, Reagan JW, Hsiu JG, Storaasli JP, Wentz WB (1982) Adenocarcinoma and mixed carcinoma of the uterine cervix. I. A. clinicopathologic study. Cancer 49: 2560–2570
Fuchs PG, Girardi F, Pfister H (1988) Human papillomavirus DNA in normal, metaplastic, preneoplastic and neoplastic epithelia of the cervix uteri. Int J Cancer 41: 41–45
Fujii S, Konishi I, Ferenczy A, Imai K, Okamura H, Mori T (1986) Small cell undifferentiated carcinoma of the uterine cervix: histology, ultrastructure, and immunohistochemistry of two cases. Ultrastruct Pathol 10: 337–346
Fung HY, Cheung LP, Rogers MS, To KF (1997) The treatment of cervical intra-epithelial neoplasia: when could we 'see and loop'. Eur J Obstet Gynecol Reprod Biol 72: 199–204
Gall SA, Bourgeois CH, Maguire R (1969) The morphologic effects of oral contraceptive agents on the cervix. JAMA 207: 2243–2247
Gallup DG, Abell MR (1977) Invasive adenocarcinoma of the uterine cervix. Obstet Gynecol 49: 596–603
Gaton E, Zejdel L, Bernstein D, Glezerman M, Czernobilsky B, Insler V (1982) The effect of estrogen and gestagen on the mucus production of human endocervical cells: a histochemical study. Fertil Steril 38: 580–585
Gersell DJ, Mazoujian G, Mutch DG, Rudloff MA (1988) Small-cell undifferentiated carcinoma of the cervix. A clinicopathologic, ultrastructural, and immunocytochemical study of 15 cases. Am J Surg Pathol 12: 684–698
Gilks CB, Young RH, Aguirre P, DeLellis RA, Scully RE (1989) Adenoma malignum (minimal deviation adenocarcinoma) of the uterine cervix. A clinicopathological and immunohistochemical analysis of 26 cases. Am J Surg Pathol 13: 717–729

Gilks CB, Young RH, Gersell DJ, Clement PB (1997) Large cell neuroendocrine [corrected] carcinoma of the uterine cervix: a clinicopathologic study of 12 cases. Am J Surg Pathol 21: 905–914
Gilks CB, Young RH, Clement PB, Hart WR, Scully RE (1996) Adenomyomas of the uterine cervix of of endocervical type: a report of ten cases of a benign cervical tumor that may be confused with adenoma malignum [corrected]. Mod Pathol 9: 220–224
Girardi F, Heydarfadai M, Koroschetz F, Pickel H, Winter R (1994) Cold-knife conization versus loop excision: histopathologic and clinical results of a randomized trial. Gynecol Oncol 55: 368–370
Gissmann L (1984) Papillomaviruses and their association with cancer in animals and in man. Cancer Surv 3: 162–181
Gloor E, Hurlimann J (1986) Cervical intraepithelial glandular neoplasia (adenocarcinoma in situ and glandular dysplasia). A correlative study of 23 cases with histologic grading, histochemical analysis of mucins, and immunohistochemical determination of the affinity for four lectins. Cancer 58: 1272–1280
Gloor E, Ruzicka J (1982) Morphology of adenocarcinoma in situ of the uterine cervix: a study of 14 cases. Cancer 49: 294–302
Glucksmann A (1957) Relationships between hormonal changes in pregnancy and the development of mixed carcinoma of the uterine cervix. Cancer 10: 831–837
Gould VE, Koukoulis GK, Jansson DS, Nagle RB, Franke WW, Moll R (1990) Coexpression patterns of vimentin and glial filament protein with cytokeratins in the normal, hyperplastic, and neoplastic breast. Am J Pathol 137: 1143–1155
Grayson W, Taylor LF, Cooper K (1999) Adenoid cystic and adenoid basal carcinoma of the uterine cervix: comparative morphologic, mucin, and immunohistochemical profile of two rare neoplasms of putative 'reserve cell' origin. Am J Surg Pathol 23: 448–458
Groben P, Reddick R, Askin F (1985) The pathologic spectrum of small cell carcinoma of the cervix. Int J Gynecol Pathol 4: 42–57
Gusdon JP (1965) Hemangioma of the cervix: four new cases and a review. Am J Obstet Gynecol 91: 204–209
Hachitanda Y, Tsuneyoshi M, Enjoji M (1989) Expression of pan-neuroendocrine proteins in 53 neuroblastic tumors. An immunohistochemical study with neuron-specific enolase, chromogranin, and synaptophysin. Arch Pathol Lab Med 113: 381–384
Hall DJ, Schneider V, Goplerud DR (1980) Primary malignant melanoma of the uterine cervix. Obstet Gynecol 56: 525–529
Hamperl H, Kaufmann C (1959) The cervix uteri at different ages. Obstet Gynecol 14: 621–631
Harnden P, Kennedy W, Andrew AC, Southgate J (1999) Immunophenotype of transitional metaplasia of the uterine cervix. Int J Gynecol Pathol 18: 125–129
Harris NL, Scully RE (1984) Malignant lymphoma and granulocytic sarcoma of the uterus and vagina. A clinicopathologic analysis of 27 cases. Cancer 53: 2530–2545
Hart WR, Norris HJ (1972) Mesonephric adenocarcinomas of the cervix. Cancer 29: 106–113
Hart WR (2002) Special types of adenocarcinoma of the uterine cervix. Int J Gynecol Pathol 21: 327–346
Hashida T, Yasumoto S (1991) Induction of chromosome abnormalities in mouse and human epidermal keratinocytes by the human papillomavirus type 16 E7 oncogene. J Gen Virol 72 (Pt 7): 1569–1577
Haswani P, Arseneau J, Ferenczy A (1998) Primary signet cell carcinoma of the uterine cervix: a clinicopathologic study of two cases with review of the literature. Int J Gynecol Cancer 8: 374–379
Hellweg G (1957) Über Schleimbildung in Plattenepithelcarcinomen insbesondere an der Portio uteri (Mucoepidermoidcarcinome). Z Krebsforsch 61: 688–715
Helmerhorst TJ, Dijkhuizen GH, Veldhuizen RW, Stolk JG (1984) Microglandular hyperplasia – a complicating factor in the diagnosis of cervical intraepithelial neoplasia. Eur J Obstet Gynecol Reprod Biol 17: 53–59
Hemminki K, Li X, Vaittinen P (2002) Time trends in the incidence of cervical and other genital squamous cell carcinomas and adenocarcinomas in Sweden, 1958–1996. Eur J Obstet Gynecol Reprod Biol 101: 64–69
Heselmeyer K, Macville M, Schrock E, Blegen H, Hellstrom AC, Shah K, Auer G, Ried T (1997) Advanced-stage cervical carcinomas are defined by a recurrent pattern of chromosomal aberrations revealing high genetic instability and a consistent gain of chromosome arm 3q. Genes Chromosomes Cancer 19: 233–240
Heselmeyer K, Schrock E, du Manoir S, Blegen H, Shah K, Steinbeck R, Auer G, Ried T (1996) Gain of chromosome 3q defines the transition from severe dysplasia to invasive carcinoma of the uterine cervix. Proc Natl Acad Sci USA 93: 479–484

Hiersche HD, Nagl W (1980) Regeneration of secretory epithelium in the human endocervix. Arch Gynecol 229: 83–90
Ho GY, Bierman R, Beardsley L, Chang CJ, Burk RD (1998) Natural history of cervicovaginal papillomavirus infection in young women. N Engl J Med 338: 423–428
Holmquist ND, Torres J (1988) Malignant melanoma of the cervix. Report of a case. Acta Cytol 32: 252–256
Hopkins MP, Schmidt RW, Roberts JA, Morley GW (1988) Gland cell carcinoma (adenocarcinoma) of the cervix. Obstet Gynecol 72: 789–795
Hopman AH, Smedts F, Dignef W, Ummelen M, Sonke G, Mravunac M, Vooijs GP, Speel EJ, Ramaekers FC (2004) Transition of high-grade cervical intraepithelial neoplasia to micro-invasive carcinoma is characterized by integration of HPV 16/18 and numerical chromosome abnormalities. J Pathol 202: 23–33
Hoskins WJ, Averette HE, Ng AB, Yon JL (1979) Adenoid cystic carcinoma of the cervix uteri: report of six cases and review of the literature. Gynecol Oncol 7: 371–384
Hurlimann J, Gloor E (1984) Adenocarcinoma in situ and invasive adenocarcinoma of the uterine cervix. An immunohistologic study with antibodies specific for several epithelial markers. Cancer 54: 103–109
Ishida GM, Kato N, Hayasaka T, Saito M, Kobayashi H, Katayama Y, Sasou S, Yaegashi N, Kurachi H, Motoyama T (2004) Small cell neuroendocrine carcinomas of the uterine cervix: a histological, immunohistochemical, and molecular genetic study. Int J Gynecol Pathol 23: 366–372
Ishikawa M, Fujii T, Masumoto N, Saito M, Mukai M, Nindl I, Ridder R, Fukuchi T, Kubushiro K, Tsukazaki K, Nozawa S (2003) Correlation of p16INK4 A overexpression with human papillomavirus infection in cervical adenocarcinomas. Int J Gynecol Pathol 22: 378–385
Jaworski RC, Pacey NF, Greenberg ML, Osborn RA (1988) The histologic diagnosis of adenocarcinoma in situ and related lesions of the cervix uteri. Adenocarcinoma in situ. Cancer 61: 1171–1181
Jones MA, Young RH, Scully RE (1991) Diffuse laminar endocervical glandular hyperplasia. A benign lesion often confused with adenoma malignum (minimal deviation adenocarcinoma). Am J Surg Pathol 15: 1123–1129
Jones MW, Silverberg SG, Kurman RJ (1993) Well-differentiated villoglandular adenocarcinoma of the uterine cervix: a clinicopathological study of 24 cases. Int J Gynecol Pathol 12: 1–7
Kaku T, Enjoji M (1983) Extremely well-differentiated adenocarcinoma ("adenoma malignum") of the cervix. Int J Gynecol Pathol 2: 28–41
Kaku T, Kamura T, Shigematsu T, Sakai K, Nakanami N, Uehira K, Amada S, Kobayashi H, Saito T, Nakano H (1997) Adenocarcinoma of the uterine cervix with predominantly villogladular papillary growth pattern. Gynecol Oncol 64: 147–152
Kaminski PF, Norris HJ (1983) Minimal deviation carcinoma (adenoma malignum) of the cervix. Int J Gynecol Pathol 2: 141–152
Klaes R, Benner A, Friedrich T, Ridder R, Herrington S, Jenkins D, Kurman RJ, Schmidt D, Stoler M, von Knebel Doeberitz M (2002) p16INK4a immunohistochemistry improves interobserver agreement in the diagnosis of cervical intraepithelial neoplasia. Am J Surg Pathol 26: 1389–1399
Klaes R, Friedrich T, Spitkovsky D, Ridder R, Rudy W, Petry U, Dallenbach-Hellweg G, Schmidt D, von Knebel Doeberitz M (2001) Overexpression of p16(INK4 A) as a specific marker for dysplastic and neoplastic epithelial cells of the cervix uteri. Int J Cancer 92: 276–284
Klaes R, Woerner SM, Ridder R, Wentzensen N, Duerst M, Schneider A, Lotz B, Melsheimer P, von Knebel Doeberitz M (1999) Detection of high-risk cervical intraepithelial neoplasia and cervical cancer by amplification of transcripts derived from integrated papillomavirus oncogenes. Cancer Res 59: 6132–6136
Koenig C, Turnicky RP, Kankam CF, Tavassoli FA (1997) Papillary squamotransitional cell carcinoma of the cervix: a report of 32 cases. Am J Surg Pathol 21: 915–921
Krimmenau R (1966) [Adenocarcinoma in situ, beginning adenocarcinomatous invasion and microcarcinoma adenomatosum]. Geburtshilfe Frauenheilkd 26: 1297–1305
Kruse AJ, Baak JP, de Bruin PC, Jiwa M, Snijders WP, Boodt PJ, Fons G, Houben PW, The HS (2001) Ki-67 immunoquantitation in cervical intraepithelial neoplasia (CIN): a sensitive marker for grading. J Pathol 193: 48–54
Kurman RJ, Schiffman MH, Lancaster WD, Reid R, Jenson AB, Temple GF, Lörincz AT (1988) Analysis of individual human papillomavirus types in cervical neoplasia: a possible role for type 18 in rapid progression. Am J Obstet Gynecol 159: 293–296
Kyriakos M, Kempson RL, Konikov NF (1968) A clinical and pathologic study of endocervical lesions associated with oral contraceptives. Cancer 22: 99–110

Lang G, Dallenbach-Hellweg G (1990) The histogenetic origin of cervical mesonephric hyperplasia and mesonephric adenocarcinoma of the uterine cervix studied with immunohistochemical methods. Int J Gynecol Pathol 9: 145–157

Lauchlan SC (1984) Metaplasias and neoplasias of Mullerian epithelium. Histopathology 8: 543–557

Lemoine NR, Hall PA (1986) Epithelial tumors metastatic to the uterine cervix. A study of 33 cases and review of the literature. Cancer 57: 2002–2005

Levy R, Czernobilsky B, Geiger B (1988) Subtyping of epithelial cells of normal and metaplastic human uterine cervix, using polypeptide-specific cytokeratin antibodies. Differentiation 39: 185–196

Lininger RA, Ashfaq R, Albores-Saavedra J, Tavassoli FA (1997) Transitional cell carcinoma of the endometrium and endometrial carcinoma with transitional cell differentiation. Cancer 79: 1933–1943

Lininger RA, Wistuba I, Gazdar A, Koenig C, Tavassoli FA, Albores-Saavedra J (1998) Human papillomavirus type 16 is detected in transitional cell carcinomas and squamotransitional cell carcinomas of the cervix and endometrium. Cancer 83: 521–527

Lombard I, Vincent-Salomon A, Validire P, Zafrani B, de la Rochefordiere A, Clough K, Favre M, Pouillart P, Sastre-Garau X (1998) Human papillomavirus genotype as a major determinant of the course of cervical cancer. J Clin Oncol 16: 2613–2619

Lörincz AT, Reid R, Jenson AB, Greenberg MD, Lancaster W, Kurman RJ (1992) Human papillomavirus infection of the cervix: relative risk associations of 15 common anogenital types. Obstet Gynecol 79: 328–337

Lörincz AT, Temple GF, Kurman RJ, Jenson AB, Lancaster WD (1987) Oncogenic association of specific human papillomavirus types with cervical neoplasia. J Natl Cancer Inst 79: 671–677

Luft F, Klaes R, Nees M, Durst M, Heilmann V, Melsheimer P, von Knebel Doeberitz M (2001) Detection of integrated papillomavirus sequences by ligation-mediated PCR (DIPS-PCR) and molecular characterization in cervical cancer cells. Int J Cancer 92: 9–17

Maier RC, Norris HJ (1980) Coexistence of cervical intraepithelial neoplasia with primary adenocarcinoma of the endocervix. Obstet Gynecol 56: 361–364

Makin CA, Bobrow LG, Bodmer WF (1984) Monoclonal antibody to cytokeratin for use in routine histopathology. J Clin Pathol 37: 975–983

Mannion C, Park WS, Man YG, Zhuang Z, Albores-Saavedra J, Tavassoli FA (1998) Endocrine tumors of the cervix: morphologic assessment, expression of human papillomavirus, and evaluation for loss of heterozygosity on 1p, 3p, 11q, and 17p. Cancer 83: 1391–1400

Martens JE, Arends J, Van der Linden PJ, De Boer BA, Helmerhorst TJ (2004) Cytokeratin 17 and p63 are markers of the HPV target cell, the cervical stem cell. Anticancer Res 24: 771–775

McCluggage G, McBride H, Maxwell P, Bharucha H (1997) Immunohistochemical detection of p53 and bcl-2 proteins in neoplastic and non-neoplastic endocervical glandular lesions. Int J Gynecol Pathol 16: 22–27

McCluggage WG, Jenkins D (2003) p16 immunoreactivity may assist in the distinction between endometrial and endocervical adenocarcinoma. Int J Gynecol Pathol 22: 231–235

McCluggage WG, Maxwell P, McBride HA, Hamilton PW, Bharucha H (1995) Monoclonal antibodies Ki-67 and MIB1 in the distinction of tuboendometrial metaplasia from endocervical adenocarcinoma and adenocarcinoma in situ in formalin-fixed material. Int J Gynecol Pathol 14: 209–216

McCluggage WG, Sumathi VP, McBride HA, Patterson A (2002) A panel of immunohistochemical stains, including carcinoembryonic antigen, vimentin, and estrogen receptor, aids the distinction between primary endometrial and endocervical adenocarcinomas. Int J Gynecol Pathol 21: 11–15

McGee CT, Cromer DW, Greene RR (1962) Mesonephric carcinoma of the cervix – differentiation from endocervical adenocarcinoma. Am J Obstet Gynecol 84: 358–366

Mestwerdt G (1947) Probeexcision und Kolposkopie in der Frühdiagnose des Portiokarzinoms. Zentralbl Gynakol 69: 326–332

Michael H, Grawe L, Kraus FT (1984) Minimal deviation endocervical adenocarcinoma: clinical and histologic features, immunohistochemical staining for carcinoembryonic antigen, and differentiation from confusing benign lesions. Int J Gynecol Pathol 3: 261–276

Michael H, Sutton G, Hull MT, Roth LM (1986) Villous adenoma of the uterine cervix associated with invasive adenocarcinoma: a histologic, ultrastructural, and immunohistochemical study. Int J Gynecol Pathol 5: 163–169

Middleton K, Peh W, Southern S, Griffin H, Sotlar K, Nakahara T, El-Sherif A, Morris L, Seth R, Hibma M, Jenkins D, Lambert P, Coleman N, Doorbar J (2003) Organization of human papillomavirus productive cycle during neoplastic progression provides a basis for selection of diagnostic markers. J Virol 77: 10186–10201

Moll R, Franke WW, Schiller DL, Geiger B, Krepler R (1982) The catalog of human cytokeratins: patterns of expression in normal epithelia, tumors and cultured cells. Cell 31: 11–24
Moll R, Levy R, Czernobilsky B, Hohlweg-Majert P, Dallenbach-Hellweg G, Franke WW (1983) Cytokeratins of normal epithelia and some neoplasms of the female genital tract. Lab Invest 49: 599–610
Moltz L, Becker K (1977) Cribriform polypoid adenomatous (atypical) hyperplasia of the endocervical glands of the uterus under hormonal contraception. Eur J Obstet Gynecol Reprod Biol 7: 331–336
Moodley M, Moodley J, Chetty R, Herrington CS (2003) The role of steroid contraceptive hormones in the pathogenesis of invasive cervical cancer: a review. Int J Gynecol Cancer 13: 103–110
Moreno V, Bosch FX, Munoz N, Meijer CJ, Shah KV, Walboomers JM, Herrero R, Franceschi S (2002) Effect of oral contraceptives on risk of cervical cancer in women with human papillomavirus infection: the IARC multicentric case-control study. Lancet 359: 1085–1092
Mulvany NJ, Nirenberg A, Oster AG (1996) Non-primary cervical adenocarcinomas. Pathology 28: 293–297
Munoz N, Bosch FX, Castellsague X, Diaz M, de Sanjose S, Hammouda D, Shah KV, Meijer CJ (2004) Against which human papillomavirus types shall we vaccinate and screen? The international perspective. Int J Cancer 111: 278–285
Munoz N, Bosch FX, de Sanjose S, Herrero R, Castellsague X, Shah KV, Snijders PJ, Meijer CJ (2003) Epidemiologic classification of human papillomavirus types associated with cervical cancer. N Engl J Med 348: 518–527
Murphy N, Heffron CC, King B, Ganuguapati UG, Ring M, McGuinness E, Sheils O, O'Leary JJ (2004) p16INK4 A positivity in benign, premalignant and malignant cervical glandular lesions: a potential diagnostic problem. Virchows Arch 445: 610–615
Nagai N, Nuovo G, Friedman D, Crum CP (1987) Detection of papillomavirus nucleic acids in genital precancers with the in situ hybridization technique. Int J Gynecol Pathol 6: 366–379
Nanbu Y, Fujii S, Konishi I, Nonogaki H, Mori T (1988) Immunohistochemical localizations of CA 125, carcinoembryonic antigen, and CA 19-9 in normal and neoplastic glandular cells of the uterine cervix. Cancer 62: 2580–2588
Negri G, Egarter-Vigl E, Kasal A, Romano F, Haitel A, Mian C (2003) p16INK4a is a useful marker for the diagnosis of adenocarcinoma of the cervix uteri and its precursors: an immunohistochemical study with immunocytochemical correlations. Am J Surg Pathol 27: 187–193
Negri G, Vittadello F, Romano F, Kasal A, Rivasi F, Girlando S, Mian C, Egarter-Vigl E (2004) p16INK4a expression and progression risk of low-grade intraepithelial neoplasia of the cervix uteri. Virchows Arch 445: 616–620
Nielsen GP, Oliva E, Young RH, Rosenberg AE, Dickersin GR, Scully RE (1995) Alveolar soft-part sarcoma of the female genital tract: a report of nine cases and review of the literature. Int J Gynecol Pathol 14: 283–292
Nielsen GP, Young RH (2001) Mesenchymal tumors and tumor-like lesions of the female genital tract: a selective review with emphasis on recently described entities. Int J Gynecol Pathol 20: 105–127
Noda K, Kimura K, Ikeda M, Teshima K (1983) Studies on the histogenesis of cervical adenocarcinoma. Int J Gynecol Pathol 1: 336–346
Nucci MR (2002) Tumor-like glandular lesions of the uterine cervix. Int J Gynecol Pathol 21: 347–359
Nucci MR, Clement PB, Young RH (1999) Lobular endocervical glandular hyperplasia, not otherwise specified: a clinicopathologic analysis of thirteen cases of a distinctive pseudoneoplastic lesion and comparison with fourteen cases of adenoma malignum. Am J Surg Pathol 23: 886–891
Oliva E, Ferry JA, Young RH, Prat J, Srigley JR, Scully RE (1997) Granulocytic sarcoma of the female genital tract: a clinicopathologic study of 11 cases. Am J Surg Pathol 21: 1156–1165
Ordi J, Nogales FF, Palacin A, Marquez M, Pahisa J, Vanrell JA, Cardesa A (2001) Mesonephric adenocarcinoma of the uterine corpus: CD10 expression as evidence of mesonephric differentiation. Am J Surg Pathol 25: 1540–1545
Östör AG (1993) Natural history of cervical intraepithelial neoplasia: a critical review. Int J Gynecol Pathol 12: 186–192
Östör AG (1995) Pandora's box or Ariadne's thread? Definition and prognostic significance of microinvasion in the uterine cervix. Squamous lesions. Pathol Annu 30 (Pt 2): 103–136
Östör AG (2000) Early invasive adenocarcinoma of the uterine cervix. Int J Gynecol Pathol 19: 29–38
Östör AG, Duncan A, Quinn M, Rome R (2000) Adenocarcinoma in situ of the uterine cervix: an experience with 100 cases. Gynecol Oncol 79: 207–210
Östör AG, Pagano R, Davoren RA, Fortune DW, Chanen W, Rome R (1984) Adenocarcinoma in situ of the cervix. Int J Gynecol Pathol 3: 179–190

Paavonen J, Vesterinen E, Meyer B, Saksela E (1982) Colposcopic and histologic findings in cervical chlamydial infection. Obstet Gynecol 59: 712–715

Palazzo JP, Gibas Z, Dunton CJ, Talerman A (1993) Cytogenetic study of botryoid rhabdomyosarcoma of the uterine cervix. Virchows Arch A Pathol Anat Histopathol 422: 87–91

Palefsky JM, Holly EA (2003) Chapter 6: Immunosuppression and co-infection with HIV. J Natl Cancer Inst Monogr: 41–46

Patel DS, Bhagavan BS (1985) Blue nevus of the uterine cervix. Hum Pathol 16: 79–86

Pater MM, Hughes GA, Hyslop DE, Nakshatri H, Pater A (1988) Glucocorticoid-dependent oncogenic transformation by type 16 but not type 11 human papilloma virus DNA. Nature 335: 832–835

Peters RK, Chao A, Mack TM, Thomas D, Bernstein L, Henderson BE (1986) Increased frequency of adenocarcinoma of the uterine cervix in young women in Los Angeles County. J Natl Cancer Inst 76: 423–428

Pine L, Curtis EM, Brown JM (1985) Actinomyces and the intrauterine contraceptive device: aspects of the fluorescent antibody stain. Am J Obstet Gynecol 152: 287–290

Pirog EC, Isacson C, Szabolcs MJ, Kleter B, Quint W, Richart RM (2002) Proliferative activity of benign and neoplastic endocervical epithelium and correlation with HPV DNA detection. Int J Gynecol Pathol 21: 22–26

Quade BJ, Yang A, Wang Y, Sun D, Park J, Sheets EE, Cviko A, Federschneider JM, Peters R, McKeon FD, Crum CP (2001) Expression of the p53 homologue p63 in early cervical neoplasia. Gynecol Oncol 80: 24–29

Quinn MA (1997) Adenocarcinoma of the cervix–are there arguments for a different treatment policy? Curr Opin Obstet Gynecol 9: 21–24

Randall ME, Andersen WA, Mills SE, Kim JA (1986) Papillary squamous cell carcinoma of the uterine cervix: a clinicopathologic study of nine cases. Int J Gynecol Pathol 5: 1–10

Richard L, Guralnick M, Ferenczy A (1981) Ultrastructure of glassy cell carcinoma of cervix. Diagn Gynecol Obstet 3: 31–38

Rorat E, Benjamin F, Richart RM (1978) Verrucous carcinoma of the cervix: a problem in diagnosis and management. Am J Obstet Gynecol 130: 851–853

Rose BR, Thompson CH, Simpson JM, Jarrett CS, Elliott PM, Tattersall MH, Dalrymple C, Cossart YE (1995) Human papillomavirus deoxyribonucleic acid as a prognostic indicator in early-stage cervical cancer: a possible role for type 18. Am J Obstet Gynecol 173: 1461–1468

Rossi G, Bonacorsi G, Longo L, Artusi T, Rivasi F (2001) Primary high-grade mucosa-associated lymphoid tissue-type lymphoma of the cervix presenting as a common endocervical polyp. Arch Pathol Lab Med 125: 537–540

Sachs H, Ikeda J, Brachetti AK (1975) [Microinvasive adenocarcinoma and adenocarcinoma in situ of the cervix uteri]. Med Welt 26: 1181–1183

Sano T, Oyama T, Kashiwabara K, Fukuda T, Nakajima T (1998) Expression status of p16 protein is associated with human papillomavirus oncogenic potential in cervical and genital lesions. Am J Pathol 153: 1741–1748

Schiffman M, Kjaer SK (2003) Chapter 2: Natural history of anogenital human papillomavirus infection and neoplasia. J Natl Cancer Inst Monogr: 14–19

Schmidt D, Horn LC, Kommoss F (2005) Neuroendocrine Karzinome der Cervix uteri. Pathologe 26: 262–265

Schneider V (2003) Symposium part 2: Should the Bethesda System terminology be used in diagnostic surgical pathology? Counterpoint. Int J Gynecol Pathol 22: 13–17

Schwartz SM, Daling JR, Shera KA, Madeleine MM, McKnight B, Galloway DA, Porter PL, McDougall JK (2001) Human papillomavirus and prognosis of invasive cervical cancer: a population-based study. J Clin Oncol 19: 1906–1915

Schwartz SM, Weiss NS (1986) Increased incidence of adenocarcinoma of the cervix in young women in the United States. Am J Epidemiol 124: 1045–1047

Scully RE, Aguirre P, DeLellis RA (1984) Argyrophilia, serotonin, and peptide hormones in the female genital tract and its tumors. Int J Gynecol Pathol 3: 51–70

Segal GH, Hart WR (1990) Cystic endocervical tunnel clusters. A clinicopathologic study of 29 cases of so-called adenomatous hyperplasia. Am J Surg Pathol 14: 895–903

Semczuk A, Baranowski W, Berbec H, Marzec B, Skomra D, Miturski R (1999) Analysis of p53 and K-ras genes and their proteins in a sarcoma botryoides of the uterine cervix. Eur J Gynaecol Oncol 20: 311–314

Shah KH, Kurman RJ, Scully RE, Norris HS (1980) Atypical hyperplasia of mesonephric remnants in the cervix. Lab Invest 42: 149

Silver SA, Devouassoux-Shisheboran M, Mezzetti TP, Tavassoli FA (2001) Mesonephric adenocarcinomas of the uterine cervix: a study of 11 cases with immunohistochemical findings. Am J Surg Pathol 25: 379–387

Smedts F, Ramaekers F, Troyanovsky S, Pruszczynski M, Link M, Lane B, Leigh I, Schijf C, Vooijs P (1992) Keratin expression in cervical cancer. Am J Pathol 141: 497–511

Smith JS, Munoz N, Herrero R, Eluf-Neto J, Ngelangel C, Franceschi S, Bosch FX, Walboomers JM, Peeling RW (2002) Evidence for *Chlamydia trachomatis* as a human papillomavirus cofactor in the etiology of invasive cervical cancer in Brazil and the Philippines. J Infect Dis 185: 324–331

Smith YR, Quint EH, Hinton EL (1998) Recurrent benign mullerian papilloma of the cervix. J Pediatr Adolesc Gynecol 11: 29–31

Smotkin D, Berek JS, Fu YS, Hacker NF, Major FJ, Wettstein FO (1986) Human papillomavirus deoxyribonucleic acid in adenocarcinoma and adenosquamous carcinoma of the uterine cervix. Obstet Gynecol 68: 241–244

Solomon D, Nayar R (eds) (2004) The Bethesda System for reporting cervical cytology. Springer-Verlag, New York

Stamm WE, Holmes KK (1984) *Chlamydia trachomatis* infections in the adult. In: Holmes KK, Mandh PA, Sparling PF, Weisher PS (eds) Sexually transmitted diseases. McGraw-Hill Book Co., New York, pp 258–269

Steeper TA, Wick MR (1986) Minimal deviation adenocarcinoma of the uterine cervix ("adenoma malignum"). An immunohistochemical comparison with microglandular endocervical hyperplasia and conventional endocervical adenocarcinoma. Cancer 58: 1131–1138

Stegner HE (1959) [On melanin-forming pigment cells and pigment tumors of the portio vaginalis uteri]. Zentralbl Gynakol 81: 1686–1692

Stein H (2000) [The new WHO classification of malignant lymphoma. After "REAL" a further step on the road to a worldwide consensus]. Pathologe 21: 101–105

Stock RJ, Zaino R, Bundy BN, Askin FB, Woodward J, Fetter B, Paulson JA, DiSaia PJ, Stehman FB (1994) Evaluation and comparison of histopathologic grading systems of epithelial carcinoma of the uterine cervix: Gynecologic Oncology Group studies. Int J Gynecol Pathol 13: 99–108

Stoler MH, Mills SE, Gersell DJ, Walker AN (1991) Small cell neuroendocrine carcinoma of the cervix. A human papilloma-virus type 18-associated cancer. Am J Surg Pathol 15: 28–32

Stoll P (1969) Gynecological vital cytology. Springer, Berlin, Heidelberg, New York

Straughn JM Jr., Richter HE, Conner MG, Meleth S, Barnes MN (2001) Predictors of outcome in small cell carcinoma of the cervix – a case series. Gynecol Oncol 83: 216–220

Talbert JR, Sherry JB (1969) Adenocarcinoma-like lesion of cervix – a "pill-induced" problem? Am J Obstet Gynecol 105: 117–120

Tambouret R, Bell DA, Young RH (2000) Microcystic endocervical adenocarcinomas: a report of eight cases. Am J Surg Pathol 24: 369–374

Tanaka T, Ohbayashi F, Shima H, Shimonaka E, Takahashi M (1984) Glassy cell carcinoma of the uterine cervix. Pathol Res Pract 178: 389–394

Tase T, Okagaki T, Clark BA, Manias DA, Ostrow RS, Twiggs LB, Faras AJ (1988) Human papillomavirus types and localization in adenocarcinoma and adenosquamous carcinoma of the uterine cervix: a study by in situ DNA hybridization. Cancer Res 48: 993–998

Tase T, Okagaki T, Clark BA, Twiggs LB, Ostrow RS, Faras AJ (1989) Human papillomavirus DNA in adenocarcinoma in situ, microinvasive adenocarcinoma of the uterine cervix, and coexisting cervical squamous intraepithelial neoplasia. Int J Gynecol Pathol 8: 8–17

Tavassoli T, Devilee P (eds) (2003) World Health Organization classification of tumours. Pathology and genetics of tumours of the breast and female genital organs. IARC Press, Lyon

Taylor HB, Irey NS, Norris HJ (1967) Atypical endocervical hyperplasia in women taking oral contraceptives. JAMA 202: 637–639

Tendler A, Kaufman HL, Kadish AS (2000) Increased carcinoembryonic antigen expression in cervical intraepithelial neoplasia grade 3 and in cervical squamous cell carcinoma. Hum Pathol 31: 1357–1362

Teshima S, Shimosato Y, Kishi K, Kasamatsu T, Ohmi K, Uei Y (1985) Early stage adenocarcinoma of the uterine cervix. Histopathologic analysis with consideration of histogenesis. Cancer 56: 167–172

Tiltman AJ (1998) Leiomyomas of the uterine cervix: a study of frequency. Int J Gynecol Pathol 17: 231–234

Trunk MJ, Wentzensen N, von Knebel Doeberitz M (2005) Molekulare Pathogenese des Zervixkarzinoms und seiner Vorstufen. Pathologe 26: 283–290

Tseng CJ, Pao CC, Tseng LH, Chang CT, Lai CH, Soong YK, Hsueh S, Jyu-Jen H (1997) Lymphoepithelioma-like carcinoma of the uterine cervix: association with Epstein-Barr virus and human papillomavirus. Cancer 80: 91–97

Tsukamoto N, Kaku T, Matsukuma K, Matsuyama T, Kamura T, Saito T, Suenaga T (1989) The problem of stage Ia (FIGO, 1985) carcinoma of the uterine cervix. Gynecol Oncol 34: 1–6

Tsutsumi Y, Nagura H, Watanabe K (1984) Immunohistochemical observations of carcinoembryonic antigen (CEA) and CEA-related substances in normal and neoplastic pancreas. Pitfalls and caveats in CEA immunohistochemistry. Am J Clin Pathol 82: 535–542

Ueda G, Shimizu C, Shimizu H, Saito J, Tanaka Y, Inoue M, Tanizawa O (1989) An immunohistochemical study of small-cell and poorly differentiated carcinomas of the cervix using neuroendocrine markers. Gynecol Oncol 34: 164–169

UICC (2002) TNM classification of malignant tumors. John Wiley & Sons, New York

Ulbright TM, Gersell DJ (1983) Glassy cell carcinoma of the uterine cervix. A light and electron microscopic study of five cases. Cancer 51: 2255–2263

Ulich TR, Liao SY, Layfield L, Romansky S, Cheng L, Lewin KJ (1986) Endocrine and tumor differentiation markers in poorly differentiated small-cell carcinoids of the cervix and vagina. Arch Pathol Lab Med 110: 1054–1057

van Dinh T, Woodruff JD (1985) Adenoid cystic and adenoid basal carcinomas of the cervix. Obstet Gynecol 65: 705–709

Vang R, Medeiros LJ, Ha CS, Deavers M (2000) Non-Hodgkin's lymphomas involving the uterus: a clinicopathologic analysis of 26 cases. Mod Pathol 13: 19–28

Vizcaino AP, Moreno V, Bosch FX, Munoz N, Barros-Dios XM, Parkin DM (1998) International trends in the incidence of cervical cancer: I. Adenocarcinoma and adenosquamous cell carcinomas. Int J Cancer 75: 536–545

von Knebel Doeberitz M (2002) New markers for cervical dysplasia to visualise the genomic chaos created by aberrant oncogenic papillomavirus infections. Eur J Cancer 38: 2229–2242

Walboomers JM, Jacobs MV, Manos MM, Bosch FX, Kummer JA, Shah KV, Snijders PJ, Peto J, Meijer CJ, Munoz N (1999) Human papillomavirus is a necessary cause of invasive cervical cancer worldwide. J Pathol 189: 12–19

Walker AN, Mills SE, Taylor PT (1988) Cervical neuroendocrine carcinoma: a clinical and light microscopic study of 14 cases. Int J Gynecol Pathol 7: 64–74

Walker J, Bloss JD, Liao SY, Berman M, Bergen S, Wilczynski SP (1989) Human papillomavirus genotype as a prognostic indicator in carcinoma of the uterine cervix. Obstet Gynecol 74: 781–785

Wang SS, Hildesheim A (2003) Chapter 5: Viral and host factors in human papillomavirus persistence and progression. J Natl Cancer Inst Monogr: 35–40

Wang SS, Sherman ME, Hildesheim A, Lacey JV Jr., Devesa S (2004) Cervical adenocarcinoma and squamous cell carcinoma incidence trends among white women and black women in the United States for 1976–2000. Cancer 100: 1035–1044

Wang SS, Trunk M, Schiffman M, Herrero R, Sherman ME, Burk RD, Hildesheim A, Bratti MC, Wright T, Rodriguez AC, Chen S, Reichert A, von Knebel Doeberitz C, Ridder R, von Knebel Doeberitz M (2004) Validation of p16INK4a as a marker of oncogenic human papillomavirus infection in cervical biopsies from a population-based cohort in Costa Rica. Cancer Epidemiol Biomarkers Prev 13: 1355–1360

Wang TY, Chen BF, Yang YC, Chen H, Wang Y, Cviko A, Quade BJ, Sun D, Yang A, McKeon FD, Crum CP (2001) Histologic and immunophenotypic classification of cervical carcinomas by expression of the p53 homologue p63: a study of 250 cases. Hum Pathol 32: 479–486

Ward BE, Saleh AM, Williams JV, Zitz JC, Crum CP (1992) Papillary immature metaplasia of the cervix: a distinct subset of exophytic cervical condyloma associated with HPV-6/11 nucleic acids. Mod Pathol 5: 391–395

Weir MM, Bell DA, Young RH (1997) Transitional cell metaplasia of the uterine cervix and vagina: an underrecognized lesion that may be confused with high-grade dysplasia. A report of 59 cases. Am J Surg Pathol 21: 510–517

Wells M, Brown LJ (1986) Glandular lesions of the uterine cervix: the present state of our knowledge. Histopathology 10: 777–792

Wentzensen N, Vinokurova S, von Knebel Doeberitz M (2004) Systematic review of genomic integration sites of human papillomavirus genomes in epithelial dysplasia and invasive cancer of the female lower genital tract. Cancer Res 64: 3878–3884

Werner R, Waidecker F (1975) [Adenocarcinoma in situ and microinvasive adenocarcinoma of the cervix uteri (author's transl)]. Osterr Z Onkol 2: 154–157

Wheeler DT, Kurman RJ (2005) The relationship of glands to thick-wall blood vessels as a marker of invasion in endocervical adenocarcinoma. Int J Gynecol Pathol 24: 125–130

Willett GD, Kurman RJ, Reid R, Greenberg M, Jenson AB, Lorincz AT (1989) Correlation of the histologic appearance of intraepithelial neoplasia of the cervix with human papillomavirus types. Emphasis on low grade lesions including so-called flat condyloma. Int J Gynecol Pathol 8: 18–25

Winkler B, Crum CP (1986) *Chlamydia trachomatis* infection of the female genital tract: pathogenetic and clinicopathologic considerations. In: Sommers SC, Fechner RE, Rosen PP (eds) Pathology annual. Appleton-Century-Crofts, Norwalk, CT

Winkler B, Crum CP, Fujii T, Ferenczy A, Boon M, Braun L, Lancaster WD, Richart RM (1984) Koilocytotic lesions of the cervix. The relationship of mitotic abnormalities to the presence of papillomavirus antigens and nuclear DNA content. Cancer 53: 1081–1087

Wyatt SW, Lancaster M, Bottorff D, Ross F (2001) History of tobacco use among Kentucky women diagnosed with invasive cervical cancer: 1997–1998. J Ky Med Assoc 99: 537–539

Yamasaki M, Tateishi R, Hongo J, Ozaki Y, Inoue M, Ueda G (1984) Argyrophil small cell carcinomas of the uterine cervix. Int J Gynecol Pathol 3: 146–152

Young RH, Clement PB (2000) Endocervicosis involving the uterine cervix: a report of four cases of a benigh process that may be confused with deeply invasive endocervical adenocarcinoma. Int J Gynecol Pathol 19: 322–328

Young RH, Harris NL, Scully RE (1985) Lymphoma-like lesions of the lower female genital tract: a report of 16 cases. Int J Gynecol Pathol 4: 289–299

Young RH, Kleinman GM, Scully RE (1981) Glioma of the uterus. Report of a case with comments on histogenesis. Am J Surg Pathol 5: 695–699

Young RH, Scully RE (1988) Mucinous ovarian tumors associated with mucinous adenocarcinomas of the cervix. A clinicopathological analysis of 16 cases. Int J Gynecol Pathol 7: 99–111

Young RH, Scully RE (1989) Atypical forms of microglandular hyperplasia of the cervix simulating carcinoma. A report of five cases and review of the literature. Am J Surg Pathol 13: 50–56

Young RH, Scully RE (1989) Villoglandular papillary adenocarcinoma of the uterine cervix. A clinicopathologic analysis of 13 cases. Cancer 63: 1773–1779

Young RH, Scully RE (1992) Uterine carcinomas simulating microglandular hyperplasia. A report of six cases. Am J Surg Pathol 16: 1092–1097

Zaino RJ (2002) Adenocarcinoma in situ, glandular dysplasia, and early invasive adenocarcinoma of the uterine cervix. Int J Gynecol Pathol 21: 314–326

Zaloudek CJ, Norris HJ (1981) Adenofibroma and adenosarcoma of the uterus: a clinicopathologic study of 35 cases. Cancer 48: 354–366

Zhang YC, Zhang PF, Wei YH (1983) Metastatic carcinoma of the cervix uteri from the gastrointestinal tract. Gynecol Oncol 15: 287–290

zur Hausen H (1994) Disrupted dichotomous intracellular control of human papillomavirus infection in cancer of the cervix. Lancet 343: 955–957

Subject Index

The manufacturer's authorised representative in the EU is Springer Nature Customer Service Centre GmbH, Europaplatz 3, 69115 Heidelberg, Germany. If you have any concerns regarding our products, please contact ProductSafety@springernature.com

Printed and bound by CPI Group (UK) Ltd, Croydon, CR0 4YY
25/09/2026
02222892-0003